HONORING THE MEDICINE

By Kenneth Cohen

The Way of Qigong: The Art and Science of Chinese Energy Healing

HONORING
~ THE ~
MEDICINE

The Essential Guide to
Native American Healing

Kenneth "Bear Hawk" Cohen

One World
Ballantine Books • New York

A One World Book
Published by The Random House Ballantine Publishing Group
Copyright © 2003 by Kenneth Cohen

www.ballantinebooks.com/one/

Library of Congress Cataloging-in-Publication Data

Cohen, Kenneth.
    Honoring the medicine: the essential guide to Native American healing / Kenneth "Bear Hawk" Cohen.—1st ed.
        p. cm.
    Includes bibliographical references and index.
        1. Indians of North America—Medicine. 2. Indian philosophy—North America. I. Title.

E98.M4 C64 2003
615.8'82'08997—dc21

                                                                2002034469

ISBN 0-345-39530-1

Book design by Susan Turner

Manufactured in the United States of America

First Edition: June 2003

10 9 8 7 6 5 4 3 2 1

To the Original People of Turtle Island

Great Mystery, I ask for your guidance. Help me to truly listen, with an open mind and a pure heart, and to speak in a way that honors the People and their teachings. May my words help to increase respect, healing, and justice for the people of Turtle Island, their children, and all of our relations. Thank you; thank you; thank you; thank you!

The Fires kept burning are merely emblematic of the greater Fire, the greater Light, the Great Spirit. I realize now as never before it is not only for the Cherokees but for all mankind. . . .

—Redbird Smith (1850–1918)
Cherokee spiritual leader

~ CONTENTS ~

‒ ACKNOWLEDGMENTS ‒

I thank my colleague and friend Joan Borysenko for her intuition and vision. After reading a very early draft of this book, she said, "You've got to publish this!" Little did she or I suspect the work and graces that would follow her encouragement.

I thank my family of birth, my father, mother, and brother, for the lessons of childhood, and my adoptive Cree family, Andy, Irene, and Joseph, for lessons that have helped shape my adulthood. I thank Cree elders Albert Lightning, Glecia Bear, and John and Steve Moosomin for their wise words and encouragement, and the many other Cree healers who have accompanied me at various stages of the journey along the Red Road, including Stuart and Yvonne, and Rose and Ric.

I thank my dear friend Tom Laughing Bear Heidlebaugh (Leni-Lenape) for his depth of understanding of Native American and African spirituality. His poetry, humor, and courage in the face of cancer and unremitting pain—and his wife's bravery in supporting and caretaking him—are an inspiration to people of all nations. The memory of my friend fills me with happy-sadness.

I thank the fine elders and healers who have been my teachers and friends: Keetoowah Christie (Cherokee), Rolling Thunder (Cherokee), War Eagle (Cherokee-Lumbee) and Helen (Comanche), Hawk Littlejohn (Cherokee), Twylah Nitsch (Seneca), Nonoy (Filipino), Fred Lee "Ingwe" (Zulu), and Dr. Aguomo Umunakwe (Igbo). *Mahalo* (Thank you) to Kahiliopua, Herb, Lahe'ena'e Gay, Abraham Piianaia, and my other Hawaiian relations for extending their hospitality and aloha. Warm gratitude to Gulli and Gudrun Bergmann for introducing me to "the Land of Fire and Ice" (Iceland) and the spirits who live there. I thank my extended family in the "Medicine": the former residents of Meta-Tantay, treasured friends Richard and Lora Dart, and my Si.Si.Wiss brothers and sisters under the guidance of Johnny Moses Whis.tem.men.knee, Vi Taqsablu Hilbert, and other elders.

Words cannot express my gratitude to N'Tsukw (Innu), who has been my friend for more than twenty-five years. I will never forget our walk up the mountain as he told me the ancient history of Turtle Island; the songs and prayers, as we shared smoke from a clay pipe; the delicious meals he served when all he could afford was an onion and a loaf of bread; visiting with his mother, who at age ninety had more vitality and wit than most women half her age; and the way he stood by me during my time of hardship. I feel blessed that N'Tsukw's good teachings became part of my life path when I was at an impressionable age.

Honor to the wise teachers who helped deepen my understanding of Western religious traditions: Rabbi Burt Jacobson, Rabbi Zalman Schachter, Rabbi Joseph Gelberman, and to the faculty of the New Seminary. After Rabbi Gelberman lost his family to the Nazis, he founded the interfaith New Seminary as a way to promote peace through appreciation and respect for *all* spiritual traditions. May this work contribute to that good vision.

I am grateful to scientists and colleagues who are bridging the illusory gap between science and spirit, between intellect and intuition, between God and Nature. To Daniel Benor, Larry Dossey, Elmer Green, and other trailblazers on the road to Knowledge and Wisdom.

For help with research or for providing impossible-to-find journal articles, I thank Rebecca Cohen, Robert Freedman, John B. Little, Fernando Pages, and Edward P. Radford Jr. The immediate and open-minded response of many scientists to my requests increases my faith in the integrity of science and convinces me that governments and corporations are more than willing to use scientists' research but rarely their ethics.

To the many other elders, teachers, and acquaintances along the Way. I thank all of these people for helping to open my mind to deeper realities. Blame me for my mistakes and misunderstandings.

To Tami Simon and associates at Sounds True, publishers and preservers of the oral traditions of many cultures. I am honored to count you as friends and colleagues.

To my agent, Ned Leavitt. How fortunate that I found an agent as dedicated to spiritual growth and indigenous wisdom as he is to integrity in business! We sealed our contract with a handshake, a pouch of tobacco, and a signature, in that order of importance. I am grateful that writing books gave us the opportunity to meet.

I thank my editor, Ginny Faber, for inspiring me with her insight, questions, suggestions, critiques, and enthusiasm. Ginny taught me that style and truth can go hand in hand—a book is great only if each word and each sentence is great. I also thank the production staff of Ballantine Books for their expertise.

Wise readers know what kind of person stands behind every good man. I thank my wife, Rebecca Turquoise Water Woman. A literary wife is even more important than a literary agent.

And to my daughter, the little Bear who became a fine young lady, who taught me the meaning of the prayer "for the future generations."

Human knowledge is like a drop of rain in the great sea of life. It is neither complete nor perfect. I welcome my readers' suggestions and criticism, so that I can improve future editions. You may write to me care of the publisher.

— AN IMPORTANT MESSAGE —
from the Author

The healing methods described in this book are presented for education, personal development, and spiritual enrichment. They should not be used as a substitute for necessary medical diagnosis, therapy, or supervision by a qualified health care professional.

Names, places, and characteristics of healing subjects have been changed to preserve confidentiality. Any similarity to specific individuals is entirely coincidental.

A Blessing from a Cree Elder

ᐊᐤ ᒪᓂᑐ ᐅᑯᓯᓯᒪᐤ, ᐅᑲᐏᒪᐤ ᐊᐤ ᑭᐱᒥ
ᓇᑐᒧᐣᑐᑎᑦ.., ᐊᐤ ᐁᔭᑯ ᐅᒪ ᒪᓯᓇᐦᐃᑲᑦ ᑲᐏ
ᐱᒥᓯᓴᐧᐦᑎᒪᑲᐦᐠ ᐅᑎ ᐃᓯ... ᐁᔭᑯ ᐅᒪ
ᒪᓯᓇᐦᐃᑲᑦ ᒥᐦᒉᐟ ᑐᐏᒋᐦᐃᑯᒋᐠ ᐃᔨᓄᐘᐠ.,
ᓇᒧᔭ ᐳᑯ ᓄᐦᐃᔭᐘᐠ ᒪᑲ ᒧᓂᔭᐘᐠ..,
ᑲᐣᑭᑌᐤᐏᔭᓯᑐᐠ., ᑲᐣᑭᑌᐤᐏᔭᓴᐠ ᒥᓇ ᐊᐳᐦ
ᒥᓇ ᒐᔨᓂᐣ ᒥᓇ ᐊᐳᐦ ᑐᐏᒋᐦᐃ ᑯᒋᐠ ᐅᒪ
ᒪᓯᓇᐦᐃᑲᑦ ᑲᐏ ᓯᓴᐧᐦᑎᒪᑲᐦᐠ..,
ᑲᐏᒪᓯᓇᐦᐊᑭᐠ., ᑲᐏ ᑭᓴᓯᓇᐦᐊᑭᐠ ᐅᒪ
ᐁᑿ....
ᐊᐤ ᒪᓂᑐ ᒪᐦᑎ ᑭᑎᒪᑭᐦᑐᐏᓇᑦ....
ᐘ ᓄᐘᔭᐠ ᑭᔭᐘᐤ ᑲᐱᒧᐦᑐᐱᔭᐠ ᒪᐏ
ᒧᐣᑐᐘᑲᓇ' ᑭᑎᒪᑭᐦᑐᐏᓇᑦ ᐅᒪ ᒪᓯᓇᐦᐃᑲᑦ
ᑲᐏ ᐅᓯᐦᑐᐟ ᑲᐏᐦᑭᓴᓯᓇᐦᐊᐠ ᐁᑿ
ᓂᐘᐦᑯᒪᑲᓂᓇᑦ ᐊᐤ ᒪᐦᑎ ᑭᑎᒪᑭᐦᑐ.,
ᑭᑎᒪᑭᐦᑐ ᒪᓂᑐ....
ᒥᐣᑐᐃ ᑐᐏᒋᐦᑯᒋᐠ ᐊᔨᓯᔨᓄᐘᐠ ᐁᔨᑯᐦᐠ...
ᐊᓀᐦ- ᑲᑭᓯᑲᐠ ᑲᐘᓂᓯᐦᑭᐠ ᓂᐘᐦᑯᒪᑲᑦᓇᓇᐠ...
ᓇᒧᔭ ᐳᑯ ᒧᓂᔭᐘᐠ ᒪᑲ ᓄᐦᐃᔭᐘᐠ ᒥᓇ ᐊᓀᐦ-
ᑲᑭᓯᑲᐠ ᐁᐘᓀᐦᑐᐦᐃᑯᒋᐠ ᓱᓂᔭᐘᐦ....
ᐊᐤ ᒪᐦᑎ ᒪᑲ, ᒪᐦᑎ ᒪᑲ, ᒪᑦᑐ
ᑭᒪᒪᐦᑕᐏᓯᐏᑦ ᑭᓴᑭᐦᐃᐏᐏᑦ ᐁᔭᑿᓂᒪ.,
ᐁᔭᑿᓂᒪ ᓂᒪ ᑲᓂᑐᑕᒪᑕᐦᐠ ᑕ ᑲᐣᑭᐦᑕᒪᑲᐦᐠ
ᑕᐏᐦ ᑕᒪᑯᒋᐠ ᐅᑕ ᑭᑿ+ ᐅᑕ ᒪᓯᓇᐦᐃᑲᓂᐦᐠ

ᑕᑲᐢᑭᐦᑕᒋᐠ ᑕᑫᐧᐢᑭ ᐱᒪᑎᓯᒋᐠ ᑕᑫᐧᐢᑭᓇᐦᑭᐠ
ᐃᐧᐢᑕᐃᐧᐤ ᐱᒪᑎᓯᐃᐧᐣ....
ᐅᑕ ᐅᒪ ᒪᓯᓇᐦᐃᑲᐣ ᑲᒪᓯᓇᐦᐃᑲᑌᐠ ᐁᑯᑕ
ᐊᐢᑌᐤ ᒪᐢᑭᐦᑭᐩ..., ᒪᐢᑭᐦᑭᐩ, ᑲᔨᓯᔨᑲᑌᐠ
ᐅᒋᐱᐦᐠ..., ᐁᑭ ᒥᔨᑯᔭᐦᐠ ᒪᒪᐤᐅᐦᑕᐃᐧᒪᐤ
ᐅᒋᐱᐦᐠ...
ᑭᒧᓱᒥᓇᐊᐧᐠ ᐁᔭᑲᐧᓂᒪ ᐁᑭ ᒥᔨᑯᒋᐠ
ᐅᒋᐱᐦᐠ...
ᑯᐦᑕᐃᐧᓇᐊᐧ ᑕᓇᓇᑕᐃᐧᐦᐅ ᐊᐧᑭᒋᐠ...
ᐁᔭᑯᒪ ᐊᓄᐦᐨ ᐅᑕ ᒪᓯᓇᐦᐃᑲᓂᐦᐠ ᑲ
ᒪᓯᓇᐦᐃᑲᑌᐠ...
ᐊᓄᐦᐨ ᐁᑲᐧ ᐱᑐᐢ ᓄᐦᑕᐃᐧᓇᐣ ᓂᑭᐢᑭᔨᐦᑎᓇᐣ
ᐱᑐᐢ ᐊᓄᐦᐨ ᐁᑲᐧ ᐁ ᐊᑎᐢᐸᔨᐠ ᐅᒪ ᑲᐦᑭᔭᐤ
ᑭᑲᐧᐩ...
ᐱᑐᐢ ᑭᑲᐧᐩ ᐃᐧᐢᑕᐊᐧᐤ ᒥᐦᒉᐠ, ᒥᐦᒉᐟ ᐊᐧᓂᓯᓇᐧᐠ
ᐅᓴᒼ ᐱᑐᐢ ᑭᑲᐧᐩ ᐁᐊᑎᐢᐸᔨᐠ...
ᐁᑯᓯ ᒪᑲ ᐅᒪ ᒪᓯᓇᐦᐃᑲᐣ ᑲᐃᐧ ᒪᓯᓇᐦᐊᐠ
ᐊᐊᐧ ᓂᐊᐧᐦᑯᒪᑲᐣᓇᐣ ᑭᔭᒼ ᑕᐊᐧᐸᐦᑕᑭᐠ
ᐁᔨᓀᐊᐧᐠ ᐁᑯᑌ ᒥᐦᒉᐟ ᐁᑲᐧᓇᓂᒪ ᑲᔨᒋᑲᑌᐠ
ᐊᓂᒪ ᓂᒪ ᓇᐣᑕᐤ ᐁᓯ ᐊᐳᐦ ᐁᑎᑫᐧ ᐊᐃᐧᔭᐠ
ᑕᑭᐦᑲᓄᓯᒪᐧᑫᐤ ᐅᒪ ᒪᓯᓇᐦᐃᑲᐣ.., ᑐᑲᓄᓯᒪᐧᑫᐟ
ᐁᑕ ᑭᑲᐧᐩ ᑭᐢᐱᐣ., ᑭᐢᐱᐣ ᐁᑯᓯᓯ
ᑕᓴᐃᐧᔨᐦᒋᑲᑌᐠ.., ᑕᐦᑭ ᑲᓄᓯᒪᐧᑫᐤ ᐊᐃᐧᔭᐠ
ᐅᒪ ᒪᓯᓇᐦᐃᑲᐣ....
ᐁᑲᐧ ᒥᓇ ᐁ ᓄᐦᑌ ᐃᑌᐧᔭᐣ ᐁᑯᑕ ᒪᐦᑎ
ᑕᑭᑎᒪᑭᐦᑕᑯᐃᐧᓯᔭᐣ ᒥᐦᒉᐟ ᐁᔨᓀᐊᐧᐠ ᑕ ᑲᑫᐧ
ᑭᐁᐧᑐᑕᐦᑭᐠ ᒪᐢᑭᐦᑭᐩ ᐁᑭ ᒥᔨᑯᔭᐦᐠ ᑯᐦᑕᐃᐧᓇᐤ
ᑕᓇᓇᑕᐃᐧᐊᐧᑭᔭᐦᐠ....
ᐊᓄᐦᐨ ᐁᑲᐧ ᑲ ᑭᓯᑲᐠ ᒥᐦᒉᐟ ᐁᔨᓀᐤ, ᐁᔭᑲᐧᓂᒪ
ᐊᐧᓂᐦᑕᐤ., ᒥᐦᒉᐟ ᐁᔨᓀᐤ ᐊᐧᓂᐦᑕᐤ.., ᑕᐣᑕᐦᑐᐢᑲᐣ

ᓱᐢᑲᐧᐨ ᐊᔨᓯᔨᓀᐊᐧᐠ ᐊᐧᓂᐦᑕᐊᐧᐠ ᐁᑲᐧᓇᓂᒪ....
ᐁᑭ ᒥᔨᑯᐃᐧᓯᔭᐦᐠ ᑕᐸᒋᐦᑕᔭᐦᐠ ᐅᑕ ᐊᐢᑭᐦᐠ....
ᐁᔭᑯᒪ ᒪᐢᑭᐦᑭᐩ ᑭᒋᑲᑌᐠ....
ᒥᐦᒉᐟ., ᒥᐦᒉᐟ ᐁᑲᐧ ᒥᓇ ᑭᒍᐊᐧᒥᓇᐤ ᐊᐸᒋᐦᑕᐤ
ᐁᔭᑲᐧᓂᒪ ᒪᐢᑭᐦᑭᐩ....
ᐁᔭᑯᒧᒪ ᐁᑭ ᒥᔨᑯᔭᐦᐠ ᐅᒋᐱᐦᐠ ᑭᒋᑲᑌᐠ
ᑯᐦᑕᐃᐧᓇᐤ....
ᒥᐦᒉᐟ ᑭᒍᐊᐧᒥᓇᐤ ᐊᐸᒋᐦᑕᐤ ᐁᔭᑲᐧᓂᒪ....
ᐁᔭᑲᐧᓂᒪ ᐳᑯ ᑕᐸᐢᐯᐦᐃᑯᔭᐦᐠ ᓂᐊᐧᐦᑯᒪᑲᐣᑎᐠ...
ᐁᔭᑲᐧᓂᒪ ᐳᑯ ᑕᐸᐢᐯᐦᐃᑯᔭᐦᐠ ᑭᐦᐃᑌᐧᐊᐧᐠ
ᑭᓭᔨᓀᐊᐧᐠ ᐃᐧᐦᑲᐢᐠ ᐅᒪ ᐁᑲᐧ ᐅᐢᐸᐧᑲᐣ.., ᐁᑯᓂ
ᐊᓂᐦᐃ ᑕ ᐸᐢᐱᐦᐃᑯᔭᐦᐠ ᑭᐦᐃᑌᐧᐊᐧᐠ
ᑭᓭᔨᓀᐊᐧᐠ....
ᑕᐯᐧ ᐁᔭᑯ ᐁᑭᐦ ᑕᐯᐧᒋᐠ ᐊᓂᑭ ᑭᓭᔨᓀᐊᐧᐠ
ᒥᐦᒉᐠ ᑕᐊᐧᓄᐦᑌᐊᐧᐠ ᐊᓄᐦᐨ ᑲ ᑭᓯᑲᐠ ᒪᑲ ᒥᐦᒉᐟ
ᒥᓇ ᑕ ᐱᒪᒋᐦᐃᑲᐧᐠ ᐁᑲᐧᓇᓂᒪ ᐊᓄᐦᐨ ᑲ
ᐃᐧᐦᑕᒪᐣ....
ᐁᑯᓴᓂᒪ ᐁ ᐃᑌᐧᐦᑕᔭᐣ ᐊᓄᐦᐨ ᐅᒪ ᐅᑕ ᑲ
ᐱᑭᐢᑫᐧᔭᐣ ᒥᓴᐊᐧᐨ, ᒥᓴᐊᐧᐨ ᓂᑲ ᐊᑲᔭᓯᒧᓇᐣ
ᒥᓇ ᑕᐃᐧᐦᑕᒪᐦᐠ ᐊᓂᒪᓂᒪ ᑲᔨᑌᐧᔭᐣ.., ᐁᔭᑯᒪ
ᑭᑕᐢᑌᐠ ᐅᒧᒪᐅᑕ., *Honoring The Medicine*,
ᐁ ᐃᑕᐢᑌᐠ ᐁᔨᑯᐦᐠ ᒥᐢᑕᐦᐃ ᐁ ᐃᑌᐧᒪᑲᐦᐠ
ᐁᔭᑲᐧᓂᒪ ᐁ ᐊᑲᔭᓯᒧᐦᐠ ᑭᔭᑦ ᒥᐢᑕᐦᐃ ᑌ
ᑎᔨᐦᑕᒥᐦᐠ ᐁᔭᑯᒪ ᐅᒋᐱᐦᐠ ᐁᑭ ᒥᔨᑯᔭᐦᐠ ᒪᐣᑐ
ᑕ ᓇᓇᑕᐃᐧᐦᐊᐧᑭᔭᐦᐠ.., ᒪᐦᑎ ᒪᐦᑎ ᑭᑎᒪᑭᐦᑎᑕᐠ
ᐁᔭᑲᐧᓂᒪ ᐊᓄᐦᐨ ᑲ ᑭᓯᑲᐠ ᑲᐃᐧᐦ ᑕ
ᑭᐃᐧᑐᑕᒪᐦᐠ ᐁᑭ ᒥᔨᑯᔭᐦᐠ ᑭᑲᐧᐩ ᒪᐣᑐ ᑐᐦ
ᓇᓇᑕᐃᐧᐦᐊᐧᑭᔭᐦᐠ ᒥᐦᒉᐟ ᐃᑎᑲᐧᐦᐳ ᐊᔨᓯᓀᐤ
ᐊᐊᐧᓯᓭᐠ ᒥᓇ ᑯᓯᓯᒥᓇᐊᐧᐠ ᑕ ᐱᒪᒋᐦᐃᑲᐧᐠ
ᐁᔭᑯᒧᒪ ᐅᒋᐱᐦᐠ ᐅᒧᒪ ᑭᐢᐱᐣ ᑲᐃᐧᐦ ᑕ
ᑭᐃᐧᑐᑕᒪᐦᐠ ᒥᐢᑕᐦᐃ ᑌ ᑎᔨᐦᑕᒪᐦᐠ ᑭᐦᑕᐧᑦ ᑕ

ᑭᐁᐧᑐᑕᒪᐦᐠ....

ᐊᐤ ᐁᑯ ᓴᐅᒪ ᐁ ᐱᒋ ᐊᐯᐁᐧᐦᐨᑕᔪᐤ ᐊᓄᐦ ᑲ
ᑲᐱᓯᑐᑕᒪᐧᐤ ᐅᒪ ᒪᓯᓇᐦᐃᑲᐧᐤ
ᑲᐃᐧᐅᓯᐦᒋᑲᐅᐧ....

"ᐊᐦ "ᐊᐦ

TRANSLATION

Oh Grandfather, Creator, Holy Woman, Earth Mother, I call on You in a sacred manner. I call on You with prayer for the sake of this book of wisdom. I pray that its knowledge be spread throughout the land. May it be helpful to many people, not only Native people but also Europeans, Africans, Chinese, and All Nations. I pray to the Spirits of the Four Winds and ask their pity that this knowledge reach out to the four directions. Pity also the calling and crying out of my adopted son, Ken Bear Hawk, who has written this book.

Many people in both our own Nation and other Nations are lost today. Money and greed have led them astray. Therefore, we request, Almighty Creator, through the power of your miraculous essence and spirit and with Your Love, that the teachings in this book bring great benefits to the people, affect them in a good way, and help them to change their lives around.

This book contains medicine, medicine from the root given by our Creator. In the past, You also gave our grandfathers and ancestors the healing medicine root. Today, everything is changing, and many young people feel lost and confused. I pray that the good words and information in *Honoring the Medicine* provide guidance for many people. May those whose hands it touches use the knowledge as medicine. This book is a spiritual medicine that will protect the people.

Creator, I pray to you for pity and blessing to help mankind return to the ways of the natural medicine placed here by our Creator for healing. Today, many people have lost their connection to Mother Earth and her spiritual gifts. We refer to these gifts as "medicine." Yet I also see that our neighbors and relatives from many nations are starting to return to the herbs, roots, and other natural medicines. My relatives, this is the only medicine that will help us to survive, as has been foretold by the elders. We will be renewed by the sacred power of the sweetgrass and the pipe.

Today, I have spoken my wishes in my Cree language. A language from across the ocean will communicate for me in this book. The wording of the book's title says so much. *Honoring the Medicine* is a tremendous concept. In the past, the medicine of the earth was understood and used for healing. Let us ask for mercy from Creator for our neglect of these medicines. This book will help us return to them. May our children, our grandchildren, and the unborn generations be given life from these medicine roots. Let us think in an expansive and good way toward the medicine so that the Spirit will live on. *Honoring the Medicine* is the kind of legacy that people should leave behind for their children. That is all I can say in praying and asking for a blessing today. *Hiy! Hiy!* (With deep gratitude)

—Prayer by Andrew Naytowhow
(Nêhiyaw—Sturgeon Lake First Nation, Saskatchewan)

- Transcribed to Cree syllabics by Mary Anne Martell (Nêhiyaw—Waterhen Lake First Nation, Saskatchewan)
- Syllabics typed by Scott Bear (Nêhiyaw—Flying Dust First Nation, Saskatchewan)
- Helpers (*Ôskapêwisak*) Joseph Naytowhow (Nêhiyaw—Sturgeon Lake First Nation, Saskatchewan) and Cheryl L'Hirondelle-Wayinohtêw (âpihtawikosisân/Nêhiyaw—Pahpahcasis First Nation, Saskatchewan)
- English translation by Joseph Naytowhow

— A NOTE ABOUT —
Cree Syllabics

Most Native American languages use English letters to represent their words. Cree and Cherokee, however, have their own writing systems. In 1819, a Cherokee man named Sequoyah, who didn't know how to read or write in any language, invented the Cherokee syllabary to represent Cherokee sounds. This was an extraordinary intellectual and creative achievement; most of the world's written languages evolved over thousands of years. Not long after Sequoyah's invention, Calling Badger, a Cree medicine man from western Canada, journeyed to the spirit world, where he learned prophecies, sacred teachings, and a unique system of Cree syllabics. The spirits warned Calling Badger that Christian missionaries would try to take credit for the syllabary. As predicted, a Methodist missionary named James Evans (1801–1846) claimed that he invented the writing system based on a combination of shorthand and common symbols from Cree art. Although many scholars support the Evans story, I am among the minority of "traditionalists" who attribute the syllabary to Calling Badger. Calling Badger's life story and teachings were passed down by the descendants of Fine Day (born sometime before 1854), the noted Cree medicine man and warrior. I heard the story of Cree syllabics directly from Fine Day's great-grandson.

The Cree system is far more flexible than the Cherokee syllabary and has been adapted to represent related Algonquin languages such as Anishinabe and Innu, as well as an unrelated language spoken by the Inuit. Thanks to their syllabaries, by the end of the nineteenth century, the Cree and Cherokee nations probably had the highest literacy rates of any nation in the world.

~ INTRODUCTION ~

In November of 1993, I was invited to speak at a small conference on complementary and alternative medicine in the Shenandoah Valley of Virginia, not far from Washington, D.C. In attendance were about twenty medical school professors, researchers, and clinicians, and representatives from several systems of healing, including acupuncture, Ayurveda, spiritual counseling, and Christian prayer healing. I represented Native American medicine. The purpose of the conference was to review these healing systems, look for common factors, and create guidelines for the conduct and evaluation of healing research.

I was surprised and delighted when the conference organizer, Wayne Jonas, M.D., a leading scientist from the National Institutes of Health, requested that I open the conference with a traditional Native American prayer ceremony to honor the medicine of America's original healers. The ceremony took place under a giant oak tree. Conference participants came from varied backgrounds and represented healing methods that seemed, on the surface, very different from one another. Yet we all stood around that oak tree with our feet planted on the same ground. This book is a branch of that tree. It is an expression of my belief that people of various healing and spiritual traditions must engage in respectful dialogue if they are to understand one another and create a strong foundation for health and peace.

At the prayer ceremony, I burned a "smudge" of sage and cedar, sacred Native American plants. We drew in the same fragrant air and mixed it with the unique breath in our own bodies. At the level of roots and breath, at the level of our humanness, there are only small differences among us. I have yet to hear a pine tree criticize the authenticity or "truthfulness" of a willow. Native American healing takes us to these roots because it is an expression of the ancient wisdom of humanity. Indigenous spirituality is the world's oldest religion. I hope that when you read this book you will trace your mind back to its own roots and reaffirm the importance of living in a way that respects our common soil.

Honoring the Medicine is about far more than "medicine" in the conventional

1

sense, about preventing or treating disease. It is about the sacred powers that, in Native American culture, are the source of life, wisdom, and healing. They *are* medicine. The medicine is in us and around us. *Honoring the Medicine* is a book for healers, which means that it is for everyone, because we are all healers. When you touch someone with your eyes or your hands, you communicate who you are. If you honor the medicine, you inspire honor and wisdom in others.

WELLNESS AND WISDOM

From the Native American perspective, medicine belongs more to the realm of healing than curing. These two concepts are not identical. Physicians aim to cure disease, to vanquish it, to make it go away. Traditional indigenous healers emphasize healing, in the sense of "making whole" by establishing, enhancing, or restoring well-being and harmony.

Imagine that you visit your physician because you have a painful cough and low-grade fever. He determines that it is bronchitis and prescribes an antibiotic, which you must take for the next ten days. The antibiotic works—your fever disappears, and the cough goes away. You are "cured." But you may feel ill in other ways—the antibiotic may have upset your digestion or weakened your immune system, making you susceptible to another infection. You certainly don't feel empowered by medication. Some drugs, such as those used in chemotherapy, have devastating side effects, such as exhaustion, depression, nausea, and death. For the patient, recovery from illness can be an impersonal and lonely battle.

Now, suppose you go to a Native American healer with the same symptoms. The healer invites your family to attend a healing ceremony. They pray with him as he holds a cup of herbal tea in his hands and asks the Great Spirit for help. You are surrounded by a community of caring human beings. Healing emphasizes your connection to people, nature, and spirit. It includes more than self-centered or personal care. The goal of healing is both wellness and wisdom.

I am not saying that Native American healers are unable to cure, only that curing is not always the exclusive, or even sometimes the primary, goal. The efficacy of a cure can be measured; it belongs to the realm of science. The effects of healing are not as easy to quantify because healing touches every aspect of a person's life—it belongs as much to spirit as to science. Though I will occasionally cite scientific research and theory to point out important parallels between Western and Native approaches to health, I believe that Native American healing goes far beyond the boundaries or capabilities of science. To accurately measure the effectiveness of Native American healing, a researcher would have to measure not only physiological or biochemical improvements but also changes in the patient's happiness and the well-being of his or her family and community. Sometimes, the result of a Native

American healing for cancer is family harmony and a more dignified passage into the spirit world.

Native American healing is America's original holistic medicine. This book explores the principles and practices of this tradition, including, most important, the underlying philosophy and values on which it is based. In Native American communities, certain individuals are born with a gift of healing or possess a particular ability to receive and carry back to us messages from the Creator or helping spirits. Nevertheless, we all have latent healing abilities that can be awakened. This is a book for all who are committed to improving quality of life for themselves and their human, animal, and plant relations. I hope that health care professionals will see themselves as "healers" and will use the principles, insights, and tools in this book to become more caring and effective.

Finally, it must be said that from the Native American viewpoint, healing, quality of life, and spiritual development cannot be separated from politics and economics. Native American healing emphasizes harmony with the Earth as an essential ingredient in personal health. But how can we find harmony with the Earth if we continue to cut her hair (the forests), steal her bones (minerals), and dump poison into her bloodstream (rivers and oceans)? We cannot preserve original healing traditions without recognizing the rights of the original people of North America to autonomy and control over their own lives and lands. The elders say that plants, swimmers, crawlers, four-leggeds, and those who fly are also "people," with God-given rights to the food, shelter, and happiness that nature provides. Throughout this book, I will not hesitate to comment on the rights of these various "peoples" whenever it is relevant to the topic I am discussing.

You will not find in these pages a linear analysis of the ABCs of healing. Such an analysis would not be possible in any event. Traditional Native reasoning and sciences tend to be nonhierarchical. All aspects of Native American healing are interconnected, and thus, one simple idea is not always the basis for a more "advanced" one. I will introduce concepts in one chapter and explore, expand, and reinterpret them again and again throughout the book.

I invite you to wander with me over the landscape of Native American healing, to view it from the perspectives of both science and intuition, to understand it as a philosophy and a lifestyle, and to hear its call for ecological and social responsibility. Sometimes, I will express my thoughts with clear dispassion; at other times, I may become ornery as hell as I recount the devastating effects of white colonialism on Native culture and describe the deficits of the Western medical establishment. I am not, however, at war with my own white ethnicity. I am at war with injustice. I hope you will join me.

The technology and power of the West can be tools of destruction if they are not balanced by earth-based, holistic wisdom. The good medicine of America's original people teaches us how to rediscover the path of beauty that was once known to all of our ancestors, whether they were born on this land or any other.

A MATTER OF METHOD

I prayed and did much soul-searching to determine the clearest and most respectful approach to this complex subject, to settle on what scientists call a *methodology*. The literature about Native American healing can be divided into four broad categories: biographies or autobiographies of Native American healers, such as Thomas E. Mails's *Fools Crow,* about the great Lakota medicine man; anthropological works, especially ethnographies, studies of individual societies; multidisciplinary studies, including books about history, art, religion, or ethnobotany that incidentally touch upon Native American healing; and New Age writings, which I believe is more than a catchall category for quasi-religious books by aging hippies. Each of these perspectives has strengths and weaknesses, but none provided the kind of format that I wished to follow in my book. I decided on an *integral methodology,* which blends multidisciplinary scholarship with personal insight. In this book, I integrate scholarship from a variety of fields—including Native American studies, alternative medicine, theology, and psychology—with my experiences as a practitioner of indigenous healing and spirituality.

— THE PROBLEM WITH ANTHROPOLOGY —

Modern anthropology emphasizes the value of participant observation, which means that the anthropologist lives with the people he or she is studying, records their culture, and may ask questions or conduct surveys. Unfortunately, participant observation does not always result in objective documentation. A researcher's personality, interests, and prejudices influence what he chooses to study, the quality of his interactions, his access to sacred or private information, the methods used to verify conclusions, and very important, the meaning and importance he attaches to conclusions. Anthropological research is usually funded by and conducted for universities. Cultures are commodified, turned into profit-making information for books or academic position. Throughout the twentieth century, indigenous cultures rarely benefited economically or socially from such research.

Early ethnographers often shamelessly lied or used other means of coercion to gain access to their subjects. Dartmouth College Professor Christopher Ronwanièn:te Jocks (Mohawk) has described the way anthropologist Frank Cushing, who lived among the Zuni during the 1880s, "threatened his way into the Kivas"[1] to gain information for his books and how other researchers stole ceremonial objects and altars to place in museums. On November 23, 1990, the United States Congress passed the Native American Graves Protection and Repatriation

Act, which requires federal agencies and private museums to return human remains, funerary materials, and sacred objects to their tribes of origin.[2]

I have personally been dismayed at how, even in modern times, protocol and common courtesy are often ignored by researchers. My own firsthand experience of such cultural arrogance involved a conversation I once had with a young archaeologist who had been hired by the federal government to survey a mountain sacred to several Pacific Northwest tribes. The archaeologist confided that after a few weeks of research, he "could find no evidence of sacred usage." I asked if he had consulted tribal elders to learn about their oral history and tradition, neither of which always produce "artifacts" for study. He brushed my suggestion aside. "I am a scientist," he scoffed. "I look at the data and analyze it. What do the elders know?" No doubt, the archaeologist told the government what it wanted to hear. The sacred mountain is now a nuclear waste repository.

Fortunately, this kind of travesty is becoming less frequent. Archaeologists like the one I just described will soon become an extinct species. Today, researchers are more accountable to Native American people than they have been at any time in the past. More important, Native American scholars are writing their own ethnographies, as much to inform tribal members as to share with other cultures.[3] Non-Native scholars are beginning to collaborate with Native elders, finally seeing them as the teachers and cultural treasures that they are, consultants rather than "informants"[4] who simply provide raw data or information. Earlier researchers often exploited their Native contacts by not explaining how their information would be used or the impact it might have on the health and political challenges of their communities.

— MULTIDISCIPLINARY STUDIES —

By "multidisciplinary studies," I mean books that are based primarily on research from a variety of disciplines rather than on personal experience. The best known is Virgil J. Vogel's *American Indian Medicine,* which draws on ethnography, history, and Western medicine. Vogel uses a *phenomenological* approach, which means that he presents only the facts. His book is a meticulously researched and well-referenced compendium of Native American beliefs and practices drawn from previously published works.

The major weakness of such text-based approaches is that they tend to give the mistaken impression that Native American medicine is frozen in the past—a museum relic, a subject for historical scholarship, or a quaint reminder of where humanity has been. There is little attention paid to it as a living system, no sense of the modern practice and relevance of Native American healing or of the important dialogue that is occurring between Indian and non-Indian culture and science.

Many multidisciplinary works also fail to engage the Native American worldview, that is, how Native Americans understand their own culture. Authors reduce their subjects to familiar and comfortable categories rather than venture into realms that question common beliefs about reality. For example, in 1964, Bert Kaplan and Dale Johnson, professors of psychology at two American universities, published an essay called "Navaho Psychopathology," in which they claimed that the effectiveness of Navaho curing ceremonies is based on suggestion or autosuggestion and on reintegration of the patient with the social group.[5] Although these are certainly important factors, the authors' conclusions are based on their own cultural assumptions that spirits are hallucinations and thus a belief in them must be purely utilitarian. I disagree, as do most practitioners of Native American healing.

A notable modern example of this reductionistic tendency can be found in scholar of religion Daniel C. Noel's book *The Soul of Shamanism*. Noel implies that the proper way for Westerners to enter the shamanic realm is by exercising their imaginations by reading novels. He states that aside from drug-induced visions, "the only direct experience of nonordinary reality we can claim as Westerners to be truly ours—and recognizably shamanic—is the experience of imagination's power in fictions and fantasies, dreams and reveries, or the arts of literature and the like."[6] Words in literature are described as "powerful peyote buttons" that can take us on magical flights.[7] Although words are indeed powerful, shamanic traditions, including both Native American and ancient European, predate the written word. Noel ignores the vast realm of Druidic, Celtic, and Norse shamanism, all of which sought wordless communion with spiritual powers, and the indigenous spirit of many early Christian mystics who saw the world as the body of Christ and sought direct contact with the Divine through communion with nature. Although shamans are imaginative, they recognize that spiritual realms can only be perceived by a quiet mind.[8]

— NEW AGE WRITINGS —

In a typical bookstore, most books about Native American healing are either in the Native American, anthropology, or American history sections. Many works that purport to be about Native American healing may also be found in the "New Age" section. The same is true in libraries. It is safe to say that their separate shelving reflects a value judgment that New Age books, generally unendorsed by academicians or Native people and rarely containing footnotes or bibliographies, are not authentic. The criteria used to determine which book goes where can be vague, however, and mistakes are often made.

"New Age" is a relatively new genre. It consists mostly of nonfiction books on a wide range of subjects, from the occult to astrology to nondenominational spirituality and inspiration. The name grew out of the New Age movement, a Western social trend that began in the 1970s, picking up where the beatnik and hippie movements of the 1950s and 1960s left off. It reflects the same dissatisfaction with materialism, conformity, and institutionalized religion, education, and government and includes a genuine yearning to find meaning, freedom, and purpose in life.

Members of the New Age movement aspire to revolutionize consciousness through meditation and other spiritual practices. They seek an alternate lifestyle, never clearly defined but generally based on communal living and sound ecological principles, such as simplicity and conservation. Some believe that an alternate lifestyle is a matter of human destiny. During the last half of the twentieth century, New Agers were anticipating and preparing for the Age of Aquarius, which astrologers predict is a two-thousand-year period, from A.D. 2000 to A.D. 4000, in which people will seek peace and community and reconcile science with humanitarian concerns. New Age writings are generally optimistic and imaginative.

Unfortunately, New Age writings are frequently overly imaginative, based on channeling from "higher" extraterrestrial sources, "memories" from past lives, or the unrestrained fantasies of self-styled experts. Authors may call themselves "medicine person" or "shaman" who have not been so designated or approved by indigenous people. Their books are often characterized by a lack of critical thinking, confusing traditional Native star knowledge with Western astrology, healing ceremonies with mediumship, and the Vision Quest with visualization. New Age books may also imply that the reader can learn Native American tradition or gain "medicine power" quickly, perhaps in ten easy lessons. By contrast, Native American healers believe that healing is a lifelong commitment that requires personal sacrifice. New Age authors do not necessarily appropriate traditions in a malicious attempt to convey misinformation; more often, they are simply ignorant of the depth and difficulty of the subject.

The problems inherent in the New Age movement are made clear by its most lucid critic, author Ken Wilber. Because there is no single or underlying New Age philosophy, he says, it is probably as correct to discuss New Age movements as a New Age movement. In Wilber's tome *Sex, Ecology, Spirituality,* he points out that "these movements fail across the board: they lack any sustained vision-logic of *both* exterior and interior dimensions, they lack a consistent technology of access to higher interior dimensions, they lack a means (and even a theory) of social institutionalization." Despite their loud espousal of "new paradigms" and quantum or post-Cartesian worldviews, the majority of New Age authors "do not engage the rational worldview in a way that can transcend and include it; rather, most of them end up regressing to various forms of mythic imperialism. . . ."[9] They reject rationality and tradition as vehemently as they believe society rejects intuition and spontaneity.

I once attended a "traditional Cherokee ceremony" in which the leader intoned Wiccan conjuring chants in Latin. He justified the mix saying that Wicca is a

European indigenous tradition and that both Wiccan and Cherokee healers use conjuring spells. True enough, but the language, intent, and geographic root of these spells are far from identical!

Books by self-appointed New Age "experts" frequently contain the same indiscriminate mixing of cultures: many wells dug but none deep enough to strike water. The quest for meaning, connection, and personal vision is taken as equivalent to "Do your own thing." Moreover, "facts" and false personal histories are sometimes created to hide ignorance. "I learned healing from my grandmother, who told me in dreams that she was a Cherokee princess and then taught me. My knowledge comes from the spirit world." Those words were spoken to me by a British teacher of "Indian shamanism." The colonial mentality is betrayed by the use of the term *princess,* a designation unknown to a people without royalty. (I have always found it odd that no one claims to have received the truth from the Cherokee emperor!)

Some New Agers are quite good actors, playing to the American romanticized image of Indians, with feathers, beads, and buckskin.[10] Claiming Indian ethnicity may mean jobs and economic opportunities that are denied real Indians, who frequently don't look the part. Tragically, many impostors are given the stamp of authenticity by publishing houses, conference organizers, and the media. This results in confusion not only for serious students of Native American culture but also for Indian people themselves.

At my lectures on Native American healing, I like to do some "reality testing." I show a slide given to me by a Cherokee elder, who said, "If you don't believe that I'm a medicine person, look at this!" It's a picture of him dressed in a full warbonnet and Plains-style breastplate, neither of which is Cherokee, surrounded by a purple glow, his "aura," courtesy of special effects. We had a good laugh the first time he showed it to me. When I present the slide at science conferences, it always draws oohs, aahs, and knowing nods of approval. And my own credibility also goes up several notches as the student of the Indian mystic. When I click to the next slide, the audience sees the elder as he normally looks—balding, crippled from diabetes, dressed in dirty overalls, and sitting in a wheelchair outside his trailer. Behind the trailer is a small storage shed where he keeps a mini-arsenal of shotguns, rifles, and pistols. I share this quote with the audience: "I used to hunt when I was younger, but now I only use weapons to scare away trespassers." With this slide, I like to shock my listeners into an alternate reality, called the reality of Indian life.

New Age books about Native American healing are frequently written by people who seem entranced by the exotic. They have learned how to talk the talk, but they don't walk the walk. It is neither easy nor fun to walk the Red Road, the path of Native American spirituality. Do you know why the grass always looks greener in someone else's yard? Because unless you're standing in it, you can probably only see the surface.

~ RESTORING SOUL ~

The *integral* approach I take in *Honoring the Medicine* blends philosophy, science, values, principles, and practice. An integral methodology is based on personal experience, dialogue with peers, and scholarship. It is also interdisciplinary because it recognizes the holistic nature of Native American thinking and culture, in which subjects such as healing, worldview, ethics, lifestyle, geography, music, dance, art, politics, and prayer cannot be divided.[11] In *Keeping Slug Woman Alive: A Holistic Approach to American Indian Texts,* University of California Professor Greg Sarris describes an approach to oral literature and storytelling that matches my own goal as an author: "[T]he writing, as much as possible, should reflect oral tendencies to engage the larger world in which the spoken word lives so that it is seen for what it might or might not be beyond the page."[12]

In sociological terms, the integral methodology emphasizes *emic* inquiry: it recognizes the internal structure and validity of culture and acknowledges that peoples have their own cultural explanations for beliefs and behaviors. This is in contrast with *etic* interpretation, which denies the inherent significance of such beliefs and assumes instead that the truth can only be seen through the lens of Western culture and its evidence-based science. The "objectivity" of science is a euphemism that often masks unconscious, culture-bound preconceptions about the criteria that determine truth.

This book is based on what I have learned in more than thirty years of study with indigenous elders and healers and on my personal experiences as a practitioner of Native American healing. It also incorporates insights and data from ethnographies and historical works whenever appropriate. However, as much as I value historical analysis, I am more concerned with the *future* of Native American healing. Native American healing has changed as Native people have adapted to new circumstances. In the past, Native American healing evolved as tribes migrated and adapted to new landscapes or as they traded goods and information with other tribes. It is a mistake to consider Native American healing only as it was practiced in precolonial times, just as it would be a mistake to presume to understand the validity of Western medicine by studying only the writings of Hippocrates. Although Native American healing practices have ancient roots and include tried and tested methods that remain unchanged over long periods of time, like scientists, Native healers adjust procedures based on clinical observation, insight, and information shared with colleagues and peers.

Native American healing is a powerful system of healing, as deserving of respect as acupuncture, homeopathy, Ayurveda, or any other great traditional method of health care. In this book, I will explore traditional, modern, and cross-cultural perspectives on Native American healing by trying to answer the following questions:

How do Native American people understand health and disease—that is, what are the principles of indigenous healing? Can the indigenous and Western communities engage in respectful, mutually enriching dialogue to the benefit of all people, Native and non-Native alike, in their common quest for healing and understanding?

The need for such cross-cultural dialogue in education and science is now being recognized by many Native Americans. Tewa Indian educator and artist Dr. Gregory Cajete puts it succinctly:

> Many aspects of American Indian culture are now being examined through more enlightened perspectives that have evolved from theoretical physics, ecology, theology, ethics, mythology, and the psychology of consciousness. This examination has great potential for American Indians. It presents a contemporary foundation for interpreting important elements of the traditional paradigms of Native America in the context of a twenty-first century world.[13]

Everett R. Rhoades, M.D. (Kiowa), of the University of Oklahoma Health Sciences Center and the Johns Hopkins School of Hygiene and Public Health, echoes Dr. Cajete's philosophy in his important essay "Two Paths to Healing: Can Traditional and Western Scientific Medicine Work Together?"

> The results of rigorous scientific evaluations of alternative healing practices, including Indian healing, may lead to major advances in our shared understanding of the nature of the healing process. While Indian people must protect our most sacred ceremonies from intrusion, we should welcome scientific scrutiny of our Indian medical practices, in the hope that all will gain from increased understanding—both western and traditional healers and their Indian and non-Indian patients.[14]

Nevertheless, I've been unable to present *conclusive experimental data* in this book for the simple reason that there isn't any. In 1992, a report to the National Institutes of Health on alternative medical systems in the United States stated:

> Formal research into the healing ceremonies and herbal medicines conducted and used by bona fide Native American Indian healers or holy people is almost nonexistent, even though Native American Indians believe they positively cure both the mind and body. Ailments and diseases such as heart disease, diabetes, thyroid conditions, cancer, skin rashes, and asthma reportedly have been cured by Native American Indian doctors who are knowledgeable about the complex ceremonies.[15]

In 1994, when I was preparing to edit one of the first scientific newsletters to look seriously at Native American healing, I put out a plea to Native American scholars and colleagues and non-Native scientists for research data. None was forthcoming. In 1997, a premier journal of alternative medicine, *Alternative Therapies in Health and Medicine,* printed my request for research documenting allopathic-indigenous medicine collaboration. Out of the nineteen thousand subscribers and many more readers of that issue, I received two responses. The first was a letter from a non-Indian physician in Canada who had been treating Indian people and participating in their ceremonies. He wondered if *I* had any experimental data. The second was from a group in New Mexico that was providing innovative treatment for HIV and AIDS patients by leading them on pilgrimages to healing places and people, including Native elders. They were unaware of any supportive research but, like the physician I described above, hoped that I had some.

What I *do* have is my clinical observations and observations and reports of other clinicians who combine Western and indigenous treatment strategies. Several hospitals located near or within Indian nations have established Indian Healing Rooms for Native healers to treat patients who are also receiving medical care.[16] There are also a few facilities where physicians, nurses, and Indian doctors work together as professional colleagues to develop culturally appropriate treatment strategies.[17] A primary focus of these collaborations has naturally been to treat Indian people for such epidemic conditions as alcoholism and diabetes. Multicultural wellness and health education programs have also sprung up across North America.[18]

There also exists a wealth of *correlative research* from healing interventions similar to those practiced by Native Americans. The scientific investigation of spiritual healing, psychic healing, and energy medicine are highly relevant to understanding Native American healing. For example, research on the effects of guided imagery (considered spiritual and psychic healing) and healing touch (a branch of energy medicine), although generally conducted by and with non-Indians, may provide insight into the mechanism of parallel Native American methods. I will discuss such correlations in later chapters.

In standard Western medicine, the intervention is considered the effective agent. It is irrelevant who prescribes your penicillin. Not so in Indian healing. The time, place, healer, and patient must be in harmony. I believe that it is impossible to avoid the personal element in writing about such a personal form of healing. In order to illustrate this personal element and to avoid violating private and privileged methods used by other healers, I have described case histories based on elements of interventions with my own clients. Name, gender, ethnicity, nationality, and other identifying characteristics have been changed to preserve their confidentiality. I describe other healers' interventions only if they have been published in works that seem to me to demonstrate accuracy, honesty, and integrity.

Some people might label my methodology as subjective or unscientific. The alternative, journalistic approach is too heartless for my taste. The decision about whether or not to report a Native American healing must be based on more than the accuracy of information. We must also consider such ethical questions as the integrity of the source and the appropriateness of information for the audience. For example, I would not wish the *New York Times* Travel Section to describe the location of my private Vision Quest site.

When the sacred is treated as an object, it becomes devoid of life or meaning. The wisdom of Native American healing may, in fact, be a way to restore meaning to a world increasingly in search of its soul.

THE LIMITS OF LITERATURE

There are certain things that this book will not teach you:

- **This book will not teach you everything important there is to know about Native American culture.**
Healing is only one aspect of culture, and spiritual healers are in the minority, no matter what their ethnicity. Let's suppose that you are speaking to a group of Native Americans, and you ask, "Will the real Native American please stand up?" Who do you suppose will stand—the doctor, lawyer, carpenter, priest, ballerina, psychologist, soldier, historian, casino owner, school administrator? "No, not them," you declare. "I wanted to see the *real* Indian." "Ah, the medicine man." "Yes, that's right." The problem with stereotypes is that they don't portray people as people. Although the continuity of Native American culture has allowed the preservation of powerful, ancient teachings, these teachings are maintained by only a small percentage of the present diverse Indian population.

- **This book will not turn you into a Native American medicine person, although it will suggest practical ways of improving your ability to heal yourself and others.**
The role of medicine man or woman is generally only open to people who are ethnically Native American and who have either grown up or spent a significant part of their lives within indigenous culture. It is a calling. The medicine powers choose their apprentices; it is not up to us. The title "medicine person" is conferred upon a man or woman by a Native American community as a token of courageous and selfless service.

Learning to become a traditional healer is hard work. It requires years of rigorous training and testing and consistent demonstration of endurance, courage, patience, generosity, and in general, character. Humor is also an essential ingredient. Elders will not teach people who take themselves too seriously or who become sullen in the face of suffering. Nor will they train a lazy person. If Native American healing is your path, you are likely to spend far more time milking goats and fixing chimneys than reading books.

- **This book will not reveal secret rituals.**

Many ceremonies are considered the property of particular Native American nations, clans, societies, and individuals. I will not discuss the details of such ceremonies. In the Indian world, you must earn what you learn. In any case, healing techniques are never blindly imitated. Individual healers often create or modify healing methods according to dreams or other forms of received spiritual guidance. Ceremonies are also kept secret for a practical reason: Native healers commonly believe that to share specific healing methods widely or indiscriminately is to dilute and weaken their power.[19] In this book, I will, however, explore the principles of the most common ceremonies, such as the Sweat Lodge and the Sacred Pipe. Both ceremonies have been written about previously by numerous Native and non-Native authors and are widely shared with people of different ethnicities and nationalities.

In *Honoring the Medicine,* I will focus on principles and methods most commonly practiced by Native American healers, such as smudging (purification with smoke), vision-seeking, counseling, massage, and herbalism. These form the core of my own work as a practitioner and an educator. Needless to say, however, in presenting specific techniques, I have had to choose from a multiplicity of individual and tribal variations. My selection is based on the answer to the question "Which methods are most likely to help Native and non-Native people deepen their understanding of Native American healing and improve their ability to heal themselves and others?" Or put in traditional terms: "Which methods can be described for the good of All Relations?"

- **One last caveat: This book is not the final, authoritative word on Native American healing.**

Diversity is the rule in Indian Country. Native Americans have practiced healing for at least twelve thousand years and possibly for more than forty thousand years. In the year 2000, there were 4.1 million Native Americans in the United States, divided into more than 700 tribes, 58 linguistic stocks, and more than 225 distinct languages.[20] If we consider the acceptance of personal innovation by individual healers and visionaries and the prevalence of cultural and intellectual exchange both today and in the past (because of trading, nomadic lifestyles, and the migration of tribes), the number of possible permutations of healing methods seems almost infinite.

No single book could represent the interests or philosophy of all Indian people. Although I will discuss common practices and shared beliefs, such as the interrelatedness and sacredness of life, there is no Indian Bible in which the fundamental tenets of sacred healing are set forth. Scholars of Native American healing and spirituality may have differences of opinion, but these are never doctrinal disputes; the closest we can come to a standard of authenticity is found in the teachings of traditional elders.

Some New Age authors, including a few Native Americans, claim authenticity because of their "lineage," referring to a specific succession of spiritual power passed down either by initiation or through the bloodline. Although lineage and training are important, a Native American healer is not considered an authority solely on the basis of these things, but only if he or she actually embodies—that is, lives—the teachings. Ultimately, a healer or an author can only represent himself or herself. It is up to the Indian community and the individual reader to determine if the words ring true.

My hope for *Honoring the Medicine* is that it will make you an appreciative student and inspire respectful dialogue with people of diverse cultures and viewpoints. I advise applying a balance of open-mindedness, humility, and healthy skepticism to *everything* you read about Native American healing, whether written by Indians or non-Indians.

TRANSLATING CULTURES: IS ENGLISH A PRIMITIVE LANGUAGE?

No matter what methodology the researcher uses, the transmission of ideas from one culture to another is always limited by his or her language. There is an element of fiction when a foreign culture is translated into an English narrative.

Throughout the world, ancient, indigenous languages are disappearing as quickly as old-growth forests. Of the three to six thousand languages spoken in the world today, 80 to 90 percent are spoken by indigenous people. According to Professor H. Russell Bernard, the ability of the human species to adapt to varied environments—such as jungle, Arctic tundra, deserts, and mountains—is due to cultural traits preserved by language. Various ethnic groups use language to communicate their understanding of weather, herbs, health, disease, survival, children, power, politics, conflict, and peace. Dr. Bernard writes in the magazine *Cultural Survival Quarterly,* "The loss of language diversity diminishes our ability to adapt because it decreases the pool of knowledge from which to draw."[21]

Books written in English or other non-Indian languages tend inevitably to convey some misinformation because our understanding is filtered through cultural perspectives embedded in the language itself. For example, words like *religion, God, healing, power, vision, nature, government, story,* or *history* carry different connotations in English than in a Native American language. To an English-speaking Christian, the word *religion* suggests sacred texts, church, and priesthood. Religion is generally something apart from everyday life concerns, though this isn't necessarily true for the very religious. To a Native American, religion is a way of life and a deep appreciation of the connection among people, Creator, and nature. The earth itself is the church, the place of worship.

As another example, to a Westerner, stories are entertaining tales, usually told to children. Although a story or parable may be used to communicate a moral or religious principle, it is not a primary way to teach culture. By contrast, to a Native American, "stories" are synonymous with "teachings." Many are shared only during the winter season, when people of all ages gather at the home of an elder to learn about history, culture, and values. Because most stories are still part of the oral tradition, rather than read or memorized from books, they are constantly evolving. Native healers do not analyze or interpret stories but rather allow stories to act on the listener so that he or she comes to understand them in his or her own way.

Misunderstandings may also occur because Native languages frequently have a multiplicity of terms for phenomena or feelings for which there may be only a single word in English. For example, Alaskans who listen to the weather report in Inuktitut (the Inuit language) are better equipped for survival and safety. Some of the most common Inuktitut words for snow are:

aniugaviniq—very hard, compressed, and frozen snow
apigiannagaut—the first snowfall of autumn
apijaq—snow covered by bad weather
katakartanaq—snow with a hard crust that gives way under footsteps
kavisilaq—snow roughened by rain or frost
kinirtaq—compact, damp snow
mannguq—melting snow
masak—wet, falling snow
matsaaq—half-melted snow
natiruvaaq—drifting snow
pukak—crystalline snow that breaks down and separates like salt
qannialaaq—light-falling snow
qiasuqaq—snow that has thawed and refrozen with an ice surface
qiqumaaq—snow whose surface has frozen after a light spring thaw[22]

In many Native American languages, orientation and place are embedded in description. For instance, a different suffix may be added to a verb if one is going to or from a cardinal direction. In the Karuk language of northern California, a few of the many common directional verb suffixes are:

-kath: hence across a body of water
-kara: horizontally away from the center of a body of water
-rina: hither from across a body of water

-rípaa: horizontally toward the center of a body of water
-ríshuk: out of a container
-kiv: out through a tubular space
-rúprav: out through a solid
-rúpuk: out of an enclosed space[23]

In some Native languages, the sense of place is reinforced by conjugating verbs according to how information is received. For instance, in the California Wintu language, "evidential suffixes" support a speaker's claim. A different suffix is used if the speaker personally witnessed an event, heard about an event, or logically deduced that an event occurred. The English phrase "I saw an eagle" lacks context and definition compared to the closest equivalent in Wintu. We can see how much more precise the practice of law could be in an Indian court. In Native American languages, discussions of culture and healing tend to be contextual rather than textual, concrete rather than abstract.

Native American languages stem from cultures that recognize interrelatedness and thus stress cooperation rather than possession. As Dorothy Lee points out in *Freedom and Culture,* a Wintu phrase that literally means "The chief stood with the people" is translated "The chief ruled the people." In English, we say, "I own that piece of pottery"; in Wintu, "I live with that piece of pottery." We also see lack of possessiveness in Indian languages' emphasis on verbs and process rather than nouns and substance. The Maliseet language spoken in Maine and New Brunswick does not contain the word *wind,* only *to blow* or *to be windy.* Natural phenomena are also represented by verbs. The Maliseet word *nipawset,* "moon," literally means "walks at night."

Indian languages thus embody a unique style of reasoning. According to Robert Leavitt, professor of Education at the University of New Brunswick (Canada):

> *Speakers of North American Native languages do not necessarily organize reasoning according to a linear sequence of cause-and-effect, or axioms-theorems-corollaries, as do speakers of European languages. Instead they may keep a number of related ideas in mind, without assigning them an order or hierarchy.*[24]

Thus, the difficulty that many Western scientists have in understanding Native American medicine may be a result of the way language tends to mold perception. Whereas a Native American healer looks at disease as a disturbance in the relationship among self, spiritual forces, community, and environment, the Western physician focuses on body parts and biochemicals. Health for the Indian is the state of *Mitakuye Oyasin* (Lakota for "We are all related"). Health for the non-Indian physician is the absence of disease and must be confirmed by laboratory tests. To foster mutual understanding, we need to do more than translate one another's languages;

we need to translate our worldview, and no matter what the language, we need to free ourselves from prejudice and preconception.

There is a contradiction and paradox inherent in the quest to learn through the written word about healing traditions that were once nonliterate and are still predominantly oral. Native Americans have always placed more value on silence and experience than on concept and dogma. To use a Zen Buddhist analogy, the only way to truly understand Indian healing may be to use the words in this book as "a finger pointing at the moon."[25] When someone points his finger at the moon, look at the moon, not at the finger. Seek the experience behind the words.

DO I JOURNEY WHERE WISE MEN FEAR TO TREAD?

I live in a small log cabin in an ancient glacial valley at an elevation of nine thousand feet above sea level. From my window, I look out on snowcapped peaks that rise another three thousand feet. Outside my home is an ancient pass over the Continental Divide, traversed by nomadic Utes, Apache, and other tribal people for at least eleven thousand years. The presence of ceremonial materials, such as obsidian and red ocher, left as offerings along the high trails, suggests that these mountains were places of prayer and vision-seeking.

The winters are long here, with the first snow falling in September and the last in May. The nearly constant wind generated by the natural tunnel of surrounding mountains frequently drops the temperature to twenty or thirty degrees below zero. During the brief spring and summer, the meadows turn into a garden of wildflowers: columbines, irises, alpine buttercups, roses. Thunder rolls across the Divide every afternoon, frequently accompanied by rain and hail. Thunderbird—the spirit of thunder, the West, and the electricity of life—lives in these mountains; I was graced by his presence during my first Vision Quest. I am grateful to the natural elements. Thunder, wind, and cold strengthen and unify the people who dwell here. I have always found that natural challenges bring out the best in people, unlike social and economic hardship, which sometimes brings out the worst. A snowstorm makes good neighbors and, for Native people, has always been a natural time for storytelling. Severe weather also provides a deterrent to anyone who would disturb the solitude of mountains and mountain people.

One snowy winter morning about fifteen years ago, my dedication to this place almost faltered. I was getting tired of both the cold and my poverty. I had just returned home from a conference presentation in Hawai'i, where I had been offered a prestigious teaching position—an inviting contrast to my mountain hermitage. I thought, "The heck with this. I'm moving to Hawai'i!" As I opened the curtains over the picture window in my living room, I saw walking over the snow-covered trail a beautiful red fox. He was not more than fifty yards off, and I knew that there

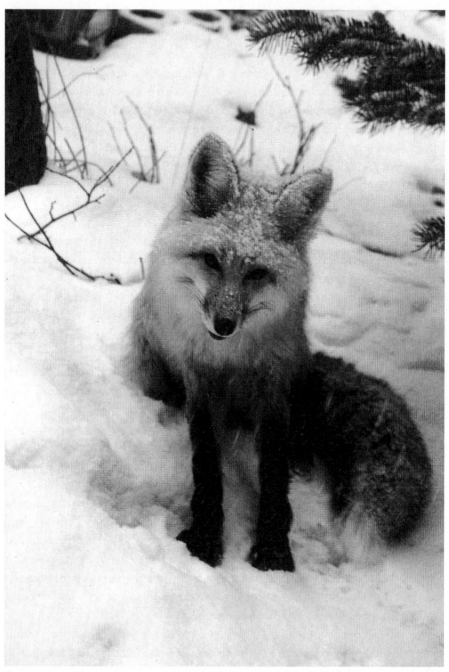

Within a week after I finished this introduction, a fox visited me again and waited patiently as I fetched my camera.

was sufficient light in the house for him to see me. Yet he kept walking toward the house, veering off the trail to pass through the garden in front of my window. When he was only two or three feet in front of me, he stopped, staring for a moment, gently and wisely, into my eyes. Then he calmly walked away. There was no question in my mind that this fox knew where he was going, that there was a purpose in his visit.

I immediately called Twylah Nitsch, a Seneca grandmother and personal friend, to tell her about the fox. "What were you thinking earlier in the morning?" she asked. I told her about wanting to leave the mountains. Grandmother quickly set me straight. "You are a Wolf Clan Teaching Lodge member. Do you think a wolf is going to come knocking at your door? No, the wolves send their little brother, the fox. That fox is a messenger and a message. You are not supposed to move away because *they* want you to stay. Native American tradition is not only for the two-legged people. It is also for the creature teachers; your prayers can help preserve the land for *their* future generations. Stop sitting on your medicine and get to work!"

When I search my soul and ask, "Why write this book?" I remember this story. I am not concerned with being known as an "authority." Creator cuts down those who use sacred knowledge for ego fulfillment or economic gain. Who can be an authority in matters of shared wisdom? The winter wind, *Keewaytin,* Spirit of the North, as my Cree relations call him, knows far more about indigenous wisdom than I ever shall. Nor am I motivated by the catharsis that every writer knows results from expressing one's truths. Rather, I am compelled to write by the lesson of that fox. If I can encourage or inspire others to listen to the voice of Mother Earth, to heal themselves and others, and to create a better world for the future generations, then I will have lived a good life. I also write because I am a parent. I would like to make the world a better place for my own children.

Like many health educators, I feel compelled to write about healing because of my personal experiences as a patient. When I was in my thirties, I developed a serious infection in my heart (see Chapter 8, pages 185–187). Native American healing—or rather, the Great Spirit's power acting through the healers—saved my life when both allopathic and alternative medicine had failed. Healing from serious illness creates obligations to be more caring for the precious gift of life and to help others navigate the storm one has weathered. I hope this book will also be of value to my Native American colleagues who are looking for new ways to understand or communicate their art.

Native American medicine and indigenous healing, in general, deserve a respected place among the world's great healing traditions. Most of the world's patients go to indigenous healers, sometimes because of better access, sometimes because of economic constraints, but often by choice. Native American medicine is certainly more compassionate than Western medicine as it is generally practiced. In the West, the separation of church and state led to a secularization of *all* knowledge.

By ignoring the sacred dimension of health, we create profanity and treat people as mechanical things, without soul or meaning. As many modern medical writers point out, we need to reintegrate healing and spirit, to realize that healing is a sacred task that involves the well-being of ourselves, our families and community, and the Earth itself. Native American healing is an example of this wisdom.

Native American healing wisdom may be needed for the survival of Indians and non-Indians alike. Its emphasis on respect, justice, and frugality with generosity is sound ecology. We need to learn these lessons if we are to prevent the widely prophesied political and economic conflicts or catastrophes and "earth changes": cataclysmic natural events that may occur as part of the Earth's attempts to rebalance the scales that Western civilization has upset. The elders say that the time is right to share sacred teachings. On August 20, 1994, a rare white buffalo calf was born on a farm in Wisconsin. Native medicine people recognized the calf as a symbol of the rebirth of the sacred in a world that has long suffered for its lack.

The urgency of sharing these teachings was confirmed for me during a Sacred Pipe Ceremony that I conducted at the turn of the millennium. The Pipe Ceremony is a way of communing with the forces of life, all of which are symbolically placed in the tobacco, ignited by the fire of transformation, and sent prayerfully up to Creator with one's breath. At the end of the Pipe Ceremony, I had a vision in which I saw, with the eye of spirit, layers of shimmering clouds hovering overhead. Eagles were flying slowly, almost meditatively, in the highest clouds. They transmitted a message to my mind: "In the Old Days, our spirits lived in and around the people. But today, people are polluting and destroying our home; few see or respect us physically or spiritually. Our spirits have withdrawn upward. We no longer dwell naturally among you but must be enticed down through ceremony and personal sacrifice."

The Eagle Spirit grants people the ability to dream and to see life from a higher, wider, and more balanced perspective. How sad that at a time when we need Eagle's inspiration the most, the Eagle is farthest away. We have made the world inhospitable to the Eagle, and like a traumatized person, his spirit has dissociated to an inaccessible realm. We can bring the Eagle back by caring for the Earth, by making the Earth a beautiful place where the Eagle will wish to nest and raise her young, and by prioritizing sacred knowledge, especially the wisdom that comes in dreams and visions, over material wealth.

I am not Native American by birth. Nor do I share Native Americans' ethnic history, though there are certainly similarities between the Native holocaust and that of my own Jewish ancestors. This work does not claim to officially represent any Native American nation or clan but, rather, expresses my personal view of Native American spirituality and healing, as learned from elders and medicine people of many nations and from the lessons of vision, dream, and prayer.

How did I come to this way of life? My training has been a matter of place, timing, and affinity. I have never sought out Native American teachers, but I gratefully listened to their wisdom when life circumstances brought us together. I have simply walked the path that Creator has set before me.

I have been involved in natural healing since my teens, when I began studying Chinese medicine and the Chinese language. I speak Chinese fluently and am the author of a book about qigong, the ancient Chinese system of healing exercises and meditations. When I was in my twenties, I met Native American healers because of our common interest in healing and spirituality. Several Native American elders accepted me as a kind of ambassador from the North (symbolizing the white race) and South (symbolizing the Chinese race) portions of the great medicine wheel of life. I do not live in China, however, and although I have immense respect for Chinese methods of healing, these do not resonate in my soul. My soul is linked to where I live and how I live.

I was an apprentice to the Cherokee elder Keetoowah, great-grandson of the famed Cherokee warrior Ned Christie, from 1976 to 1981. Keetoowah gave me my Indian name, "Bear Hawk" (*Yonah Tawodih*), and the sacred pipe, taught me legends and songs, and trained me in various healing methods. An invitation by the Canadian Ministry of Culture to teach natural healing in Saskatchewan in the 1980s resulted in meetings with respected Cree elders. In 1987, I was formally adopted by Andy Naytowhow, a Cree pipe carrier and spiritual counselor from Sturgeon Lake First Nation, Saskatchewan. I was on the road much of the time during the 1980s and continued studying with medicine people from several Indian nations. I discuss some of these journeys in "Meetings with Remarkable Elders," one of the appendixes to this book.

While following my interest in the common roots of indigenous spirituality, I became a close friend and student of healers among the Zulu people of South Africa and the Igbo of Nigeria. I feel blessed beyond any personal merit of which I am aware to have been given teachings and permission to share teachings from all four quadrants of the Great Wheel: the Red, Yellow, White, and Black. I know that all four colors are spokes from a common hub, and that hub, the Great Mystery, is ultimately beyond knowledge. If my words even hint at where to look, then perhaps this book will accomplish something good. "God is never a matter of distance, but of direction or orientation," a wise man once told me. If you have the courage to look within and without, you may find that you also have an indigenous soul.

Indian relations recognize my work as congruent with and often representative of their values and practices. The teachings are expressed with their encouragement, guidance, and support. I have tried to live according to the advice of traditional Native American elders for most of my adult life. I pray that this book honors their gifts.

NATIVE AMERICAN OR AMERICAN INDIAN
Can You Be Politically Correct?

Although Shakespeare said, "A rose by any other name would smell as sweet," you are less likely to want to see, smell, or buy a rose if a florist offers to show you "a blood-colored outgrowth of a thorny shrub." Names do make a difference.

Minorities and oppressed people are especially sensitive to the terminology used to describe them or their culture. The same words may mean different things to Native Americans or to white people, or they may be insulting in one language and either meaningless or used inappropriately in another. For example, no Native American woman wants to be referred to as a *squaw,* an Algonquian-based insult. A Native American physician does not expect to be called "chief." Some tribes are designated by strange foreign terms like *Gros Ventre* ("Big Bellies"), *Nez Perce* ("Pierced Noses"), or *Apache* (a Zuni Indian word meaning "enemy"). Native cultural and religious terms are sometimes appropriated by Western businesses for their commercial value. Would you feel comfortable riding in a Jeep Jew or drinking Communion Beer?

I have also seen people go to the other extreme: they try so hard to make every word polite and politically correct that they become tongue-tied, like a centipede that is asked, "How do you move all those legs?" I once met a young white man who had learned Indian sign language from a book and planned to use it when he visited an Indian reservation. He believed that this would demonstrate his respect for tradition. I was sorry to disappoint him: "When Indian people don't speak one another's languages, they communicate in English. People are likely to think that you are 'signing' because you're deaf." I don't wish to scare you from talking with or about people who are unfamiliar. If you speak with a Native American and are unsure about appropriate terminology, simply ask. Your question communicates respect.

AMERICAN INDIAN OR NATIVE AMERICAN?

There are problems inherent in any of the terms commonly used by both indigenous and nonindigenous people to designate the original inhabitants of Turtle Island (an ancient indigenous name for North America). In precolonial times, a general term for aboriginal Americans was unnecessary and did not always exist.

Today, as in the past, Native Americans identify themselves by family, community (or band), clan, and nation. A Native American clan is a group of people who recognize kinship because of a special relationship to or descent from a common ancestor or ancestral group. Clans may be named after a deed, characteristic, or *totem* (Algonquian for "helping spirit") of the ancestor—for example, the Bad War Deeds Clan, Long Hair Clan, Bear Clan, Wolf Clan, Caribou Clan, Wind Clan, Salt Clan, or Yucca Fruit Clan.[1] The words *nation* and *tribe* are often used interchangeably, though the term *nation* is generally more appropriate. The word *tribe* means a social group of numerous families and generations that share a common history, language, and culture. A nation is a tribe that is also a politically distinct entity and has the right to self-determination.

How would an ancient indigenous American identify himself or herself? A Cherokee woman living five hundred years ago would not call herself an American Indian. She might say, "I am Saloli [a common personal name, meaning "Squirrel"], an *Ani Wahya* [Wolf Clan member] *Ani Yunwiya* [Cherokee], from Kituwah [an ancient town site, near present Bryson City, North Carolina]." Saloli's people call themselves Ani Yunwiya, the Principal People, in their own language. In other Indian languages, a tribal designation might refer to the tribe's lodges (Haudenosaunee, "People of the Longhouse"), a sacred animal (the Absarokee, "Children of the Long-Beaked Bird," the Raven or Crow), or their lands (Tsimshian, "Those inside the Skeena River" in British Columbia).

Christopher Columbus, a lost sailor discovered by the Taino tribe of the Antilles in 1492, called the indigenous people he encountered *los Indios,* "Indians," because these gentle and generous people were *una gente en Dios,* "a people in God." Some scholars believe that the term *Indian* may reflect Columbus's belief that he had landed in India, an apt indication of his lack of orientation. The English, French, and Italian colonial invaders who followed him lumped all of Turtle Island's original inhabitants together as "savages" or other similar terms derived from the Latin *silvaticus,* meaning "a person of the woods" (*silva*). By the seventeenth century, *Indians* became the common designation, although the French continued to use *sauvage* through the nineteenth century. In 1643, Englishman Roger Williams summarized the common range of nomenclature in *A Key into the Language of America; Or, An Help to the Language of the Natives in That Part of America Called New-England:* "Natives, Savages, Indians, Wild-men (so the Dutch call them Wilden), Abergeny men, Pagans, Barbarians, Heathen"—terms that reflected and reinforced the Europeans' belief in the moral, theological, cultural, and biological inferiority of America's original inhabitants.[2]

The tone soon shifted. The new Euro-Americans began to refer to the Native

Americans as wild animals rather than wild men. In *Indians of California: The Changing Image,* James J. Rawls, Ph.D., history instructor from Diablo Valley College in Pleasant Hill, California, writes that "whites often compared California Indians to creatures that they regarded as especially repulsive": snakes, toads, baboons, and hogs.[3] Supported by an anthropocentric theology that placed man at the center of creation, Christians could exterminate "pests and vermin" without compunction. Similarly, modern soldiers find it easier to wage war against labels—"Nips," "Gooks"—than against human beings with souls and families. Generalizations and stereotypes also serve political ends, as they allow legislators to promote laws that manipulate the fate of widely divergent people with unique needs and lifestyles while emphasizing American unity and nationalism.

Today, it is virtually impossible to find a universally satisfactory or politically correct term for the original people of this continent. When one of my Cherokee elders was referred to as an "American Indian," he exclaimed, "I ain't no damn Indian! I'm a Native American." Yet most of America's original inhabitants do call themselves "Indians" among themselves. A Cree friend calls himself "Indian" but reminds me that in Canada, the preferred generalization is "First Nations." "Yet," he tells me, "I prefer *Native American* in literature. The term feels more elegant." So he becomes an "Indian" in everyday life and a Native American in books.

A consistent designation is important for clarity. I do not wish to perpetuate confusion by referring to the "aboriginal, indigenous, Indian, Native Americans of the First Nations." Frankly, I like to call the indigenous people "the People," a term consistent with the words used for original Native nations in their own languages. In the Cree language, indigenous North Americans are collectively referred to as *iyiniwak,* "Peoples." The names of many individual tribes, when translated, also simply mean "the People." An Innu ("the People" of Labrador, Baffin Island, and Québec) elder and friend, N'tsukw, has a definition that is a real gem: "We call ourselves the People because we know that we are only just people, two-leggeds, not better or higher than any other form of life or any other aspect of Creation."[4]

In this book, I have opted for elegance and generally referred to the People as Native American. I will, however, sometimes use the terms *Indian, First Nations* (when referring specifically to Canadian Indians), or *indigenous* (when my discussion is relevant to indigenous people of other lands).

WHO IS NATIVE AMERICAN?

What makes a person a Native American? This is an important and controversial topic. Is a person a Native American because of his or her ancestry, culture, or political status, or because of self-identification, which may or may not be verifiable? Who is entitled to live on tribal lands or share tribal revenue? Whose voice must be heard when consensus decisions are made either within Indian nations or between Indian nations and foreign governments? Who has the right to carry a Native American passport?

Criteria that establish Indian identity may include membership in or adoption by a recognized Indian family, a specific percentage of Indian "blood" (*blood quantum,* in legal terms),[5] or residence on tribal lands. Among some tribes, to claim tribal membership, you need only trace your genealogy to a Native American ancestor. (By this definition, former American President Bill Clinton is Cherokee.)

The United States government has frequently issued statutes that attempt to define Native ethnicity in order to clarify the rights of its "domestic dependent nations." The results have been uniformly disastrous. For example, during the early nineteenth century, many Native people did not register on U.S. government–sponsored tribal rolls. They did not recognize United States jurisdiction or care about the government's attempts to quantify them. Today, their descendants are clearly Native American, though not in the eyes of the U.S. government. Entire tribes, such as the forty-thousand-member Lumbee of North Carolina and the Duwamish of Washington (tribe of the famous Chief Seattle), remain unrecognized and are defined by the United States as nonexistent, often because of ignorance of a tribe's history and continuity; a lack of distinct, treaty-guaranteed lands; and greed for title over contested tribal homelands and their resources.

The Native American identity issue was highlighted in 1990 with the passage of the United States Indian Arts and Crafts Act. The act made it illegal for non-Indians to sell goods that are labeled "Indian-made." The law was designed to protect both consumers and Native Americans and has a clear application when you turn over an "Indian-made" pottery bowl and discover that it was "made in Japan." The law, however, also allows the U.S. government to prosecute Native Americans who do not meet *United States definitions of identity.* A descendant of a nonenrolled Native American or a member of a Native American community who does not have the requisite blood quantum can no longer legally sell "Indian-made" jewelry at a pow-wow.

The real issue here is not *what* determines Indian identity but *who* determines it. The question of Indian identity should not be in the hands of United States courts in the first place but rather decided by Native American nations and communities. Kanien'kehaka (Mohawk) scholar Taiaiake Alfred brings wisdom and clarity to the issue:

> *Respecting the right of [indigenous] communities to determine membership for themselves would promote reconstruction of indigenous nations as groups of related people, descended from historic tribal communities, who meet commonly defined cultural and racial characteristics for inclusion.*[6]

TERMS FOR NATIVE NATIONS

Many of the English names for Native American nations are based on derogatory terms used by the enemies of those nations. For example, the names *Iroquois* and *Sioux* are derived from words that mean "enemy." The word *Mohawk,* one of the six nations that comprise the Haudenosaunee Confederacy (Mohawk, Seneca, Onondaga, Oneida, Cayuga, Tuscarora), is based on an Algonquian word that means "cannibal monster." They call themselves Kanien'kehaka, People of the Flint. Some tribal designations are based on insulting remarks about a tribe's way of life, such as *Eskimo,* derived from a phrase meaning "eaters of raw meat," or *Naskapi,* meaning "uncivilized." In this book, I use tribal names that are widely recognized by both Native and non-Native scholars as respectful designations (see the accompanying table). I hope that other people who refer to Native American nations will continue this custom and adopt designations preferred by the tribes. In order not to confuse the reader, however, I will sometimes use less exact terminology when referring to peoples who have distinct words for each of their many bands or who use common tribal names among outsiders but different, more personal terms among themselves. (The Apache, Arapaho, and Comanche, for example, call themselves the Inde, Inunaina, and Nerm, respectively.)

Names of Native American Nations

COMMON TERM	PROPER TERM
Cheyenne	Tsistsistas
Crow	Absarokee
Delaware	Leni-Lenape
Eskimo	Inuit, or Inupiaq
Iroquois Confederacy	Haudenosaunee, or "Six Nations"
Montagnais or Naskapi	Innu
Navajo	Diné
Nootka	Nuu-chah-nulth
Ojibwa or Chippewa	Anishinabe
Papago	Tohono O'Odham
Sioux	Lakota, Dakota, or Nakota
Winnebago	Ho Chunk

EARTH PEOPLE

In Native American literature, the term *white man* is frequently a designation of colonial values—the need to dominate, divide, and acquire—rather than of ethnicity.[7] People who superficially imitate Native Americans while denying their own ethnicity, perhaps by wearing Native American clothing and jewelry and imitating speech patterns and mannerisms, are called by an equally derogatory term: *wannabees.* There are also wannabees among Native American people: "red apples," who are red on the outside but white on the inside. In the past, red apples were called "loafers around the forts," because they hung around the soldiers' forts to receive handouts rather than fight against injustice or live in a way that affirms Native American freedom, sovereignty, and values.

Today, we have an entirely new fruit, one with a white skin and a red heart. What should we call people who identify with Native American values and behave in a way consistent with those values? A person can be born Indian but act like a colonizer. A person can also be born white or Asian or black and act like a traditional Native American. Yes, it is possible. Not through imitation but by having the courage to follow the guidance of the heart. I have met many non-Native people who have shed colonial assumptions and learned to live lightly and respectfully on the earth. Native American elders recognize that in today's mixed-up world, race is no longer a guarantee of culture. The Creator has revealed his wonderful sense of humor in putting so many red souls in multicolored bodies!

People who respect Native American people, culture, and land and who are willing to make a personal and political stand for them deserve a proper term of respect. I like the designation suggested by a Lakota acquaintance: *Maka Oyate,* Earth People. The term is similar to a Cree phrase that is sometimes used by spirits (who speak through a ceremonial leader) to refer to Indian people: *aks-ju-aski-wes-skin-hagun,* "Earth-Made People." In the Holy Bible, the first human being is called Adam, meaning "Earth Person," because this androgynous being was formed of earth infused with God's breath.

You cannot become an Indian if you were not born one. But you *can* be an Earth Person.

WHAT NATIVE AMERICANS MEAN BY "MEDICINE"

To an English speaker, a "medicine" is something used to treat disease or enhance well-being. Native Americans accept this definition, but in the context of traditional culture, the word *medicine* has a much broader and richer meaning. Medicine means the presence and power embodied in or demonstrated by a person, a place, an event, an object, or a natural phenomenon. In some tribes, the word for medicine may connote spirit, power, energy, or mystic potency. For example, in the Wyandot (Huron) language, the word *arendi* (sometimes spelled *orenda*) means "spiritual power" or "medicine." The "medicine man" is the *arendiwane,* a compound of *arendi* and *wane*, meaning "powerful" or "great." Thus, the "medicine man" is someone whose spiritual power is great. His medicine, whether a prayer or an herb, affects more than illness; it establishes or restores a state of harmony and positive thinking.

A medicine may be something you have, a "medicine object" that has the power to affect your or another's well-being. For example, I have a beautiful piece of granite with a small amethyst crystal embedded in it. It was given to me by a dear friend, and whenever I look at it or hold it, I feel happy. I discovered that when I allow a client to hold it, he or she also feels happy. This is a kind of medicine.

More important, if you live a life of integrity and kindness, then medicine (spiritual potency) will become part of you. The elders teach that some medicine is inborn. The Great Spirit gives each person a medicine, a unique spiritual gift or talent. What a tragedy when people do not take the time to explore those gifts or do not have the confidence to express them!

Medicine may be good or bad according to the intent with which we use it or how it affects people. A kind word is good medicine, and an insulting or a discouraging word is bad medicine. A natural herb received from a compassionate healer is good medicine. The same herb, offered by an angry person, is bad medicine. A stethoscope is good medicine when used by a caring and wise physician. A stethoscope is an instrument of evil if the physician is demeaning to the patient.

Your feelings, intuition, and culture may determine whether a medicine is good or bad. For example, the owl is good medicine to some Northern Plains peoples, who often consider it a symbol of change and spiritual transformation. Yet my Cherokee friends won't allow an owl feather in their homes because they consider it to be an omen of death. Tobacco is a powerful healing ally to Native Americans who use it in prayer. However, to a white person who lost a loved one to emphysema or cancer, just the thought of tobacco may create feelings of anger and bitterness. Dreams may also be good or bad medicine. Dreams of healing or helping advice or dreams that have beautiful images are good medicine. Nightmares may also be good medicine if they are sources of personal insight or if they provide warnings that lead to positive change. Native Americans believe, however, that some nightmares are bad medicine inflicted by malicious spirits, people, or sorcerers.

Good medicine always gives you a sense of sacredness or sacred power. Good medicine is healing.

MEDICINE PEOPLE AND SPIRIT POWERS

The terms *medicine man* and *medicine woman* are ambiguous. Many Native languages have specific words for various healing specialists, including snakebite doctors, midwives, conjurers, diviners, bone-setters, wound-healers, and herbalists. Various types of healers may identify themselves by wearing symbols of their specialty. For example, a Seminole healer who wears an owl feather in his hat is a "general practitioner" and can treat many types of disorders, symbolized by the many bars on the owl feather. If he wears a yellow-flicker feather, he is a headache specialist and can get at the root of the problem the way a flicker probes a tree for insects.

Some healers are associated with specific animals, elements, or powers that they invoke or with which they commune, variously called dream helpers, spirit helpers, spirit powers, spirit guides, tutelary spirits, totems, guardian spirits, or animal allies. For instance, a healer might be a "bear-dreamer" because she dreams of bears, or a "water-doctor" because she uses water in healing ceremonies. Because Native Americans recognize that all phenomena exist in physical and spiritual dimensions, there are an infinite number of spiritual powers, and no person can name or understand them all. Powerful Cree healers may commune with *Asinapewiyiniw*, Old Man Stone Spirit, or with the spirit of an emotion such as Love or the spirit of an activity—for example, the Song Spirit. These powers may grant healers the ability to treat a limited or wide range of problems. Healers may increase their repertoire as they acquire new powers or spiritual visions. The following three examples illustrate a typical range of categories of healing practitioners as well as the similarity of these categories from one tribe to another:

Yurok (*Northwestern California*)[8]

- **Meges:** Herbalist.
- **Kwes?oye?ey:** Prayer Doctor.
- **?umelo:yik:** Brush Dance Doctors, who perform the child-curing Brush Dance and practice steaming patients with herbal infusions.
- **Kegey:** The High Doctor, Indian Doctor, or "Sucking Doctor." From the verb stem *key(chek'in-)*, "to sit," and an internal element (infix), e.g., meaning "an intensive repeated action or practice," probably referring either to the practice of sitting on a redwood stool and smoking a pipe while diagnosing a patient or to the sacred place for healing training high in the mountains, known as a "prayer seat." The Kegey can cure serious disease by sucking out disease-causing objects or spirits. The Kegey is usually a woman, and the potential to become one is frequently passed from mother to daughter.

Lakota[9]

- **Pejuta Wicasa, Pejuta Winyela:** Herb Man, Herb Woman.
- **Heyoka:** A Sacred Clown or Contrary, who may heal with the power of thunder.
- **Wapiya:** Literally, "to make good," translated sometimes "Conjurer." The Wapiya is a ceremonial leader who may use clairvoyance and spiritual powers to locate healing herbs or to suck or draw out disease-causing objects or spirits.
- **Wicasa Wakan, Winyan Wakan:** Holy or Sacred Man, Holy or Sacred Woman, who can cure, prophesy, conduct ceremonies, and talk to the spirits in nature and people. This beautiful term may also imply someone who serves the Wakan, the Sacred and Divine.[10]

Anishinabe[11]

- **Maskikiwinini:** Herbalist.
- **Wabeno:** "Dawn Men," who use the power of fire and hot coals to heal and make charms.
- **Jessakid:** Healers who receive from the Thunder Spirit the gift of seeing hidden truths and sucking out disease.
- **Mide:** The High Healers and Priests of the Midewewin Grand Medicine Society. *Mide* commonly means "the sound of the drum" (related to the Penobscot term for healer, *medo'olinu,* "drum-sound person").

Without understanding the special meaning of the word *medicine,* English readers might assume that *medicine man* or *medicine woman* refers to an herbalist (for example, *pejuta wicasa*). Frequently, however, the term *medicine man* is used to translate an indigenous term for holy person (for example, *wicasa wakan*). A holy person is the highest and most diverse kind of healer, someone who has such deep knowledge of spiritual forces that he or she can discover whatever kind of medicine is most suitable for the patient's well-being, whether it be herbal, psychological, or ceremonial. I use the terms *medicine man* and *medicine woman* in this sense, as synonyms for "holy person." I sometimes preface the name of a medicine person with "Grandfather" or "Grandmother." These are terms of respect and an expression of my feeling of personal affinity rather than a suggestion of blood relationship.[12]

Any type of Native healing practitioner, whether a holy person or a specialist, may also be called a "healer" or an "Indian doctor," and I will sometimes also use these terms. Their practice is naturally called "healing" or "doctoring." Among Native American people, it is common to speak of a healer's "doctoring" someone—that is, performing a healing intervention. A healer can also "doctor" or "doctor up" an object—that is, imbue it with spiritual power.

The title "medicine man" or "holy person" is an honorific conferred by a community in recognition of a person's wisdom and service. It is not generally used by a healer in reference to himself or herself. Many healers refer to themselves as "spiritual interpreters." Floyd Looks for Buffalo Hand, Lakota full-blooded grandson of Chief Red Cloud, writes, "I have been told that there are no holy men on this earth, only gifted men. They are called spiritual interpreters."[13] If someone says, "I am a holy person" or "I am a medicine man," I take this as equivalent to saying, "I just typed up a Ph.D. degree, signed it, and hung it on my wall."

CEREMONIES

I will devote an entire chapter to ceremonies later in this book. However, because I use the term *ceremony* frequently, it is important to give a brief definition here in order to prevent misunderstanding. A ceremony is a prescribed sequence of actions that enables one to experience and communicate with a spiritual realm or to influence events—for example, a rain-making or planting ceremony. Ceremonies may be personal, inspired by visions and dreams, or they may be tribal traditions, passed down from generation to generation. They may be performed individually or, more commonly, by the tribe or community. Ceremonies are conducted by a "ceremonial leader," a medicine man or woman trained in the protocol. To attend a ceremony is to participate in it, even if you are not assigned a role to play. Native American ceremonies may occur in a variety of settings, including ceremonial lodges, ordinary homes, outdoor arbors, or in the wilderness. Healing interventions are generally considered ceremonies, as are "teachings," traditional Native American lectures about sacred subjects. Speaking about sacred subjects invokes the attention and presence of spirits, requiring the speaker to perform ceremonial actions that demonstrate respect.

SHAMANS AND SANGOMAS

Many books use the word *shaman* instead of *medicine man,* especially when referring to spiritual practitioners among the Inuit and northwestern peoples. The term *shaman* properly refers only to indigenous people from Siberia, Manchuria, and central Asia. It is derived from a Manchurian or Siberian Tungusic word that means a person who contacts spiritual forces while in an ecstatic, aroused, or altered state of consciousness. The shaman retrieves information and power that are useful to her community—for example, divining the location of a herd or learning how to heal a mental or physical disease. Shamans in many Asian traditions, including China, were primarily female.

There are certainly important similarities in belief and practice between Asian shamans and Native American medicine people. We can also find similar parallels between Native medicine people and healers from Africa or Australia. Yet we do not call Native medicine people *sangomas,* a Zulu word for healer. I do not feel comfortable applying an Asian word to Native American healers or holy people. The English term *medicine person* seems to be a better generalization.

COMPLEMENTARY AND ALTERNATIVE MEDICINE

Conventional, or allopathic (from Greek words that mean "other than disease"), medicine[14] consists of the methods of diagnosis and treatment of disease that are part of the politically dominant culture and thus considered standard practice in that culture's medical schools and clinics. Other methods of healing are frequently labeled unconventional or nontraditional. Of course, the meaning of the word *traditional* depends on one's point of view. To most of the world's peoples, indigenous healing is traditional, and all other systems are "alternative." In 1993, the World Health Organization estimated that at least 80 percent of the world's population relies on some form of traditional—that is, nonallopathic—medicine as the primary source of health care.[15] If we eliminate Western countries, the figure jumps to 90 percent.[16]

During the 1970s and 1980s, the most common broad terms for nonallopathic interventions were *holistic* and *alternative.* The holistic medical movement began in the 1970s as a philosophy and collection of practices that intended to treat the whole person—body, mind, and spirit. During the 1980s, clinicians, scholars, and journalists began to promote the concept of "alternative medicine." I do not like the term *alternative.* Although it can imply a patient's right to choose between viable alternatives, it may also suggest that the patient *must* choose one or the other, allopathic or unconventional. This phrase goes against the intent of many "alternative" practitioners who recognize that different healing modalities can work well together. If a patient is suffering, we should not deny him or her any therapy that works.

Today, the accepted and politically correct designation—and the one that I prefer—is complementary and alternative medicine (CAM). This phrase has been officially endorsed by the United States National Institutes of Health. It avoids altogether the ambiguous and controversial phrase *nontraditional.* CAM aptly suggests that various healing modalities, whether alternative or allopathic, can complement one another. CAM, unlike allopathic medicine, places an equal emphasis on disease prevention, therapy, and health promotion. Many CAM practitioners are more concerned with health care than sick care and with qualitative factors such as patient satisfaction rather than quantities measured in the laboratory. They also tend to recognize that it is important for the provider to follow his or her own advice and to be a model of commitment to health.[17]

There is an extraordinary variety of CAM modalities, including acupuncture, dance therapy, homeopathy, massage therapy, music therapy, therapeutic touch, herbology, psychic healing, pastoral counseling, and spiritual healing (including prayer and worship). Native American medicine is the oldest method of CAM practiced in the West and certainly the only one that has grown out of and truly belongs to the American landscape.

THE GREAT SPIRIT

Native American healers are unified in their belief that the Great Spirit is the source of healing and life. I use the terms *Great Spirit, Great Mystery, Creator,* and *God* interchangeably. Some Native people call the Great Spirit "Grandfather," in contrast to the Earth, which is called "Mother" or "Grandmother." Many consider the Great Spirit beyond or inclusive of all gender and may thus use masculine and/or feminine forms of address. Examples of specific terms used among various tribes include:

- **Acbadadea:** Maker of All Things Above (Absarokee)
- **Hesákádum Eseé:** the Maker of Breath (Muskogee)
- **Kitchi Manitou:** the Great Mystery (Anishinabe)
- **Shongwàyadíhs:on:** the Creator (Haudenosaunee)
- **Si Cel Siam:** the Creator (Samish)
- **Wakan Tanka:** the Great Sacred or Great Spirit (Lakota)
- **Wiyôhtâwîmâw:** the Father (Cree)

Do Native Americans worship God? Yes. Equally important, they seek ways to *experience* God.

According to Francis La Flesche's *Dictionary of the Osage Language:*

[T]his great power [Wa-kon-da] resides in the air, the blue sky, the clouds, the stars, the sun, the moon, and the earth [including all living things]. . . . Sometimes the Osage speak of a tree, a rock or a prominent hill as Wa-kon-da, but when asked if his people had a great number of Wa-kon-das he would reply, "Not so; there is but one God and His presence is in all things and is everywhere. We say a tree is Wa-kon-da because in it also Wa-kon-da resides."[18]

Part I

PRINCIPLES
– AND –
VALUES

— THE NATIVE AMERICAN — PHILOSOPHY OF LIFE

Native American healing is based on a spiritual philosophy of life, which I outline below. Even if you have never learned healing techniques, you can be considered a healer if you follow the philosophy and let it become the basis for a good way of life.

- There is a Creator or Great Spirit. The Great Spirit is the creator of all life. Because the Great Spirit formed all life out of the same elements, human beings are interconnected and related to all of nature. Harmonious relationship with nature promotes health; living out of balance with the web of life promotes illness.

- Nature is alive. Natural phenomena exist in both the physical and spiritual dimensions. The physical and spiritual realities interpenetrate and influence each other. Human beings have the ability to become aware of and communicate with both realities.

- In varying degrees, life energy and power are in all natural phenomena and in some man-made objects. This energy is associated with wind and breath; it is the breath of life.

- Holiness is an attribute of spirits, places, natural phenomena (including all living beings), objects (amulets, medicine bundles, and so forth), and the Great Spirit. Holiness can be attained by people or imparted to activities or objects.

- Spirits may be helping or harming, good or evil. Evil may be attained by people or imparted to activities or objects. Sorcerers (also called "witches") use their powers to cause harm.

- Nature is an important source of health and wisdom. (There was little sickness long ago, compared to the present day. People who lived in nature were always walking and exercising and ate the healthy foods that nature provided.)

- A spiritual person is intimate with nature and knows the names, characteristics, and stories associated with local plants, animals, waterways, and mountains. He or she also understands and communes with "the Four Winds," the sacred power of the directions East, South, West, and North.

- Silence is the foundation of truth. Words are most meaningful when they emerge from silence and when they are received by a quiet mind.

- Prayer is communication with the Great Spirit and/or the wise beings or powers that he created. It includes both listening and speaking. To pray to the Great Spirit is to seek unity with the Great Spirit. It is good to begin and end each day with prayer. Pray before eating and before all important activities.

- Ritual gestures, objects, and "symbols" (such as the Four Winds) do not have meaning; they *are* meaning. To say of two related spiritual phenomena "*A* symbolizes or represents *B*" is not always accurate. The Bear does not simply represent the West; he *is* the West. The healer does not dance like the Eagle; she *is* the Eagle dancing. The swan feather on the altar does not represent the swan; it *is* the swan medicine power.

- A spiritual person embodies spiritual values such as honesty, honor, respect, humility, courage, patience, generosity, and humor. A spiritual person inspires and teaches these values by example. He or she has what Native Americans call "a Good Mind."

- To live a meaningful and happy life, we must find our purpose. People can deepen their connection to the Creator and discover their purpose through prayer, fasting, dreaming, and other spiritual practices. A healer helps patients to find their own dreams, visions, and purpose in life.

- Elders are keepers and transmitters of sacred knowledge.

- Children are sacred. People should consider the effects of their thoughts, words, and behavior on the future generations.

- Men and women have equal but different power and responsibilities.

- Human knowledge is limited. Many things cannot be known.

I

— THE POWER OF SILENCE —

*Ah my brother, you will never know the happiness of thinking nothing
and doing nothing. This is the most delightful thing there is next to sleep.
So we were before birth; and so we shall be after death.*
—A Pueblo tribesman speaking to Carl Jung[1]

Silence is the universal language. It is a common human experience that the deepest communication occurs when nothing needs to be said: in silence, one hears the language of lovers or close friends and senses the understanding that flows between people and their pets or between parent and child. According to Native American teachings, we can have this quality of silent communication with anyone, with any place, and with any aspect of nature.

The first time I met the Cherokee medicine man Rolling Thunder, we sat without speaking for about ten minutes under a willow arbor in the desert. In this way, we could listen to the place from which words arise, to each other's silence. It was a good introduction, a good foundation on which to build a friendship. Years later, I heard Rolling Thunder say, "In the old days, if two Native people met on the trail, they could communicate through silence. They just *knew* each other's heart and intentions without words."

Similarly, one of my elders used to say, "We are born with two ears and one mouth because we should listen at least twice as much as we speak. A healer should be like the fox. The fox has big ears because he is a good listener." Native American healers affirm that only a silent mind can assess the health of a patient. Silent listening is the key to understanding. You cannot understand or heal yourself or others if you are unable to listen or if the only thing to which you listen is your own thoughts. Without silence, you are looking at yourself in a mirror, even when you think you are looking outside.

In Native American culture, the spiritual person is, most importantly, a good listener. But the word *listening* implies more than hearing sounds or comprehending

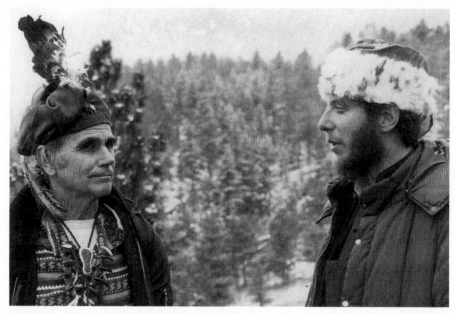

Rolling Thunder and the author, 1982. Photo by Paul Orbuch.

language. It includes the intuitive impressions received by a silent mind. It allows room for input uncolored by preconception and prejudice. "The *wicasa wakan* [holy person] loves silence," writes the Lakota holy man Lame Deer, "wrapping it around himself like a blanket—a loud silence with a voice like thunder which tells him of many things. Such a man likes to be in a place where there is no sound but the humming of insects."[2] The Arapaho believe that silence is the mark of maturity. Having earned the right to withdraw from the noise of public activities, the seven wisest men of the tribe, known as "the Seven Old Men," retreat to a quiet life (*tei-itoniine'etiit*). Their silence guards sacred knowledge and ensures the continued life of their tribe.

Silence is the essence of the Vision Quest, the solitary period of fasting and communion in nature to discover one's life purpose and, sometimes, healing power. The greatest challenge of the Vision Quest is not fasting from food and water; it is fasting from words and thoughts, what the ancient Chinese called "the fasting of the mind." Only through profound inner fasting can one perceive and commune with the Sacred. If the quester's mind is unquiet, he will attach meanings or symbolism to his experience prematurely. Thinking about an experience stops experience. You cannot be in an experience and outside of it at the same time. The highest purpose of the Vision Quest is to touch a mystery beyond words, perceived only in silence, solitude, and darkness. Many years ago, Inuit shaman Najagneg told the Danish explorer Knud Rasmussen, "I have searched in the darkness, being silent in the great lonely stillness of the dark. So I became an *angakoq* [shaman], through visions and dreams and encounters with flying spirits."[3]

— DREAMING OF SILENCE —

When I was thirteen years old, many years before I began training with Native American elders, I had two dreams that taught me the power of silence. When I later discovered that silence was at the heart of Native American spirituality, I knew that I had come home.

I dreamed that I was at the ocean, standing alone in sand dunes, listening to the rhythm of the waves. My mind was utterly quiet. In the silence, I knew the meaning of the ocean in a way that words could never communicate. I looked up and saw all the stars of the galaxy glistening in a clear sky. A shooting star fell, and then another, and another. Soon all the stars were shooting across the sky, leaving only black space behind. Gazing into the immensity, I was filled with a profound peace. Out of that blackness, an eagle emerged, slowly flapping its wings. I knew that the world I had previously known had ended.

In the second dream, later that year, I was also near the ocean, looking out, this time, over a quiet evening sea. I inhaled deeply, drawing in the ocean with my breath. My separate self and all the thoughts and belief systems that maintained it disappeared. I became the ocean. I awakened ecstatic, knowing that the dream had shown me a reality deeper and more expansive than the everyday.

In the most sacred places, we do not perceive spirits, but only the silence of the Great Mystery. We go to those places to touch the deepest wisdom and to renew our being. I still enter a silent state when I am near the ocean. Silence can awaken the Eagle of wisdom, allowing him to emerge from even the darkest skies. When we breathe with a silent mind, we share the breath of life with nature. We can inhale and exhale the ocean, a tree, or a cloud. Like listening to the ocean waves, breathing also puts us in touch with the energy and rhythm of life. Perhaps the crashing waves and retreating tides *are* the breathing of the ocean.

Listening puts us in touch with the energy, vibration, and spiritual forces that lie at the heart of creation. As author Maureen Trudelle Schwarz, Ph.D., writes in her beautiful book *Molded in the Image of Changing Woman,* "All entities in the Navajo world consist of the primary elements of moisture, air, substance, and heat, which are permeated by vibration. . . ."[4] Sound moves slowly enough that we are aware of its pulse and the way it issues from and returns to silence. We can hear sound because it vibrates the eardrum; we can feel it more physically and dramatically when the sound of a drum vibrates the body's resonant bones and tissues. Listening provides ample evidence that life consists of energy and rhythm. Light, by contrast, moves so quickly both in space and through our optic nerves that we cannot sense its rhythm. Interestingly, the Holy Bible provides a clue to the relationship between sound and sight. "God *said,* 'Let there be light,' and there was light." In other words, the vibratory power of God's word created light. Sound and light are both holy, but sound came first.

DON'T SPEAK TOO MUCH

Native American elders like to listen to what people don't say, to the spaces before, between, and after words. Words can lie, but silence tells the truth. Anishinabe scholar and author Dr. Basil Johnston says that using only as many words as the occasion demands—sometimes no words at all—is "the first principle of credibility and trust."[5] When I visited the great Cree medicine man Albert Lightning at his home, he greeted me with a warm handshake. We sat together in silence for about twenty minutes, neither of us speaking a word. Then *Mosom* ("Grandfather") began sharing stories and teachings that lasted through the night. I had passed his "test." In all indigenous cultures, silence is a token of respect, self-control, patience, and humility.

In all settings, economy of speech encourages truthfulness. The speaker is careful not to warp or exaggerate the truth or to go beyond the limits of what he knows. Economy of speech also shows common courtesy and respect for the listener. In Apache society, one of the basic ways of displaying courtesy is *laago yalti',* "not speaking too much." Attempting to fill silence by "making conversation" or by asking many questions is rude. People who speak too much are too preoccupied with their own ideas to act in cooperation with others. Keith H. Basso, professor of anthropology at the University of New Mexico, writes in his brilliant work on Western Apache culture *Wisdom Sits in Places:*

> *A person who speaks too much—someone who describes too busily, who supplies too many details, who repeats and qualifies too many times—presumes without warrant on the right of hearers to build freely and creatively on the*

speaker's own depictions. . . . In other words, persons who speak too much in-
sult the imaginative capabilities of other people. . . .[6]

LISTENING TO DISEASE

The virtues of silence are implicit in the Apache concept of *igoya'i,* "wisdom."
Igoya'i is a state of heightened awareness and sensitivity that allows one to detect
and avoid potential sources of harm. To a traditional Native American healer, listening to a patient means silencing one's thoughts to gain a more direct perception
of the patient's physical, mental, and spiritual health. The native healer forms a kind
of intuitive and spiritual first impression against which the relevance of knowledge
and clinical experience can later be weighed. Inner silence creates an outer state of
"active listening," in which the healer can pick up messages hidden in the patient's
words, tone of voice, and body language.

The value of listening is known to good doctors in any culture. As cardiologist
Bernard Lown affirms, "[L]istening is the most complex and difficult of all tools in
the doctor's repertory. One must be an active listener to hear an unspoken problem."[7] A healer with this capacity can detect health problems while they are still sub-
clinical—that is, without obvious or measurable symptoms.

The patient, too, must listen. Silence puts us in touch with the presence of the
Great Mystery within, the quiet depths from which healing insight and power
emerge. (Similarly, in the Holy Bible, Ezekiel 1:4, God is called *Chashmal,* "the
Speaking Silence.") Silence allows a patient to detect his or her own imbalances. On
the other hand, speaking, thinking, or worrying about disease gives power to the
disease. This is true whether you are thinking about your own illness or another's.
Native American healers believe that thoughts are a form of subtle energy that can
influence physical reality, even at a distance.

Words, say the elders, have power. They can create reality. The Absarokee (Crow)
term *dasshússuua* literally means "breaking with the mouth." Rodney Frey, in his important work *The World of the Crow Indians,* explains it this way: "Words, brought
forth through the mouth, have the ability to break, to alter or to bring about, a situation. One may hesitate to discuss an illness, fearing that the use of words describing it may inadvertently cause the affliction."[8] Many Native healers believe that
diseases are either caused by or *are* offended spirits. Speaking about, or even naming, a disease may attract these spirits' attention, thereby intensifying symptoms or
making the disease more difficult, if not impossible, to cure. If non-Indian doctors
realized the power of their words, they would be far more circumspect in their discussions of disease either with patients, with patients' families, or with other doctors. Patients would also be careful not to allow disease labels, negative thoughts, or
just too much talking to interfere with their healing.

Native healers also recognize that talking about disease strengthens a patient's identification with the disease. The more the patient says, "I have diabetes," the greater the cognitive and energetic rut. Silence, on the other hand, helps foster a state of peace, tranquillity, possibility, and hope.

SURVIVAL OF THE QUIETEST

Like the meditative traditions of Asia, the Native American appreciation of silence probably began with the need for stillness, silence, and attentiveness while hunting.[9] Gary Snyder, the Pulitzer Prize–winning poet, writes, "The personal direct contact with the natural world required of hunters and gatherers—men and women both— generated continual alertness."[10] Words were few and to the point, lest they be carried by a sudden gust of wind to the hunter's prey, thus alerting it to danger. Stepping on a twig or breaking a branch could mean the difference between feast and famine.

Native American hunters learn to move silently yet invisibly through the woods. An extraordinary description of this skill can be found in the writings of the celebrated director of the Tracking, Nature, and Wilderness Survival School in the Pine Barrens of New Jersey, Tom Brown Jr., a white man who learned his art from the Apache spiritual teacher Stalking Wolf. "We learned the principles of passing unobserved. Be still. Be silent. Conform to the shape of what surrounds you. Take advantage of the shadows and places where the light makes things uncertain."[11] Stalking Wolf taught Brown to "move as the wind moves," fluidly and in harmony with the environment. Animals notice movements that are erratic or eccentric. To demonstrate his skill, Stalking Wolf would sometimes creep up on a deer and let his arm dangle over the deer's back like a tree branch. The deer might scratch himself against his outstretched fingers. Or Stalking Wolf, after standing tree-like for a period of time, might give the deer a smack for being so careless around a potential predator.

PRACTICING SILENCE

The power of silence echoes in many works written about diverse Native American cultures. According to Gerald Vizenor (Anishinabe), professor of Native American Studies at the University of California, Berkeley, "the Anishinaabe were driven to silence"[12] that was filled with song, poetry, and story. Creek Medicine Man Bear Heart says, "The beauty of silence . . . helps us collect our thoughts and center our lives so we can maintain a sense of calm when we return to the hectic society and resume our work."[13] In a booklet published by the Seneca Indian Historical Society, Seneca elder Twylah Nitsch discusses a Native American term for meditation, *entering the silence.* "Living in harmony with the peace and quietude of Nature taught the Seneca self-discipline. They moved slowly, spoke softly, and developed a natural quietude. This silence was acquired and signified perfect harmony in spirit, mind, and body. Being silent was an earned virtue and revered as an honorable trait."[14] In *Inuksuit: Silent Messengers of the Arctic,* researcher, photographer, and student of

---

Practicing silence is not a matter of doing but of not-doing. Thinking is a physiological process that induces electrical and biochemical changes throughout the body. If we pay really close attention, we find that the process of thinking always corresponds to a subjective feeling of tension, most often centered in the face, jaw, and tongue. When we think, we are, in effect, speaking to ourselves. The metabolism speeds up. The heart beats quicker, the body breathes faster, and the mind literally races into the quickest brain-wave pattern, called *beta waves.*

Achieving silence requires you to relax and slow down, to stop doing and start being. You can practice silence from any position. It is easiest, however, to learn how to be mentally quiet from a seated or supine posture. Let tension drop away into the ground. Enjoy the feeling of the ground supporting you. Pay attention to your breath. Take seven deep breaths in and out. Each time you inhale, imagine fresh energy coming in, and when you exhale, imagine stale energy, tension, and mental distraction departing. Now breathe naturally and without force. Notice your breathing rate. Deep breathing has freed up the muscles of the diaphragm and allowed relaxed and unhurried respiration. If your air passages are healthy, you should not be able to hear your breathing. As the breath becomes silent, the mind becomes silent.

If there are sounds in your environment, let them play upon your eardrums without wondering what they mean. Sounds cannot disturb inner silence. Be a still pond without the ripples of thought.[15]

When you come out of the silence, you will find that your mind is much sharper. The mind, like the body, needs periods of rest. Reasoning is dulled through excessive use and honed by silence.

---

the Inuit Norman Hallendy quotes Osuitok, an elder from Baffin Island, who describes a deep state of awareness called *inuinaqtuk* that brings more insight than dreaming. It is related to solitude, peace, and silence and "is like a window through which one can see into things as never before. It's as if you moved out of the tiny space you occupy in this world and can see the whole world and can see past its shadows."[16]

Today, both Native and non-Native people recognize that in our noisy, stressful, and excessively busy world, the need for silence is greater than ever before. Taking occasional "silence breaks" can also help you understand the teachings in this book at a deeper level.

2

— THE FOUR WINDS —
Getting Oriented in
the Realm of the Sacred

Among Native Americans, the Four Directions, or more commonly, "the Four Winds," are considered powerful spirits. Wind, the breath of the Great Spirit, is the sacred force that permeates the natural world. To the Diné, it is *nilch'i*, "holy wind." The Lakota speak of *ni,* the sacred breath, the source of life and strength. The sacred sweat lodge, called *initipi,* is a tipi, the well-known Plains Indian dwelling, for cleansing the *ni.* When the *ni* is strong and clear, we are healthy. When the *ni* is gone, we are dead. Anishinabe elders teach that the Great Mystery created the world by breathing life into rock, water, fire, and wind. According to Diné tradition, Changing Woman created human beings by breathing on a mixture of skin from her body with white shell, turquoise, abalone, jet, and corn of all colors. In the Bible, God breathed his or her *ruach,* "sacred breath," into the earth (*Adama*) to create the first human (Adam). Adam was not a man but an androgynous Earth Person. All ancient traditions agree that air is the same as spirit.

Breath is invisible and immaterial, yet it is the most powerful force in nature. We can live without it for only a few minutes. We live immersed in air. We breathe in air to create the metabolic fuel that keeps the cells alive. Breath literally flows through our bodies, yet the only way we can feel air's power is when it is in motion. We sense its presence subtly when we breathe or speak. It is most obvious in the form of wind. The Great Spirit speaks through the wind. The wind is his or her messenger.

The Four Winds remind us of the importance of knowing not only who we are but where we are. A person who explores the meaning and power of the Four Winds has a sense of direction on the earth and in life. Each of the Four Winds represents qualities that contribute to psychological and spiritual health, and a person who understands them feels in harmony with the universe. For example, the East, where the sun rises, symbolizes inspiration and spiritual renewal. The West, where the sun sets, is, by contrast, a place of dreams and introspection.

The Four Winds are commonly represented as a cross or a cross within a circle, the *cangleska wakan,* "sacred hoop," as it is called in Lakota.[1] To explore the meaning of the Four Winds, we must learn about the symbolic meaning of the circle, the number four, and the directions. These concepts are central to all facets of Native American culture. As you deepen your understanding of the Four Winds, you will deepen your understanding of Native American healing. The Four Winds are a model and map that can help you find your way in many situations in life.

THE CIRCLE:
WHERE THE END IS THE BEGINNING

The universal symbol of wholeness is the circle. Life is a circle that moves from birth to old age to death to new life. When we are at the end, we are also at the beginning. All learning occurs along the circle of the Four Winds, from the place of inspiration (East) to development (South) to application (West) to maturity (North). Ideas take shape and acquire meaning as they move along this great circle. An old person becomes an elder in the Native American sense if he or she has journeyed mindfully around the circle, from the direction of birth in the East, through growth in the South, to the mature autumn of life in the West, and finally to old age in the North. The direction is not, however, always a one-way, clockwise progression. There are times in people's lives when they jump from one position to another: grandparents and children, for example, seek wisdom from each other.

The circle is the most common shape in nature.[2] In contrast to many man-made objects, everything in nature appears to be at least partly round. In one of the most beautiful passages in all of Native American literature, the Lakota sage Black Elk says, "Everything the Power of the World does is done in a circle. The sky is round, and I have heard that the earth is round like a ball, and so are all the stars. The wind, in its greatest power, whirls. Birds make their nests in circles, for theirs is the same religion as ours."[3]

Science agrees that the circle or variations on it—such as the sphere or spiral— are the essence of life. Cells are round. The DNA in them consists of spirals: the "double helix." Bones are round and show curving lines of flow in their interior. Plant stems and trees are also round. We judge the age of a tree by the number of rings in the trunk. Even water curves as it meanders and swirls. Throw a pebble in a lake and watch the rippling circles. A stream tends to flow in snakelike patterns, unless, on its way down a hillside, its nature is overpowered by the linear force of gravity. Theodor Schwenk, former director of an institute for the study of water and air movement in Germany's Black Forest, writes in his book *Sensitive Chaos: The Creation of Flowing Forms in Water and Air,* "Wherever water occurs it tends to take on a spherical form. It envelops the whole sphere of the earth, enclosing every object in a thin film. Falling as a drop, water oscillates about the form of a sphere; or as dew fallen on a clear and starry night it transforms an inconspicuous field into a starry heaven of sparkling drops."[4] Water and air *circulate* in the human body and cycle through the body of the earth.

The circular shape occurs often in traditional Native American culture. Tipis, wickiups, wigwams, Inuit winter homes (iglus or igloos), sweat lodges, and other traditional dwellings or ceremonial lodges are round. I have heard Native American healers complain that they lost a great deal of their spiritual power and efficacy when they began to live in square or rectangular homes. When Indian people gather for a ceremony or to discuss important matters, they sit in a circle so that everyone is equal. Ceremonial objects such as the sacred pipe are turned in a circle to invite the powers of the Four Winds or to send out blessings in all directions. The drum is round, as is the gourd rattle. Round stones—such as the obsidian "Apache tear" or small anthill pebbles placed in ceremonial rattles—have a special power and suggest unity.

Native American sacred and social dances are performed in a circle. In the beautiful intertribal *fancy dance*, the dancer may twirl or hop in a circle. Native American hoop dancers express the unity of life by acrobatically twirling a dozen or more hoops around their waist, legs, arms, and entire body. The most basic dance of all, and the one that non-Natives usually learn first, is the "round dance," in which participants move in a circle as their feet pat the ground in rhythm with the drum. Dances may be practiced as personal contemplative exercises as well as in a group. In one of the most powerful personal dances, the dancer dances to each of the Four Winds, one after the next, praying with body and mind for guidance and help.

THE FOUR WINDS MEDICINE WHEEL

A familiar Native American circle is the *medicine wheel,* a representation of Native American philosophy, beliefs, and values in the shape of a wagon wheel. The hub and the points on the circular perimeter may carry a wide array of symbolic associations. The hub of the medicine wheel represents a core principle, commonly the Great Spirit. The points on the circle represent particular qualities. The spokes demonstrate that the points are interconnected because they emerge from and flow back to a common center.

There are two kinds of medicine wheels, symbolic and physical. The symbolic medicine wheel is drawn on paper or imagined and used by Native educators to teach values and culture. The Four Winds Medicine Wheel, which has four spokes, is one of these. Other wheels used to communicate other teachings may have a different number of spokes. For example, I sometimes teach my students how to draw a wheel with twelve spokes, one for each of the twelve months of the year. The center of the wheel represents where they live. Each circumference point is named for a seasonal occurrence, such as "Aspens Yellow, First Snow, Great Wind, Bitter Cold." Creating or contemplating this *Medicine Wheel of the Seasons* sensitizes students to their local environment and to the unique beauty and spirit of each month.

The physical wheel—generally made with stones, pebbles, posts, or lines etched in earth or sand—marks a permanent or temporary ceremonial site from a few feet to hundreds of feet in diameter. There are nearly two hundred ancient stone medicine wheels throughout North America. Many medicine wheels are sacred calendars used to predict astronomical events, such as the equinoxes and solstices, and to determine the proper timing for seasonal ceremonies. These include the stones at the Bighorn Medicine Wheel in Wyoming, the wooden posts at Cahokia Mounds State Historic Site in Illinois, and the spiral "Sun Dagger" etched on a stone wall at Chaco Canyon, New Mexico. Medicine wheels were part of the everyday life of Native peoples. For example, the fifteen poles that form the circular frame of the Northern Plains tipi is a medicine wheel representing fifteen traditional values: Obedience (to tradition), Respect (for all), Humility, Happiness, Love, Faith, Kinship, Cleanliness (in mind and body), Thankfulness, Sharing, Strength, Good Child Rearing, Hope, Protection, and Interdependence.[5]

One of the most interesting medicine wheels I ever visited was a distinct ringlike impression in a field of wild grass that marked the place where the tipi of the great Cree medicine man Fine Day had once stood. There had been no lodge on this land for more than a hundred years, yet the grass grew differently where the rim of the tipi had touched the earth. I don't remember now if it was the length or color of the grass that was different, but there was no mistaking the spot. John Moosomin, a wonderful old Cree medicine man, now departed, told me that Fine Day's spiritual power had left a permanent mark on the ground. We commemorated and honored it with a pipe ceremony.

FOUR AND SEVEN:
WINNING NUMBERS IN THE GAME OF LIFE

In all of the world's religions, numbers are far more than units of measurement; they symbolize values and powers and give people the security of knowing that the world is orderly and intelligible. The Greek philosopher, mystic, and mathematician Pythagoras (circa 532 B.C.) said, "All things are numbers." Plato (circa 428 B.C.) believed that God was a geometer. To discover hidden meanings in the *Torah*, ancient Jewish philosophers sought the numerical values associated with Hebrew letters.

Christians attach special significance to the Holy Trinity and to the quaternity symbolized by the Cross. In Chinese philosophy, three has the power to create harmony among the Three Powers (San Cai) of Heaven, Earth, and Human. Qigong healing exercises practiced three or nine times (three squared) are considered far more efficacious than sets of two or eight. African Zulu diviners communicate with the ancestors and with the Divine *Nkosi Yezulu* by tossing and interpreting animal bones numbered from one to thirteen. For example, if *Kune,* which means both "Unity" and "Four," falls faceup, it suggests cooperation. Among Native Americans, four and seven are the most important sacred numbers.

Four generally indicates the presence of the Great Spirit's power in the four directions—in other words, through all of space. In *Psychology and Religion,* Swiss psychiatrist Carl G. Jung points out that "the four is an age-old, presumably prehistoric symbol, always associated with the idea of a world creating deity. . . ."[6] Jung explains that in mystical traditions throughout the world, the number four represents the God within both the human soul and the world. The ancient Greek god of revelation, Hermes, was sometimes called "the Four-Headed Hermes" because of his association with the four directions and four seasons. The Mandukya Upanishad, an important Hindu text from approximately the eighth century B.C., says the sacred syllable *om* is composed of four parts: A, which symbolizes the waking state; U, the dreaming state; M, dreamless sleep; and Silence, also known as *Turiya,* which symbolizes blissful unity with God. In the Osage language, the quartered circle is called *Ho'-e-ga,* a term that also means the sacred space between the dual powers of Father Sky and Mother Earth.[7] And as we have seen, the Great Spirit is present in the four quarters.

The number four is symbolically drawn by the Great Spirit on the crown of all human infants. It is the cross formed where the skull bones meet at the fontanel, the soft spot. The Great Spirit's breath—the soul—enters the body at birth through the fontanel and leaves at death through this same point, now hardened. The Hopi believe that the fontanel, *kópavi,* is a vibratory center that communicates with the Creator.[8] In the Lakota language, the fontanel is called *pe'wiwila* and *peówiwila,* "little spring on the top of the head," suggesting the sacred springs through which spiritual powers can enter or leave the earth.[9]

There are four races of man: the red (Native American), yellow (Asian), black (African), white (Caucasian), and shades of color in between. There are four roots to the great Tree of Peace, the symbolic heart of the Haudenosaunee Confederacy, because peace and justice should extend to the four quarters of the earth. A year consists of four seasons: spring, summer, winter, and fall. Life also has four seasons: infancy, childhood, adulthood, and old age. We experience four qualities of being and knowing: physical, mental, emotional, spiritual. Seneca elder Twylah Nitsch says that these four qualities correspond to four stages of life. From birth through

51

age twelve, we learn primarily through and about the body. From age twelve to age twenty-four, we learn through the mind. Age twenty-four to age thirty-six is the stage of emotional learning. After age thirty-six, we explore the realm of spirit.

Four elements were known to ancient people throughout the world: earth (or rock), sky (sometimes called "wind" or "air"), water, and fire. Nature has four realms—mineral, plant, animal, and human—which may be visualized as four concentric circles, in which mineral, the oldest, is in the center. Some Native Americans add to this list four sacred animal spirits guarding the four directions, four plant spirits, four stones, or four sacred mountains. In Lakota mythology, a four-legged buffalo represents four ages of the world. Each year, the buffalo loses one hair, and each age, he loses one leg. The Buffalo is now on his last leg; when that is gone, the world will perish in a flood. People who follow the Great Spirit's guidance can help forestall or prevent this disaster.[10]

Like four, the sacred number seven symbolizes wholeness and circularity. Seven includes the four directions as well as above, below, and the seventh direction, the Great Spirit, who is everywhere at once. Or seven may symbolize space and time: the four (East, South, West, and North) combined with the three (Past, Present, and Future). Ceremonies and ritual actions are performed in numeric units of four and seven. A sacred pipe presented to an elder four times in succession signifies a sacred request. A chant or ceremony repeated four or seven times or a dance that completes four or seven circuits attracts attention from the spirits. In some Cree Sweat Lodge Ceremonies, four elders offer healing advice or other kinds of therapy to a patient. Many Native American healers prepare herbal teas with four or seven ingredients and recommend a four- or seven-day course of treatment. Spirits once requested that I return to a particular sacred site four times, once every seven years. I did not begin writing this book until that cycle was completed. Even *saying* the sacred numbers four or seven can have an effect. Cherokee poems and chants may include the word *Gahlgwogi!*, "Seven!," to increase their power. I wrote the following poem to my dear friend and elder the Cherokee medicine man Hawk Littlejohn, shortly after our first meeting. In the poem, I use several words that have a special meaning among the Cherokee. *Tawodi* is Cherokee for "Hawk." "Long Person" is the traditional way to address a river when seeking its help for healing or purification. *Wado* means "Thank you" in Cherokee. The "Beloved Mountains" are the Smoky Mountains of North Carolina, ancient home of the Cherokee.

Tawodi

Long Person, I come to pray with you
Where life begins at the edge of earth and water.
You have been flowing since before I was born;

You will sing long after I am gone.
Hear now my voice and stretch it back
And onward so it moves, like you, beyond time.

Wado! I am thankful for this old friend returned
Brother Tawodi, who stood with me on similar banks
In our Beloved Mountains, long ago.
We were brothers, not only in spirit.

Our friendship is sacred.
These words are True.
Gahlgwogi!

DIRECTIONAL SYMBOLISM:
IS THERE A STANDARD?

Among different Native American peoples, there is considerable variance in animals, colors, elements, ethical values, and other natural phenomena and principles associated with the Four Directions. For example, to invite the presence of the West Wind to a healing ceremony, a Seneca medicine man would invoke the Cougar Spirit, while a Lakota healer might pray to the Thunderbird. A Lakota artist would depict the East yellow, South white, West black, and North red, whereas an Anishinabe artist would use yellow to represent the East; red, the South; black, the West; and white, the North. Among the Cherokee, East is red, South is white, West is black, and North is blue. The Tewa represent the East as white, the South red, the West yellow, and the North blue-green. In Pawnee tradition, the Four Winds are associated with the four *semicardinal* directions: Northeast black, Southeast red, Southwest white, and Northwest yellow.

That said, tribal associations are rarely considered absolute, and exceptions abound. Native Americans recognize the importance of personal expression and intuitive vision in healing ceremonies. For example, in Cherokee tradition, red is the color of the East; yet an individual Cherokee may choose a different color to symbolize the East when following the instructions of dream helpers. Lee Irwin, in *The Dream Seekers,* his masterful study of Plains Indian visionary experience, explains that every dreamer "has his or her own associations with colors and various powers. . . . Although the use of color symbolism is pervasive and an intrinsic feature of ritual behavior, it was determined not by ritual sanctions but through dreams."[11]

I learned an important lesson about the balance of prescribed cultural forms and personal creativity in the 1980s when I conducted a Sacred Pipe Ceremony in honor of two respected Lakota elders. Generally, before a Pipe Ceremony, the leader prepares an altar that includes a particular number of "tobacco ties." These are pinches of tobacco individually wrapped in colored cloth and tied in a row to a string. The colors of the cloth symbolize the Four Winds. The tobacco is a representation of prayer; when it burns, its smoky breath rises to the Great Spirit.

I wished to honor Grandmother and Grandfather by offering the Pipe Ceremony according to their tradition. Knowing the specificity of some Lakota rituals, I asked Grandma which colors of cloth I should use to make the tobacco ties. She asked, "What are *your* colors?" I told her my personal colors, received during dreams and visions: red cloth for the East, yellow for the South, black for the West, and white for the North—coincidentally, the colors used by some of my Cree relatives when they conduct ceremony. I also add green for earth, blue for sky, and one more secret color that represents the healing power of the Great Mystery. Seven colors in total. Grandma said, "*Wasté.* That's good."[12]

I try to model and teach the qualities that I associate with each of the Four Winds in my work as an educator and a healer. I am not the first to assert that there are common, though not universally held, associations with the Four Winds. During the last thirty years of the twentieth century, many Native American educators created Pan-Indian medicine wheels of the Four Winds that affirm common, shared values across Indian Country.[13]

The accompanying table is a summary of basic directional correspondences that form the basis of my discussion. I start with the East and proceed clockwise, following the natural cycle of the year.[14] The sun rises in the East, corresponding to spring, comes to fullness in the South or summer, sets in the West—autumn, and sleeps in the North—winter. Our lives follow the same cycle, from birth in the East to growth in the South, old age in the West, until finally we return to our ancestors in the North. In the Lakota language, a newborn is called *icimani,* "traveler," because life is a spiritual journey from one unknown to another. On the wheel of life, everything changes and passes, except for the Great Spirit, the center of all that is.

THE FOUR WINDS

EAST	SOUTH	WEST	NORTH
Morning	Noon	Afternoon	Evening
Spring	Summer	Autumn	Winter
Red	Yellow	Black	White
Earth	Air	Water	Fire
Eagle, Mouse	Deer, Coyote	Bear, Thunderbird	Buffalo, Owl

THE EAST:
WHERE THE SUN RISES

As the sun rises in the East, the mystery of the night fades. The East is thus early morning and springtime. It is the direction of spiritual renewal and the birth of new ideas. Although the primary symbol of the East is the Eagle, which, like the sun, rises high into the heavens, the Bear is also related to the East Wind. The Bear goes to sleep in the West, the autumn. In the spring, the she-bear emerges from her den with her cubs, born during hibernation. The East Wind teaches us to look out on the world like a bear cub, with fresh, innocent eyes.

The East is the direction of rebirth for people who have overcome difficult challenges. During times of life change—when aspects of the body, emotions, or spirit are in transition—we may feel lost in chaos. The old order has not yet ended, and the new one is not yet in view. As we travel around the wheel of life, we learn to die to the past, to release that which is no longer needed for our growth. We learn that we have no obligation to be who we were, nor should we expect others to be who we want them to be. In life, nothing is fixed; the world is different from moment to moment. By letting go of beliefs and belief systems, we are able to experience life directly and *immediately,* without the mediation of concepts. The best strategy for happiness may be to have no strategy at all. Expect the unexpected; be ready for surprises. Step out into the light of day in the East.

The ability to commune with nature, a person, or spiritual forces requires a quiet, open, and receptive mind. A person who can achieve this quietude is walking the Native American path to truth, commonly called the Red Road. Red is the color of the East Wind, the color of blood and life. Among Northwest Native nations, a person who wears red clothing to a ceremony is saying, "I make a commitment to life. I will try my best to leave the world a better place at the end of life than when I entered it."

The East is also represented by the earth element. Just as the East Wind teaches us to see life in a new light, without preconceptions or bias, it teaches us that the whole world is sacred. Each blade of grass, every insect, every star in the sky deserves respect and has a lesson to teach. People who walk the Red Road are Earth People. Earth People are those who make harmony with nature and respect for life their priorities. Being an Earth Person is not a matter of skin color but rather of the character of the heart and of having the courage to behave in ways consistent with its wisdom. Earth People include all aboriginal and tribal people worldwide who have maintained their values and traditions. Euro-Americans can also be red Earth People.[15]

White Buffalo Calf Woman, an ancient holy being who taught sacred ceremonies to the Lakota and other Northern Plains tribes, advised the Indian people to "[m]ake every step a prayer." Prayer is two-way communication. We not only express our truth to the Great Spirit; we also listen to the Great Spirit's messages. Prayerfulness is symbolized by the Eagle, the spirit of the East Wind. The Eagle teaches us to soar above mundane, petty concerns and to have a grand, panoramic vision. He is the highest-flying bird. When we feel bogged down or stuck in a rut, the spirit of the Eagle can lift our spirits up. Because he flies so close to the Creator, the Eagle is considered a messenger, carrying our prayers upward and bringing blessings down. In ceremony, the Eagle is invoked with song and visualization. A Cree healing song says, "Golden Eagle gives you his wing feathers. He gives you his tail feathers." In a waking dream, the medicine man ascends with the Eagle, seeking guidance, the answer to a personal question, or healing power for a patient. I have been in sacred Sweat Lodge Ceremonies in which participants felt themselves fanned and purified by the wings of an invisible Eagle or in which the Eagle, as the power of the Wind, shook the willow-framed sweat lodge to announce his presence.

The Eagle is also a protector, a powerful spirit who illuminates our path, looking out for negative or disruptive forces, so we can either avoid or, when necessary, battle them. One of the symbols of the Haudenosaunee Confederacy is an eagle perched on the top of the Tree of Peace. The eagle warns the allied member nations of approaching danger. By keeping a high, spiritual perspective, we can find the appropriate course of action. We are less likely to be reactive or aggressive. This does not, however, mean that we must be passive or weak in the face of evil. A spiritual person uses strength as necessary; he or she would not hesitate to throw greedy merchants out of the temple!

Like the rising sun, the Eagle also represents creativity and inspiration. To Native Americans, the most important form of creativity is the freedom to follow one's own path while maintaining respect for other spiritual paths. The Eagle leaves no tracks in the sky and follows no trail. Yet the flight of the Eagle has direction and intent. Isn't this the paradox of the spiritual life? We follow a path without signposts; we balance courage, commitment, and trust, journeying from, through, and toward the Unknown.

In the East, the world emerges from the darkness, symbolically reborn from day to day. Such rebirth teaches us the importance of hope and renewal, of blessing and being blessed, the virtue of *holy joy*. During my first Vision Quest, described in Chapter 4 of this book, an eagle taught me that holy joy is an important attribute of the East.

The Inuit of Baffin Bay say that evil tends to avoid places where people are happy. In the 1920s, Aua, an Iglulik shaman, told Danish explorer Knud Rasmussen that after trying unsuccessfully to achieve shamanic power through asceticism and solitude or with the help of other shamans,

[F]or no reason all would suddenly be changed, and I felt a great joy, a joy so powerful that I could not restrain it, but had to break into song, a mighty song, with only room for the one word: joy, joy! And I had to use the full strength of my voice. And then in the midst of such a fit of mysterious and overwhelming delight I became a shaman, not knowing myself how it came about.[16]

Aua later described how he learned to call his spirit helpers, the shark and shore spirits, by singing a song in which he repeated the word *joy* numerous times, until he burst into tears. Aua's joy emerged "for no reason at all," unbidden, rather than as a result of pain and deprivation. It makes sense that spiritual powers prefer mirth to misery.

I am not trying to deny the role or importance of suffering in spiritual growth. One of the most touching compliments I ever received was when Leni-Lenape spiritual teacher Tom Laughing Bear Heidlebaugh said in front of a group of Native American associates, "Ken has sinned and suffered enough to have learned something." I have my battle scars, and I know that profound and joyous realizations sometimes grow from life's testing ground. It is a mistake, however, to believe that suffering is, of itself, spiritual or ennobling. I have known both Christians and traditional Native Americans who pride themselves on the depth of their scars. We all experience times of difficulty. Suffering can be accepted as a passing season that is not rejected, but certainly not encouraged, pursued, or prolonged. Life brings enough suffering without having to make a virtue of it.

The lesson of the East Wind and the new day is to stay focused on the Now, to live in the present. The majesty and grand vision of the Eagle is balanced by another totem of the East, the humble Mouse, who sees only what is directly in front of him. The Mouse teaches us that life is always changing. Because the same moment never returns, we should keep the senses open and pay attention. The beauty of spring flowers is fleeting. If we look but are too preoccupied to see, we will miss it. And while we can neither hold on to beautiful experiences nor expect them to stay forever, we need not mourn their loss. With an open heart, we can trust that beauty, like spring flowers, will always return.

THE SOUTH:
WHERE THE LIGHT SHINES

In Native American prayer, the South is frequently called the direction "where the light comes from." Light is a symbol of life. For people who live in the Northern Hemisphere, to travel South is to go toward light and warmth. The Innu, Cree, and other northern tribes observe how southern winds melt the long snows and drive back the cold. They say that the South, like the East, brings renewal. Grandmother Twylah Nitsch (Seneca) calls the South-North axis the "life line." The South Wind, she says, can teach people about their destiny, how to journey with grace and wisdom from where the light is fullest, in the South, to where the light is dimmest, in the North. The axis also represents the balance of heart (South) and mind (North), feeling and intellect, movement and stillness.

South is thus the direction of the heart. If you face a gentle South Wind, you may find that your heart begins to smile. The South Wind can bless you with purity of heart and innocence, qualities symbolized by the Deer. In the North, we must turn inward to conserve our warmth. It is a direction of strength, severity, and testing. But in the South, we can be gentle and vulnerable and give ourselves permission to express our feelings. We pray to the South Wind to release obstructions, confusion, resentment, stubbornness, and hardness of heart.

In the seasonal cycle, the South Wind brings summer. In the South, the seeds that were planted in the East rise from the ground and reach fruition. Life is in full bloom. The South is a time of balance in our lives. We are in the fullness of our being. We can look back toward the playfulness of childhood (East) and forward toward the introspection of the coming fall (West) and winter (North).

The Lakota say that the South Wind, *Okaga,* creates beauty and is the husband of the beautiful woman *Wohpe,* "Falling Star." Okaga made the first flowers and seeds and is associated with the gentle beauty of waterfowl, meadowlarks, and cranes. The Lakota sacred tale of the courting of Wohpe highlights the maturity of the South Wind. Each of the Four Winds tried to please Wohpe and win her favor. The North went hunting and brought back game, but the meat was icy and cold. The West, the direction of the thunder spirits, took out a drum and sang and danced, but the power of his song shook the tipi so hard that it collapsed. With the enthusiasm of youth, the East Wind talked so much and so foolishly that Wohpe felt like crying. But the South brought Wohpe warm, beautiful things and won her heart.

The South Wind awakens the senses and teaches us to appreciate music, art, food, and our bodies.[17] It is the direction of love, sensuality, and sexuality. The latter quality is represented by the Elk, a close relative of the Deer. A person with "Elk Medicine" has the power to attract the opposite sex and may counsel people who have questions about courtship. Love and sexual passion, however, must be balanced with intellect and spirit, lest the emotions of the South burn like a fire out of control. Traditional Native American elders stress the importance of balancing sexual passion and spontaneity with intelligence and modesty. We should express sexual feelings with sensitivity, honor, and respect for a partner, always considering the harmony between two people more important than personal needs. *Ma-na'-ji-win',* "respect," say the Anishinabe, is the foundation of all unions between men and women.

The sexual passion symbolized by the South Wind is very important to indigenous healers, who are both physical and spiritual. They are passionately involved with life, yet through the gifts of the East, they maintain the spiritual perspective of the Eagle. Many indigenous healers, including Native American, believe that a strong sexual drive may indicate the potential to become a spiritual teacher or healer. When former Harvard University professor of education Richard Katz, Ph.D., analyzed the psychological differences between healers and nonhealers in African Bushman (*Kung San*) society, he found that the healers were more passionate about life. This suggests that the emotions may be a key to assessing health and focusing healing power.[18]

The South represents air, the breath of life in the body, and meditative breathwork, including Yoga *pranayama* (breath control) and Chinese *qigong* (breath-energy healing).[19] Air reminds us that life is not about us alone, but it is a process of give-and-take, sustained by a fundamental exchange of elements. We inhale the oxygen exhaled by plants and exhale the carbon dioxide that plants need to breathe. If we were to hold the air in our lungs, we would die, as would other forms of life with which we are interdependent. We live by letting go, not by holding on.

The South is the color yellow, which represents the warmth of the sun and the "yellow" Asian peoples, including Han (Mongoloid) Chinese, Japanese, and Tibetans. Some readers might wonder, "How could ancient Native Americans have known about China, Japan, or Tibet?" I can answer this in two ways. First, archaeologists and historians have found evidence of ancient Asian-American contact, such as the presence of Japanese pottery thousands of years old along the coast of Ecuador, Chinese jade in Central America, and three-thousand-year-old Chinese travelogues that describe the geography of the Americas.[20] Second, and, in my opinion, more important, Native American oral history speaks about Chinese and other ethnic "colors" because of the clairvoyant vision of medicine people. They just *knew* that other races existed.[21] In accord with the teachings of the South Wind, the "yellow" people are masters of breath control and breath meditations.

The South reminds us to have faith. Faith is different from intellectual belief. It requires that we trust that which cannot be described. The trouble with descriptions is that we often tend to substitute them for experiences. We become caught by the words and forget the reference. The word "stone" is not the same as the experience of seeing or holding a stone. A strong *belief* in the Great Spirit is necessary only if we feel separated or alienated from him or her. Humility is required to admit that there are things one cannot know or believe in; it requires courage to have faith in the Great Mystery.[22]

The South is also associated with Coyote, the trickster and spirit of humor. Perhaps the most difficult belief to give up is the belief in a separate, independent "I." We take ourselves too seriously. Coyote is there to remind us that we are just a speck, a small drop in the ocean of life. Why get so wrapped up in our personal melodramas? Have we forgotten that angels can fly because they take themselves lightly? Humor helps us to cope with, gain power over, and heal from pain, frustration, loss, and suffering. In his book *The Healing Power of Humor,* author and humorist Allen Klein cites many well-known comedians who experienced difficult and painful childhoods, including Charlie Chaplin, W. C. Fields, and Jackie Gleason. Yet they emerged relatively unscathed because they learned, through laughter, to see themselves from different and perhaps larger perspectives.[23] All the Native American medicine people I have known have had wonderful senses of humor and would sometimes crack jokes at what at first seemed the oddest moments—in the middle of a healing or during a counseling session. I have even seen an elder use humor to test prospective students. If they have a good sense of humor, they pass and are considered capable of learning about Native American culture; if they are too serious, they fail. When guests came to visit the Cherokee medicine man War Eagle, he would lower his voice and speak with trepidation of his audiotape of "sacred and secret Indian music." I always enjoyed the guests' expressions as they were privileged to hear this tape of Alvin and the Chipmunks singing powwow songs! To this day, I remember War Eagle's jokes as much as his "medicine teachings." Perhaps they are one and the same.

A Dakota friend wisely advises, "Take the work seriously, not yourself." Native Americans understand that both humor and mystical insight arise from a flexible consciousness, the ability to perceive in a new way or from multiple perspectives. Flexibility is also the essence of harmonious relationships and conflict resolution. If we hold too rigidly to our opinions, then Coyote might push us even more deeply into our ruts, until our stubbornness or errors are glaringly obvious. In his *Proverbs of Hell*, the poet William Blake said, "If the fool would persist in his folly, he would become wise."

The South represents the power of the feminine: gentle intuition instead of cutting intellect, a prioritizing of relationship over control, and wisdom found in patient receptivity rather than impulsively aggressive action. Native American cultures have always recognized the different but equally important nature of men's and women's medicine. Each gender has its own teachings, ceremonies, and power. A Cherokee elder once suggested to me that women and men might be able to heal themselves more effectively if they did healing and spiritual practices while facing South and North, respectively.

Like the Chinese *yin* and *yang,* feminine and masculine energies pervade the universe. The northern Pawnee (the *Skiri*) call the planet Venus *cu-piritta-ka,* "female white star," and describe her as a beautiful and powerful woman. She married the great warrior Mars, *u-pirikucu,* "big star" (which may also refer to Jupiter). The earth was created to be a home for their child.[24] In the book *Profiles in Wisdom,* Oh Shinnah Fast Wolf, a spiritual teacher of Native American and Scottish descent, writes:

> *For five thousand years, we have been strongly influenced by the red, masculine-charged ray that emanates from the planet called Mars. . . . Mars' reputation is his love of war; he'll go out and create wars just for the fun of it. . . . At the turn of the [twentieth] century we began to be influenced by the violet ray, which emanates through the planet Venus, which we call the gateway to the above and beyond.*[25]

In order to tune in to this feminine power, Oh Shinnah recommends gazing at Venus and thinking the word *surrender.*

Other Native Americans have similarly found Venus to be a source of inspiration and guidance. Black Elk rose early each day to greet the rising of "the daybreak star," which he called "the star of understanding."[26] According to Michael Crummett's book *Sundance,* once during a Vision Quest, an ancient Absarokee warrior rose at four in the morning to gaze at the Morning Star and pray to the Creator. "The Indian's response came when the four-pronged Morning Star twinkled four different colors, alternately sparkling in red, green, yellow and white."[27]

Long ago, say the Haudenosaunee, the great holy man known as the Peacemaker advised warring nations to bury their weapons beneath the Tree of Peace, symbolically declaring that reasonableness and trust are the foundation of peace. I believe that the Peacemaker reminds us of many qualities associated with the South; he affirmed that people must rid themselves of greed, aggression, power, and domination. But of course, trust must go two ways. Without reciprocity and respect, the trusting person becomes a victim of the patriarchal bully, a lesson that Native Americans know too well.

THE WEST:
WHERE THE SUN SETS

The West corresponds to sunset, to autumn, and to the autumn of one's life, old age. The setting sun symbolizes the mind's sinking below the horizon of everyday consciousness; it is the quality of introspection. The spirit of the West Wind is the Bear when he enters his cave to hibernate and sleep through the long, cold nights. The Bear leads us into the dream world. He helps us to remember our dreams and reminds us that dreams are important. People who open their spirits to the power of the West learn to dream while awake, to sense the mythic, spiritual, and narrative elements of everyday experiences, the way life events fit together into a meaningful whole. The West also teaches them to be more awake in their dreams: to intentionally find answers to waking problems while dreaming.[28] The Turtle, another symbol of the West Wind, also helps us understand our dreams by teaching us to go within, to find strength in solitude, and to be steady and persevering in our quest for self-understanding.

The West Wind reminds us to release attachment to past events, to let the past drop, like falling leaves. It is important to honor the past and our ancestors, but being preoccupied with the past is unhealthy. It interferes with present enjoyment of life. Hawk Littlejohn, a Cherokee medicine man and friend, once remarked that most people go through life like a squirrel with a very long tail that keeps getting tangled in the underbrush. At some point, we need to go back and release the knots that keep us bound to old, inefficient, and outmoded ways of thinking and behaving. The introspective power of the West Wind is often the first stage in this process. You cannot change an unhealthy habit unless you are first aware of it.

The West is commonly represented by the color black. Black absorbs all frequencies of light and represents a person who is seeking illumination. The greatest beauty is always beyond knowledge and hidden in the darkness of the unknown. Hold up a candle in a bright room, and little is accomplished; hold it in a dark room, and you can see a great deal. Black means facing the shadow, the dark places within. Native Americans understood the concept of a hidden "shadow" side of human nature long before it was popularized in the West by Swiss psychiatrist Carl G. Jung. As I have heard elders say time and time again, "Life is a balance of opposites. All things have a light and shadow side. A spiritual person seeks to understand and accept both." A person who does not acknowledge the "black" condemns in others precisely the qualities that are most disliked in himself. "When you point your finger at someone," says Twylah Nitsch, "look where the other three fingers are pointing."

The black of the West Wind represents the black people of Africa and the water element. Water connects us to the ancient energies of the earth. The same water that flowed through the bodies of the dinosaurs has been recycled for millions of years to flow through our own bodies today. Water links people to their ancestors and to Africa, one of the ancient cradles of culture. The power of water to cleanse, bless (for example, baptism), and heal is recognized throughout the world. *Agbara Miri*, "the Spirit of Water," is a powerful helping spirit for the Igbo shamans of Nigeria. Ancient Chinese Taoists tossed water to the four directions to cleanse a temple. In the Vision Quest tradition of some Native American tribes in the Pacific Northwest, the quester contacts spiritual powers during a pilgrimage that includes bathing in every river, lake, or stream he or she passes. In the sacred Sweat Lodge, people are purified by the steam rising from water tossed on red-hot stones.

For many Native American tribes, the Water Element is controlled by another

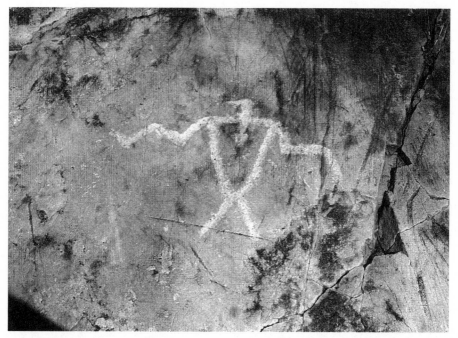

Thunderbird, with a "heart-line" showing the source of breath and power. Jeffers Petroglyphs Historic Site, Minnesota.

totem of the West Wind: the Thunderbird, a mythological being who lives in the high mountains. Thunderbird speaks in rolling thunder and rumbling earth; in rain, hail, sleet, and snow; in flashes of light that blind the eyes and supercharge the air. Thunderbird creates the electricity that links sky and earth and teaches us how to use its power to heal ourselves or others. According to Lakota mythology, Thunderbird (*Wakinyan*) is the messenger and active power of an even older spiritual power, Stone (*Inyan*). Thunder is the voice of the Mountain and the power of the West Wind. Thunder and Wind are spirits that purge the world of impurity.

In the Lakota tipi, the West is the place of honor. When we sit in the West, we look toward the East, the tipi opening, the place of new light. In old age, we also look toward the East, the light of youth. We think not only of our own mortality but of our obligations to leave something good for the coming generations. The West teaches us the folly of waste, whether this be wasted resources or a wasted life. In the West, you wonder, "How will I be remembered after I am gone? What have I done to create a better world? Have I made an impact that will be felt by the seventh generation?" The West is linked with the East as elders or grandparents are linked with children. Native Americans frequently address all elders as "Grandfather" or "Grandmother." Those who have passed through three-quarters of the great medicine wheel of life have much to teach their "grandchildren."

In the West, we learn the gift of trust—not the emotional trust of the South but rather a spiritual trust of the unknown. When a light is turned on, we can see objects; we are aware of distinctions and differences. In the black darkness, we are in a unified, nondifferentiated reality. We feel closer to the Great Mystery. In Native American tradition, the Vision Quest is a way of reclaiming our connection with this Mystery. The search for sacred meaning reorients us toward the center of the circle. In the words of fifteenth-century Christian mystic Nicholas of Cusa, the wise person is "a sphere whose center is everywhere."[29]

But spiritual lessons carry a price. The West is also the direction of sacrifice. We must give up something in order to receive. The sacrifice may be food (fasting), flesh (small pieces of flesh are ritually cut from the arms, chest, or back in the sacred Sun Dance, a yearly ceremony of social and spiritual renewal, which honors the Sun, the Four Winds, and the Creator), words (the fast of silence), possessions (the "Giveaway" ceremony, in which possessions are distributed to the community to honor a vision, a healing, or some other special occurrence), or it can be the giving up of egotism and pride. Even popular sports such as running, conventionally considered secular by non-Indians, have for Native Americans a spiritual significance. The runner sacrifices sweat (water) and breath (air), thereby returning to the Creator a portion of the gifts that sustain life. Giveaways are expressions of gratitude. In the autumn of life, we learn to be grateful for the lessons we have received, and we prepare for the great giveaway, the return of the body to Mother Earth. Facing West, we learn that generosity is a key to happiness. It comes from the recognition that we own nothing and that we owe everything to the Creator. In the West, we learn to stand humbly, nakedly, without possessions before the Great Mystery. We offer up our spirits and souls to become, in the words of the Lakota holy man Fools Crow, "a hollow bone" for the Creator's power.

The West is the place of spiritual vision and transformation. It reminds us of the beauty of earth and sky and of our duty to take care of our home.

THE NORTH:
WHERE THE COLD WINDS BLOW

The North is the most mysterious and challenging direction. The North is the winter season and the cold, purifying, and strengthening winds. It represents austerity, hardship, and the strength, fortitude, and wisdom we gain by meeting and overcoming adversity. Thus, the North is also the direction of our personal difficulties and spiritual tests. It may be the dark night of the soul, the time of suffering that prepares us for new direction.

Turning North, we face the Polestar, the unmoving pivot of the constellations, the still point amid change. The North symbolizes balance, moderation, and the importance of connecting with our wise and tranquil depths no matter what the surface disturbance. The North is the resting place between West and East, the setting and rising sun, the fall and spring. The autumn leaves have fallen, and life is waiting to be reborn. We have shed old attitudes, beliefs, and outmoded ways of being and are at a crossroad, waiting for new direction. Standing in the North requires patience and prayer; we need to let life unfold rather than try to make hasty decisions or force action prematurely.

The strength of the North is represented by the Buffalo, particularly the White Buffalo, a symbol of spiritual renewal. The Buffalo is a great nourisher; his meat, hide, and bones were the primary source of food, clothing, and tools for Native Americans of the Great Plains. Thus, the spirit of the Buffalo sustains us and helps us overcome our challenges. As my old friend Keetoowah (Cherokee) used to say, "If I sing the buffalo song, you'd better watch out. Nothing can stop me!"

In Christian terms, the North teaches us to die to what Saint Paul calls "the flesh"—that is, limited perceptions and concepts that maintain our consensus reality—in order to be reborn in "the Spirit." The North is also the land of the ancestors and those who have passed into Spirit. When we wish to ask forgiveness, understanding, or advice of the spirit of one who has died, we make an offering to the North. This aspect of the North is represented by the Snowy Owl. Many Native peoples believe that the Owl takes the soul to the land of the dead or helps a person "die" to an old self.

The Cree say that the North is white like snow or the hair of the elders. The North is old age, but it is not simply the accumulation of years. It is rather the accumulation of wisdom that makes one an elder. I once entered a sweat lodge with a Dakota friend, who wisely reminded me to "be the elder part of yourself." Even though the North generally means elder wisdom, we may discover such wisdom in greater or lesser degree at any stage of life.

I stood on a mountaintop with an Innu elder one spring morning. From this high vantage point, we were able to see traditional camping, fishing, and hunting areas used for millennia by his people. Saying that he wished to thank the Great Creator for the beauty and teachings of this place, he took some tobacco from his pouch and began to offer it to the directions, starting in the South and then turning to face the West, North, and East. When he faced North, I noticed that he seemed to make his prayer and offer the tobacco more quickly. When the ceremony was over, he replied to my unspoken question, "North is the direction of tests and hardship. I don't want the North Wind to take much notice of me, lest I invite any more!"

Yet Native Americans feel that it is important to be thankful for the lessons that life presents, whether these be easy or difficult, whether they bring pleasure or pain. I often recite a Native American prayer that translates, "Creator, my Friend, whatever hardships befall me, I will not fear." It is important to realize that our challenges make us stronger. People who survive illness and hardship with an open mind and without bitterness are frequently the best healers. It is important to remember that the hardship of the North does not last forever, though it may certainly seem so at times.

For early Native Americans, the transition from autumn to winter always meant a change of lifestyle. Although hunting, trapping, and fishing might continue all year long, most subsistence patterns changed depending on the climate, the migration of game, the fluctuation of maritime resources, and the availability of seeds, nuts, fruit, or other plant parts. Spring, summer, and fall were times for planting, cultivating, harvesting, and gathering crops, drying fish and game, laying up food and supplies for winter, and visiting distant friends. Winter was a time to enjoy crafts, games, and storytelling. It was also the spiritual season, when spirits made their presence known to the community. Winter is, for many traditional peoples, the only time when sacred stories are told. If an elder is asked in the spring to recount the Creation story, he may remark, "It is not the right time." In the Spirit world, the seasons are the opposite to our own. Spirits sleep during the spring, summer, and fall, the time when people are most "awake" and active. But in the winter, as we rest and spend more time indoors, the spirit powers awaken to teach us. We honor their lessons with ceremonies and prayers of gratitude and respect and a commitment to living with integrity.

The North Wind corresponds to the Fire Element and the color white. It represents the white European race, whose gift is the intellect. But the intellect is a gift that, like fire, can burn out of control, leaving destruction in its wake. It must be balanced by the earth wisdom of the East, the feminine heart of the South, and the quiet introspection of the West. The intellect is our curse and our blessing. Western society's reliance on intellect and technology has led to people's alienation from nature and created a wall between the mind and the heart. The North can also be a source of mental clarity. The North can teach us to use the mind wisely. Among the many gifts of the North Wind are memory; the capacity to understand and organize; concern for freedom and justice; and finding detachment from anger, fear, jealousy, and other negative emotional states. The ability to reason and calmly think things through is essential for peace.

The North is sometimes represented by a mountain. According to *The Sacred Tree,* "The higher we climb its slopes, the steeper and more difficult the way becomes. And yet the higher we go, the more we can see and the stronger we can become."[30] We never reach the top of the mountain; we are always on the journey.

A Winter Prayer

I am grateful to you, Snowy Owl.
Take me from the West, where the sun sets,
Where my mind sinks into its depths,

To your home in the North,
Cold northern winds that test and strengthen.
And on to the East, place of new light.
May I have the courage to make this journey
To face my tests with dignity and grace,
To see through my places of darkness
And release what is old and unneeded.
Snowy Owl, you are beautiful!
Fly by me with still, silent wings.
I know that you bring not death,
But spiritual rebirth—
May I be renewed as a child,
From moment to moment.
Winter is, after all, only a point
On the Great Circle of Life.
And whether it be difficult or easy,
I know that it is good.

Many Native American elders feel that today the Earth and its people are in the North, the place of Purification. Like an organism that has been invaded by viruses and toxic chemicals, the Earth has been assaulted. She is fast approaching a critical mass at which the only recourse may be a radical purge of the antigens. The Purification may lead to a cataclysmic destruction of life as we know it through earthquakes, floods, massive fires, and hurricane-force winds, or it may be a spiritual cleansing, a return to balanced behavior facilitated by awareness. I have heard Native elders express both the pessimistic and optimistic viewpoints. They all agree, however, that whatever occurs will be a result of our own actions; mankind will reap what it sows.[31]

A PERSONAL VISION

The Four Winds brought me to my home in the Colorado mountains. After I completed graduate school in Berkeley in the late 1970s, I had had enough of cities. I knew I wouldn't be content simply to visit nature: I wanted to live in it. I fasted, prayed, and asked the Great Spirit for guidance.

One day, a beautiful Native American woman dressed in white buckskin came to me in a waking vision. She stood with her arms resting gracefully at her sides and her palms facing outward. A white light that seemed to emanate from her palms surrounded her entire body, and a round mirror hung, like an amulet, around her neck. She silently communicated to me that I must look into the mirror to find the answer to my questions. As I did so, I saw snowcapped mountains that I immediately recognized as the ones in which I had camped several years earlier. I knew at once that these were *my* mountains. Then the scene changed; it "zoomed in" on one special mountain, red like red sandstone or the sacred red pipestone, the spiritual heart of the mountain range. I saw myself standing on its peak, looking out on limitless vistas in all directions. Then, with a sound that was an expression of my whole being, a prolonged vowel between "Oh" and "Ah," I called out my gratitude to the Four Winds. I could feel the sound being carried infinitely far in the four directions, all the way to the home of the Four Winds.

I moved to those mountains within a month. I continue to see them in both waking and dreaming reality.

ASKING THE FOUR WINDS TO HELP YOU

Among Native Americans, the Four Winds are more than metaphors. They are also Four Spirits and teachers to whom one may pray for guidance, healing power, or protection from misfortune.

— CLEANSING —

The elements of nature represented by the Four Winds can be called upon to cleanse your body of impurity. The healing practices described below are found in various forms among indigenous cultures throughout the world.

Earth Element (Gift of the East Wind)

As mentioned earlier in the chapter, White Buffalo Calf Woman instructs us to make every step a prayer. Her words may be interpreted figuratively (every step in life) or literally (every step on the Earth). The Earth can heal you through the simple act of walking in a natural environment, if you walk mindfully. Give yourself permission to let go of the day's worries. Practice awareness and appreciation of the sounds, sights, smells, and feel of nature.

Grandmother Twylah Nitsch suggests a beautiful method of communing with the Earth in her book *Entering into the Silence*. First, find a secluded, special place that does not infringe on the property rights or privacy of others. "Open a small hole in which to talk with Earth Mother. Tell her about the reason for this counseling. Talk it out. Thank her for listening. Return the earth covering so that it is not noticeable. Thank the GREAT MYSTERY for the Gifts of Beauty that help all creation function in a positive manner."[32] I have found that if my mind is quiet, I can hear the Earth replying to my concerns. The Earth is truly a living being and wise counselor. Ask the Earth about needs rather than desires, about deep concerns rather than material objects. It wouldn't be appropriate to ask your counselor for a new car or a million dollars. You should not hesitate, however, to discuss health or the welfare of your children.

You are most likely to have the strength to follow the Earth's advice and to overcome challenges if you visualize and express that your goal is already accomplished. Instead of saying, "I hope I can cure my depression," say "I accept the Earth's wise advice and am grateful that I have found the way to overcome depression." Grandma Twylah suggests that while practicing entering into the silence, get rid of the word *hope* and substitute words that express gratitude and acceptance that the guidance you need is already in front of you. Instead of thinking, "I hope that my asthma will be cured," think "I trust that my asthma has been cured. Thank you."

You can strengthen your connection to the Earth and to the East Wind by being kind to the Earth. Remember these rules: recycle, don't waste, use earth-friendly products, and most important, simplify your life by reducing consumption of fuel and resources.

Air Element (Gift of the South Wind)

Stand in a pleasant breeze or wind. Imagine that your body is light and porous like a cloud, so that the wind can blow *through* you. As the wind passes through your body, be grateful that the wind is carrying away stagnation, blockages, and toxins.

We breathe the wind. Pay attention to your breath to deepen your awareness of the Great Spirit. Many Native American songs involve specific methods of breathing or use the sound of the breath in one of the song's verses. Inhalations draw in strength; exhalations send blessings or the good message of a song out.

Practice breath awareness outdoors whenever possible, sitting either on the ground or on a comfortable log or chair. Feel how, with every inhalation, you allow the breath of nature to enter your body and refresh it. With every exhalation, you release the unneeded and old air. Each cycle of breathing renews you with the Creator's life-giving power. Breathe in through your nose and out through either your nose or your mouth. Breathe naturally, like a child, using the abdomen rather than the chest. Abdominal breathing is and was practiced by hunters throughout the world. It is the slowest and quietest way of breathing and thus the least likely to scare away prey. When you inhale, the abdomen gently expands. When you exhale, the abdomen retracts. Don't pull the breath in; don't push the breath out. Let nature breathe you!

If you show respect to the Air Element, the South Wind will be your ally. Do not support industries or businesses that discharge toxins. Do your part to minimize air pollution. Drive your car less. Reduce airplane travel. (Jet planes are more polluting than cars and very ugly to look at when you expect to see clouds.) Harness wind power. (I buy 100 percent of my electricity from wind power sold by my local electric company.) Slow down, be silent, and stop wasting your breath.

Water Element (Gift of the West Wind)

Among the ancient Cherokee, virtually every important undertaking—going to war, preparing for a healing, getting married—was preceded by ritual plunging in water. Many Native people go to hot springs for purification. Songs to the spirit of water have healing power. Some Salish chants end with the word for "sacred water," while the singer imagines his or her body cleansed with waters flowing from crown to feet.

Here is a simple yet effective way to use water to heal yourself. When you bathe in a river or lake, thank the water and ask for cleansing. One of Rolling Thunder's (Cherokee) favorite methods of purification was to stand barefoot in a gentle stream or river while respectfully and gratefully asking the stream to carry away the things he didn't need.

Water is sensitive to our thoughts and feelings. If you want the water and West Wind to help you, you must help the water. Do not contaminate the water. Petition the government to stop chlorination and fluoridation. Here's a novel thought: since water is for drinking, why are we urinating in it? Unfortunately, considering the present urban population of the United States, it may be impossible to avoid using toilets. You can mitigate the harm by buying a low-flush toilet.

Fire Element (Gift of the North Wind)

The smoke from a campfire cleanses the body of scents and negative energies picked up during the day. Smoke was the original form of incense, used by hunters to mask human smells. Allow the sound, sight, feel, and smell of a natural campfire to cleanse your senses. Imagine the heat and healing energy of Grandfather Fire or of the sun entering your body and burning away impurity.

Indigenous people throughout the Americas have used the energy of the sun directly to purify and energize their minds and bodies. Sit outdoors in the dawn sun, with your hands on your lap, palms facing upward. Sensitize yourself to the light and warmth of the sun on your body and hands. Then reach up as though grasping the sunlight. Bring the sunlight toward the crown of your head with an inward, gathering motion. As your hands descend slowly to your lap, imagine the golden light flowing through your body. Alternately, you may gather the sunlight and direct it to specific areas of your body that need healing. Place your palms either a few inches above or directly on that body part and imagine your body nourished by the sun's healing energy.

There are many ways of demonstrating gratitude to Fire and thus attracting blessings from the North Wind. Each morning, be thankful for a new day and new light. Learn how to make a fire in the old way, with flint or a wooden drill. Appreciate the patience, focus, and skill that all human ancestors required in starting or tending a fire. You will be less likely to take fire for granted. Never spit or urinate into a fire or toss anything into a fire in a disrespectful way. Make a prayer whenever you start or see a campfire. As much as possible, convert to solar power. Lastly, use your mind, the fire within, in a good way. Think good thoughts, and if you're not, then devote yourself to finding out why. Pollution begins in the mind.

— ASKING FOR GUIDANCE —

Any kind of question that you might ask a spiritual healer or pastoral counselor can be put on the framework of the Four Winds, from personal relationships to advice about overcoming a disability. Simply meditate on one or several attributes of each of the Four Winds, receiving spiritual wisdom while meditating. For example, mediators in Vancouver, British Columbia, use the Four Winds Medicine Wheel with First Nations' clients during mediation of social and legal problems, including alcoholism and criminal misbehavior, helping them to find guidance about the reasons for their problems and what can be done about them.[33] Elders sometimes use the Four Winds Medicine Wheel to help offenders, their victims, and their communities to find a form of healing, restitution, and when necessary, punishment, that is agreeable to all. Michael Tlanusta Garrett (Cherokee), assistant professor in the Department of Counseling, Special Education, and Child Development in the University of North Carolina, suggests that to find greater life harmony and self-understanding, think of each of the Four Winds while asking the following questions, looking for the answers within yourself:

East: Who or what am I a part of; where do I belong?
South: What do I enjoy doing or do well?
West: What are my strengths; what limits me?
North: What do I have to contribute or share?[34]

A simple way to seek guidance from the Four Winds is to stand outdoors in a place that is special to you. Close your eyes and respectfully ask each of the Four Winds in succession for guidance and help in solving a problem. You can either stand in place or, as I prefer, turn to face each of the Four Winds. The Four Winds can be petitioned in an open and nondirected way, a simple call for help. Or you can ask specific questions that are in harmony with each wind's attribute. Be open to the possibility that the reply may come in a variety of ways. Some people see the answer in images; others hear a sound, feel a sensation, or intuitively know the reply. Don't forget to express your gratitude to the Four Winds when the meditation is over.

To find the solution to a patient's health problems, I ask the following questions:

- **East:** What is the illness, and what is its cause or origin? (Sometimes, while I am asking the East Wind about causes, the North Wind adds information about parents or ancestors whose genetics or behavior may have contributed to the illness.)
- **South:** How did the illness develop? What emotions have caused or are caused by the illness? How is the illness affecting family relationships?
- **West:** Are there fears associated with the illness? What does the patient need to release or sacrifice to allow healing? What do I need to know about the patient? What does the patient need to know about himself or herself?
- **North:** What are the obstacles to the patient's healing? How can the patient find strength and health? What is the best way to facilitate the healing process? How can I help the patient return to clarity and wisdom?

When appropriate and necessary, I may also ask the North Wind how to help a patient make a transition into the Afterlife.

— FOUR WINDS VISUALIZATION TO BUILD SPIRITUAL — STRENGTH AND SELF-ESTEEM

The following visualization is adapted from Thom Henley's beautiful book *Rediscovery: Ancient Pathways, New Directions*. The Rediscovery Program consists of youth wilderness camps throughout the world that focus on the spirituality of all of life by "drawing from the strength of native traditions, the wisdom of Elders, a philosophy of respect and love for the land and each other. . . ."[35] The program began in western Canada and receives strong support from indigenous elders, who contribute their stories and skills to youth education. The activities, games, and teachings in the original Rediscovery Program are based on Haida Indian culture. Thus, the visualizations described in the *Rediscovery* book use the Raven, Sea Otter, Grizzly Bear, Cedar Tree, and other Haida imagery. The imagery I present below is based on features appropriate to the mountains and Northern Plains area where I live. You should similarly modify the imagery to make it suitable to your environment.

The script is most effective if someone reads it to you.

Imagine that you are walking through a beautiful pine and aspen forest on a clear spring morning. As dew evaporates from the trees, grasses, and wildflowers, the air is filled with a fragrant scent. The sound of birdsongs mingles with the murmur of small rivulets that bubble out of the moist earth. The sun is shining on the base of a particularly alluring tree, a giant old pine tree, a grandfather tree. You can feel the tree's presence as you approach it. You see a red backpack leaning on the tree and are amazed to find your name sewed on it. You reach in to receive a very special, sacred gift, a gift from the East. It is an Eagle feather. As you hold it, you know that you have the power to see and speak the truth. The Eagle gives you the courage to be who you are and to express yourself in your own way, but always with respect.

You reach into the backpack again to receive your gift from the South. It is a beautiful rattle with a deer-foot handle and a strip of coyote fur wrapped near the top. As you shake the rattle, you know that life can be light and enjoyable, like a dance. The deer gives you the ability to move with grace and to speak from the heart. The coyote reminds you always to look for humor when life seems difficult or dark. Don't take things too seriously. The coyote is also self-reliant and able to survive in any terrain. You have what it takes to survive and to live a long and good life.

You reach into the backpack to receive a gift from the West. It is a bear-claw necklace. You place it around your neck. You know that you have been given the strength and courage to follow your dreams. The necklace also reminds you that, like a bear, you love nature and are healthiest when you are in touch with nature's healing power.

There is another gift waiting for you. You reach into the red backpack and bring up a gift from the North. Like a magician pulling a giant cloth out of a little hat, you are amazed to take out an entire buffalo robe. You wrap yourself in it and feel protected by its warmth. The buffalo makes you a warrior for peace and a provider for your family. You can overcome your challenges and travel a good pathway through life.

Is there something else in the backpack? You reach in and feel on the bottom of the pack a small copper medallion. On one side, you see an engraving of your face; the other side is shiny but blank. The two sides represent your ability to say yes or no. You have the confidence to show the side of the medallion with your face—to say yes to things that are right and good for your life. You also have the courage to wear the blank side—to say no to anything that is unhealthy for you. There may be times in your life when people judge you unfairly or when they try to influence you to do things against your will or good judgment. Remember that you can say no. You have permission from the spirit world to be just who you are. You are a unique, special, and caring person.

Now, return each of the gifts in reverse order, one by one, to your special backpack while thinking of their meaning: the medallion, the buffalo robe, the bear-claw necklace, the deer and coyote rattle, and the eagle feather. You lift the backpack onto your shoulders. It is light and comfortable. In fact, it is so light that you hardly know it is there unless you think about it. That's good, because you will be wearing this backpack or remembering and using the things in it throughout your journey through life.

Let the image go. These special gifts of the Four Winds will always be with you, and you can imagine them again at any time. Return to awareness of where you are. Be aware of your body, of your breath, of the environment around you. Open your eyes with gratitude to the Four Winds.

It is also possible to practice a less scripted and more creative version of the Four Winds visualization. Build on the following script.

Reach into a medicine bag, red cedar box, or other sacred container for your gift from the East, the direction of creativity and inspiration. What is it? Now receive your gift from the South, the direction of love and the heart. Hold it in your hands. Learn its message and teaching. As you reach in again, you receive a gift from the West, symbolizing your dreams and your ability to know yourself. What have you received? Reach in for a gift from the North, a gift of spiritual wisdom and strength, including the strength to overcome challenges. Finally, with respect and gratitude, return each object to the container.

You may wish to keep the results of these visualizations private. Native people feel that sacred knowledge sometimes needs to mature in silence. Speaking about it too early freezes and limits the experience in a conceptual grid. Wind is subtle; it cannot be held in your hands. Perhaps the same is true of the lessons of the Four Winds.

3

— THE CYCLES OF TRUTH —
Wisdom from the Wolf

When people ask me, "What is Native American spirituality?" I usually discuss the Cycles of Truth, a twelve-pointed medicine wheel like the face of a clock that represents fundamental Native American values such as gratitude, respect, and acceptance. These values are the foundation of integrity (or "wholeness"), balance, and happiness. The Cycles of Truth clearly shows that Native American spirituality is not a matter of doing this or that ceremony or wearing buckskin and beating a drum but is, rather, a state of mind and heart. It is, very simply, being a good person and living in harmony with nature.

No one knows who created the Cycles of Truth. The first person known to speak about or teach it was the early-twentieth-century Seneca medicine man Moses Shongo. Although it was created by a Seneca Indian, the wheel expresses principles common to all Native peoples. Why "cycles" and "truth"? I can only speculate, since neither Moses Shongo nor his well-known granddaughter Twylah Nitsch ever explained why these English words were used. "Cycles" suggests ebb and flow, movement and return, change, and process. "Truth" suggests an immutable principle. Cycles of Truth conveys the idea that life is movement and stillness; we must adapt to the changing circumstances of life. The question is not how you can understand "respect" as an abstract principle but how you can be respectful in actual situations.

The values represented on the Cycles of Truth are generally called "gifts." In contrast to the Christian assumption of original sin, Native Americans believe that all people are born with spiritual values; they are gifts from the Creator. To Native Americans, people are not born with "original sin" but with "original sanctity."[1] Native American spirituality models virtuous behavior rather than restricting "bad" behavior. There is no Native American equivalent to the Ten Commandments. Instead of saying, "Thou shalt not covet," Native elders say, "An honorable person is generous." Elders "focus on teaching and on counselling,"[2] writes Rupert Ross in *Dancing with a Ghost: Exploring Indian Reality*. "By offering their assistance and counselling, they demonstrate their belief in each person and their faith that they can get themselves back on the path to a good life."[3]

Ross explains that Native Americans "focus upon prescribing states of mind, states to be attained in a progression towards ultimate self-realization."[4] The elders' teachings are meant to awaken our innate goodness; a person who attains a spiritual state will naturally behave in a good way. Implicit in this philosophy is the notion that Native American values are not rules that must be obeyed but, rather, good words that are meant to inspire, guide, and instruct. Elders also teach values by modeling them; they "walk the talk."

A way of life based on an assumption of innate *goodness* is important because it leads to personal happiness and healthy communities. In Native American healing, goodness has special significance because it is contagious. A healer with a good heart inspires goodness in the patient. During Native American massage therapy (see Chapter 10, "Massage and Energy Therapies"), the healer transmits kindness

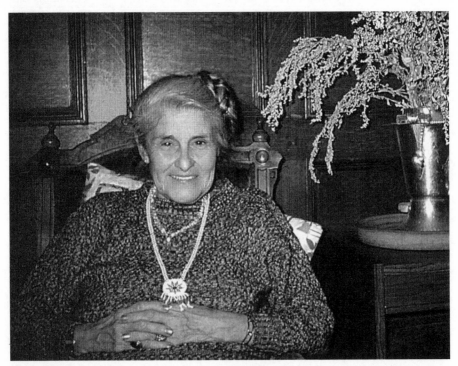

Twylah Nitsch, 1987.

and wisdom through his or her hands. For example, in the Apache Sunrise Dance (*náíees*), a rite of passage for young girls entering puberty, after the initiate dances for as long as six hours, she lies on a blanket and is massaged by a woman elder. "It's believed that as the godmother touches the girl with her hand and foot, some of the godmother's personality and character is transferred to the young woman," writes reporter Deenise Becenti (Diné) in the journal *American Indian*.[5] What is true of massage therapy is also true of other Native healing methods. Whether conducting a ceremony or offering an herbal tea, a healer who has a good mind is a good healer.

HOW THE CYCLES OF TRUTH BEGAN

Twylah Nitsch, a member of the Seneca Wolf Clan, was born in 1912 in the Seneca Nation, Cattaraugus Reservation, near Buffalo, New York. Like many Native Americans, in addition to her common English name, Twylah also has a spiritual name in her Native language: *Yehwehnode,* "She Whose Voice Rides on the Wind." A spiritual name, usually conferred on a young person by an elder or a helping spirit, is the name by which spirits recognize a person and is generally reserved for ceremonies.

Twylah's initiation into the healing practices of her people began with a near-death experience that happened when she was three years old. She remembers playing in the yard and suddenly feeling as if she was choking. She passed out. By the time her mother and grandfather, Moses Shongo, found her lying on the ground, her breathing had stopped and she had no pulse. There was no apparent reason for the child's collapse; nothing was stuck in her throat, and she had not been suffering from any disease. Bending over her limp body, the medicine man prayed and breathed into Twylah's mouth. He was not trying to administer mouth-to-mouth resuscitation—this technique was unknown to him—but rather to transfer life breath and healing energy into his granddaughter. It worked. Twylah revived, and as she opened her eyes, Grandfather said, "Now my breath is her breath. In the future, she will be deaf, blind, and crippled yet will heal from all of these afflictions. She will carry on where I leave off." In essence, he foretold Twylah's future as a spiritual teacher. All of his predictions came true.

Not long thereafter, Grandfather began teaching Twylah the Cycles of Truth, the foundation of Native American wisdom. He would place twelve stones in a circle on the ground and describe the symbolic meaning of each. This medicine wheel became the foundation of Grandma Twylah's lifetime of work as an educator, a counselor, and director of the Seneca Indian Historical Society and the Wolf Clan Teaching Lodge, an educational organization devoted to sharing traditional Seneca Wolf Clan teachings, stories, songs, and dances with people from diverse cultures.[6]

From 1984 to 1987, I visited Grandma Twylah's home on the Cattaraugus Reservation twice a year.[7] I learned the Cycles of Truth from her. Gradma Twylah was still actively teaching the Cycles of Truth and other aspects of Seneca wisdom through the 1990s, and when I spoke to her at the end of 2001, she was lucid, full of wisdom, and as she put it, "still kicking butt."

Wolf Clan teachings are especially pertinent in today's mass culture. The Cherokee healer Eli Gatoga said that human beings should be wary of blindly following in the footsteps of others. "We are in the Age of the Wolf,"[8] said Grandfather Eli. The wolf is a trailblazer, unafraid of wild or dark places. The wolf also reminds us that human beings are part of the natural world; we belong to it in the same way that the wolf belongs to the forest. In the Anishinabe Creation Story, Wolf was Original Man's first companion. Together, they walked across the newly created earth and realized their kinship with all of life.[9]

The wolf also symbolizes cooperation, protection, loyalty, and communication. The social behavior of wolves is more like man's than any other animal. The wolf works and hunts cooperatively, in a pack. Wolves mate for life, and both the male and female wolf care for the young. The wolf communicates over long distances, howling to other wolves that he has located prey or senses far-off danger. Extremely sensitive to the environment, a wolf can smell a single caribou three miles away. Like humans, wolves are playful and love to celebrate, sometimes gathering for no reason other than to howl together, wag their tails, and frolic. Wildlife biologists believe that such jubilation may be a form of "mood synchronization."[10] The same could be said of both Western and Native American religious celebrations.

THE CYCLES OF TRUTH AS I TEACH IT

My interpretations are based on the guidance I have received from Grandma Twylah and many other elders, as well as my own life experiences. As you contemplate each gift, you may develop your own associations and interpretations.

The easiest way to visualize the Cycles of Truth is to imagine the face of a clock, as shown in the accompanying figure. Starting at one o'clock, the twelve gifts are: (1) learning, (2) honoring, (3) acceptance, (4) seeing, (5) hearing, (6) speaking, (7) loving, (8) service, (9) living, (10) working, (11) walking, and (12) gratitude. Remember that any point on the circle may be considered the beginning. The "clock" is only a metaphor, and there is no inherent reason to start our discussion at number one. The values are numbered simply to help you remember them.

THE CYCLES OF TRUTH

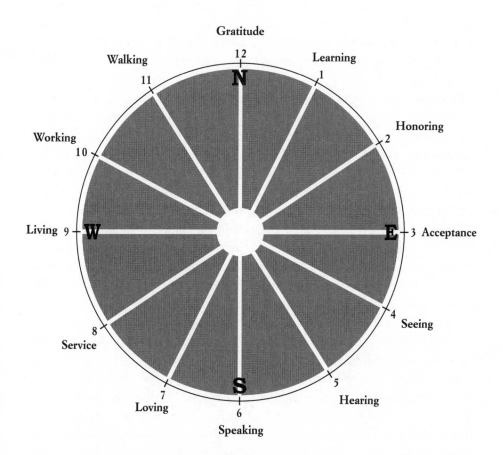

1. LEARNING

Whenever anthropologists were seen near Seneca territory, Moses Shongo would say, "Be careful; the Bigheads are coming!" Native Americans are wary of people who accumulate information for information's sake. This is considered a form of greed not unlike greed for land, resources, and power over others. Learning is more than memorizing facts and gathering data. Native Americans recognize that learning is based on sensory input and the most important "text" is nature. The gift of learning means learning from all experiences: we learn from the natural world, where every leaf and track has a lesson to teach; from people, the children and the elders; from our hardships and joys; from dreams and artistic creation; and yes, even from books. Intellect must be balanced by intuition and caring, so that information will be used appropriately, for the good of all and for the future generations.

In other words, learning requires balance and open-mindedness. The mark of a great teacher is his or her enthusiasm for learning, which manifests itself as enthusiasm for teaching and draws students into the learning process. We will not always have our teachers at our sides. If the teacher teaches us the importance of learning and *how* to learn, she has done her job. Similarly, healers learn from their patients. A great healer is one who teaches, inspires, and models how a patient can heal himself or herself.

From the Native American viewpoint, learning requires silence and awareness. Elders stress the importance of observation, listening, and patience rather than the questioning and analysis that are the hallmarks of Western education. The Cree language has no word for "why." Answers eventually come to a good learner, framed in his or her own words and style of reasoning. For example, when a Cree trapper tans a moose hide in the traditional manner, he makes it soft and pliable by pulling and stretching it tautly while rubbing it with the moose's own oily brains; hence, it is "brain-tanned." By paying close attention to the trapper's actions, the student learns how vigorously and for how long to stretch and rub the hide to make it tough for moccasins or soft for a vest. Sometimes, by the time a teacher answers the question "why," the student already knows the answer. When a kayak is about to roll in a freezing Arctic wave, you don't ask why it is rolling, you just follow the lead of the more experienced kayaker. Questioning for the sake of clarification or to clear up misunderstanding is good, but we must be careful not to stunt our own creativity, problem-solving ability, or survival by asking questions too soon.

Learning is related to another principle called kinship. Knowledge is good if it makes us feel connected to other people and to nature. In Native American culture, learning is frequently cooperative and interactive. Knowledge does not flow only from a teacher to the student; it moves in a web of connections among teachers, students, and the tribe. Here's a concrete example. My wife, Rebecca, wanted to learn how to prepare a traditional Saskatoon berry and venison stew for a feast she was hosting among our Cree relatives. A friend who heard about the feast brought her a side of venison that he had hunted. The next day, we were visiting a Cree elder whom I had doctored a few days earlier. She told us how to make the stew and also informed us, in no uncertain terms, that she would enjoy making it with her feisty eighty-year-old sister. Later that day, as news spread on the "moccasin telegraph," a Cree medicine man called us to offer prayers and songs at the feast. By the day of the feast, we had learned not only how to make the stew but how to prayerfully enjoy it!

Modern Native Americans also value university education, but they recognize where it fits in the big picture. The intellect is only one faculty, and a mischievous one at that, with a talent for self-deception. If we are going to use the intellect, let's use it well, with clarity and social and ecological responsibility. Native Americans who respect their old traditions follow two paths of learning—in the words of Cherokee elder Andrew Dreadfulwater (1908–1984), "one from God, the Spirit, and one from the schools."[11] But whether learning from a moose or a mathematics text, Native Americans value cooperative learning that benefits family and community. Unfortunately, this value is at odds with the approach of modern educational institutions, which prioritize the individual learner. When a Native or white child takes a test in school, she is expected to know all the answers. If she asks a classmate for the answer, it is called cheating. But is it really right to reward individual problem solving and punish students who seek answers from the group? Human survival depends on group collaboration. Learning should promote ethical values, not erode them.

2. HONORING

Honor is respect for the Creator, Creation, yourself, and others. It means both self-esteem and esteeming others because we are all children of the Great Spirit. With honor, we respect our differences, including religious and spiritual ones. Elders across Indian America agree that respect is the foundation of a happy and satisfying life.[12]

An honorable person walks tall, with courage and pride, yet without losing his modesty or humility. An honorable person brings pride to his or her family, community, and nation. The elders teach that the honor of one is the honor of all. The highest reward for honorable or courageous acts is not personal glory but rather the respect of one's relations. Honorable acts are also rewarded by spiritual powers, who give the worthy person rich dreams and visions.

Honor is not reserved for special occasions. According to Native American tradition, it should be a part of everyday life. Honor guests by showing them hospitality. Always give them your best food and bed, and if they are poor, offer some traveling money before they depart. When someone does something good for you or your community, honor him or her with kind words, food, or gifts. Native Americans offer special honor to tribal members who have served in the U.S. military. Few non-Indians realize that Native Americans' fight for sovereignty does not preclude them from defending the land we all share. Seneca Wolf Clan *sachem* (traditional political and spiritual leader) Donehogawa (1828–1895) was better known by his English name, Brigadier General Ely S. Parker, military secretary to General Ulysses S. Grant during the Civil War. It was Parker who transcribed the surrender agreement signed by Robert E. Lee at Appomattox. In 1921, Absarokee Chief Plenty Coups attended the dedication of the Tomb of the Unknown Soldier in Washington, D.C., to honor the Absarokee soldiers who fought in the First World War. He laid his war bonnet and coup stick[13] on the casket. In 1944, there were 21,756 Native Americans

81

serving in the military. Navajo "code talkers" transmitted Allied messages in an unbreakable code, their own Diné language. After the September 11, 2001, terrorist attacks on the World Trade Center and the Pentagon, Native Americans volunteered once again to defend the United States.[14] Today, at intertribal powwows, audiences stand in respect as the color guard of Native American veterans leads dancers into the arena.

Native people sometimes host an honoring feast or dance to express gratitude. Songs can be dedicated to the honor of a person or an event. During a winter healing ceremony in the Swinomish Nation, near LaConner, Washington, I watched an elder dance to honor his spirit power, the helping spirit who appears in visions and dreams. At the end of the ceremony, participants shared their prayers and thoughts with one another. When it was my turn, I stood up and asked the elder to stand with me as I read the following poem, which I had composed in his honor.

Spirit Dance

For the sake of the future and unborn generations,
To provide a spirit trail for them to follow,
The old man dances.
In a candlelit cedar-planked room,
Wooden benches along the walls
Filled with the community of prayer helpers,
The old man dances.
He is beyond age.
He breathes calmly as his feet stomp
   to the strong drumbeat.
His eyes are penetrating, already looking
   through this reality to the next.
The old man dances.
Though dressed in poor work clothes,
I see him in what he has earned—
Red and black flowing cape, with shell-button totems:
They are dancing with him.
The old man dances
To honor the Creator's gift.
He knows that a gift not honored
         a gift not given
Is quickly lost.

The Ho Chunk (Winnebago) spiritual leader Reuben Snake said that it is good to honor even those who curse you. "Kill them with kindness," he advised. The

Cherokee elder Keetoowah was fond of saying, "I used to hate my enemies. Now I'm going to love them to death." Love is a powerful defense against negativity, preventing aggressive and reactive people from causing similar negative reactions in your consciousness. It is easiest to honor others when there is love in the heart. Love creates unity and acceptance, whatever the surface differences. My Native relations agree with a tenet of all the world's great religions: "God is Love," and darkness cannot live in its light.

3. ACCEPTANCE

The gift of acceptance means seeing and acknowledging the spiritual beauty in all beings, appreciating them for what they are rather than trying to manipulate or mold them into what one would like them to be. I once learned a beautiful lesson about acceptance and respect from an unexpected source. A friend invited me to his home to attend a reception for a great Qu'ranic scholar and holy man from Pakistan. The room was filled with nearly a hundred people: Muslim scholars and practitioners, Sufis, and both young and old students of mystical and religious traditions. At one point during the reception, the holy man sat next to me. His dark wrinkled skin, long gray-white beard, and white kaftan made him look as though he had just emerged from the pages of the *Arabian Nights*.

Knowing little about the Muslim faith, I chose not to join the discussion but rather maintained a respectful silence. At one point, the elder took my hand in his and closed his eyes. The room became quiet. After a few minutes of reflection, he opened his eyes and asked me, "What is the great message of the Qu'ran?" I said, "I do not know, sir, but I would like to know." He responded, "The words that Allah has written in your heart are different from what he has written in the heart of the person sitting across from us. We are each unique. Find out the message that he has written in your heart and you will have understood a great teaching of the Qu'ran." In this sage I saw an affirmation of a principle taught by Native American elders: there are unique and divine truths hidden in the human heart. We must learn to recognize and accept them.

Acceptance also means not being a perfectionist and forgiving the faults we see in ourselves and others. It is important that we accept our weaknesses, even as we know our strengths. Without doing so, we are likely to ignore our problems or to blame others, making it more difficult to change or improve. Sometimes, acceptance requires supreme patience. In order to make wise decisions, there are times when we have to accept criticism or when we need to listen dispassionately to angry words. The Haudenosaunee *Great Law of Peace* says that a chief should have "skin seven spans thick" as proof against negativity. This does not mean, however, that acceptance is blind or passive. It has limits. We should seek to change any situation

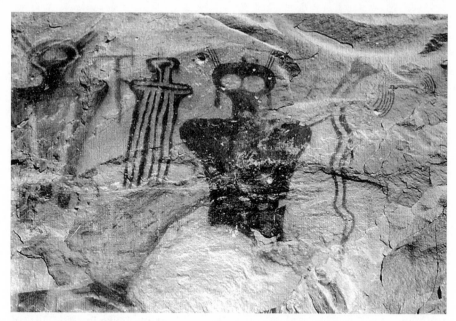

Medicine person or spirit with large eyes, antennae, and a snake spirit helper. Rock art, approximately fifteen hundred years old, from Thompson Wash, Grand County, Utah.

that is harmful or unjust. The gift of acceptance is thus balanced by "response-ability," the ability to respond appropriately: with fortitude, courage, wisdom, and compassion.

4. SEEING

The gift of seeing is spiritual insight, the ability to perceive subtle or hidden truths with the eye of spirit. In many indigenous languages, healers are called "seers." Among the Igbo of Nigeria, the highest *dibia,* "shaman," is called "one whose eyes see the spirit." The Copper Inuit term for medicine person is *Elik,* "one who has eyes." Petroglyphs along Utah's Colorado River portray holy people with large circular eyes and surrounded by animal spirits. Some Cherokee healers diagnose a patient by looking for his image in a quartz crystal, a stone that throughout the world represents clear light made visible and solid. Among the Muskogee (or Creek), originally from Alabama and Georgia, a hunter carried a powerful crystal called *sapiya* with some pigment (red ocher) in a deerskin pouch. "When applied to his face, the pigment was believed both to enhance his eyesight and to attract game," writes University of Georgia professor Charles Hudson in *The Southeastern Indians.*[15] In hunting cultures, the ability to see clearly, and perhaps to see beyond the physical reality, was essential for survival.

Throughout the world, "illumined" or "enlightened" people are believed to be acutely sensitive to the translucence of the physical world. They see the forces and powers that animate it, especially light. Native Americans consider light to be an attribute of the Great Spirit. Author Jay Miller writes in his *Tsimshian Culture: A Light through the Ages,* a work about the Tsimshian Nation of northern British Columbia, "[L]ight (*goypah, goypax*) was and is the mediator with universal potency, a manifestation of the divinity, called Heaven, that pervades everything."[16] He also observes that many objects or beings sacred to the Tsimshian are associated with light, including abalone shells, quartz crystals, copper plaques, and even the iridescent quality of salmon skin.

In the Wolf Clan Teaching Lodge, the gift of seeing is symbolized by the hawk, a bird known for its speed and sharp vision. Grandma Twylah says that the hawk teaches us to appreciate the importance of imagery, dreams, stories, and myths. The hawk, like the eagle, reminds us to view life from a higher and wider perspective and realize that, as in a dream, all events in our lives are connected in mysterious and meaningful ways. We can use our intuition to discover life's plots and subplots.

5. HEARING

The gift of hearing means sensitivity to the vibrations or energy of life and clear-minded receptivity. In Christian terms, the gift of hearing means the practice of obedience (from the Latin *ob,* "near," and *audire,* "to listen"). An obedient person keeps his spiritual ears open to the Truth and follows its guidance. When we cease listening, life is meaningless and absurd (from *ab surdus,* "completely deaf").

The gift of hearing includes the appreciation of all kinds of music, both instrumental and natural, and the ability to perceive harmony or disharmony. A walk in the forest is refreshing because the sounds of nature always create a beautiful harmony. The oriole's song blends perfectly with the murmur of the brook and the whisper of the wind in the pines. The more time we spend in nature, the more sensitive we become to harmony and the more adept we become at understanding disharmony, including dissonant behavior, omens, or sounds. A powerful healer can hear health or disease in the tone and timbre of a person's voice. The Chinese, whose healing system also depends on careful listening, have a wonderful saying: "The physician writes the prescription as the patient steps through the door." His or her diagnosis is based on the sound of the patient's footsteps!

Among musical instruments, the drum and rattle have the greatest power to tune us to life energy. The surface of the earth and the vault of the sky are like drumheads. The steady drumming that accompanies Native American songs causes earth and sky to resonate, like the heartbeat of nature. The rattle or shaker also expresses vibratory power. In *The Mishomis Book: The Voice of the Ojibway,* Anishinabe elder Edward Benton-Banai writes that the sound of the rattle (*she-she-gwun*) is like the primal sound at the beginning of Creation.[17]

Many Native Americans believe that pierced ears augment the power of listening and represent wisdom and understanding. Piercing the ears of a male or female child is a rite of passage that, for some tribes, requires a special ceremony. Interestingly, the Tsimshian sometimes call white people or anyone insensitive to their ways "no ears" (*wah 'tsmuu*).[18] I would add that a person who listens with a closed mind is also a "no ears," because he will hear only what he wants to hear.

6. SPEAKING

The gift of speaking is connected to the gift of hearing. It is important to speak *from* our listening, to speak with a quiet, humble, and open mind, whether we are communicating with people or nature. A basic rule of traditional Indian oratory is never to try to persuade or coerce other people into believing your own truth. Speak with strength but without arrogance. If your words are true, listeners will accept them. If you try to compel belief, listeners will mistrust your message. (Missionaries are only successful with the insecure.) If you feel the need to be forceful, ask yourself why. Do you doubt your own words? In this southern, six o'clock portion of the wheel, we are reminded of faith, a gift of the South Wind. Speak with faith in the intelligence of your audience and you will be surprised at how often they rise to meet your expectations.

Speaking is communicating with other humans, with the Great Spirit in prayer, and with the spirits of stones, plants, and animals. Some animals, such as the wolf and the whale, are especially skilled at communicating with one another and with human beings. A wolf howl can be heard six miles away, but this is nothing compared with the whale. Whales make the lowest-pitched yet loudest sounds of any animal. At twenty cycles per second (hertz), a blue whale's song is a deep moan that is almost below the threshold of human hearing. Yet it is so loud—155 decibels—that it is as if you were standing three feet from a jet engine at full power. The acoustical properties of water allow whales to communicate *across* the oceans and marine biologists to track them from a distance of one thousand miles.[19] Having gone swimming many times in sacred Hawaiian waters, I can attest to the fact that whales can also communicate by subtle, nonacoustical energies. Even if a human cannot physically hear or see a whale, it makes its presence known from miles away.

Native Americans in the Pacific Northwest say that, of the various whales, orca ("killer") whales have the closest connection with wolves. They both hunt in packs or pods and use acoustical signals to stay in touch; their herd is a "heard." A person who has a close spiritual affinity with the wolf or orca has the power to telepathically contact people who are very far away, even in other continents. The wolf carries a person's thoughts through the forest, becomes an orca in the sea, and then a wolf again on land. Wolf and orca transform one into the other; they are, in Jay Miller's words, "dual aspects of the same supernatural being."[20]

Many Native American traditions say that sound is a creative force. When a thing is named, its being is evoked. To say *wind* is to call on the power of the wind. This is especially true of indigenous languages because they are direct expressions of the land from which they arose. Words are carried by sacred breath. They have power and must always be spoken with care. Hurtful thoughts and words may have harmful consequences. Loving words can heal.

7. LOVING

Loving is love of the Great Spirit and love of the earth and all who dwell upon her. Its symbol is the sun. The sun shines on all unconditionally, and it is always present, even when we can't see it. All beings long for love, and we grow by giving it. Love reminds us of the Great Spirit's limitless and mysterious power, because the more we give love, the more love we have. Even so-called unrequited love is repaid by a deepening of spirit. All forms of love are sacred: love of Creator, personal love, and sexual love.

Love gives meaning to life, yet we cannot create or attract it intentionally. Love is not a matter of effort. It comes as a grace when we prepare ourselves day by day by living in a good way. The human mind divides subject from object and thus exiles us from nature. Love intimates the way back. It reminds us that happiness is found when we surrender to forces that are unknown and unknowable.

Native healers use the power of love in their work. Nuu-chah-nulth healer Johnny Moses says, "God's love is the greatest power." No personal totem or spirit power can heal a patient as strongly as God's love. A healer tries to put a patient in touch with that love. Grandfather Moses Shongo used to imagine a patient's illnesses or toxic energies releasing and dissolving into "the light of love." Lakota holy man Fools Crow sometimes diagnosed a patient by first touching the patient with love through his eyes, then placing his hand on the patient's shoulder. "I rub the shoulder gently so they will know the love I have for them. I care about them, even if some people don't have enough faith. . . ."[21] In Steve Wall and Harvey Arden's *Wisdomkeepers: Meetings with Native American Spiritual Elders,* the late Haudenosaunee chief Tadodaho Leon Shenandoah, a man of great wisdom and love, says, "We [human beings] were instructed to carry a love for one another and to show a great respect for all the beings of this earth."[22] In other words, love and respect are the essence of the Creator's "original instructions."

8. SERVICE

Euro-Americans often think of knowledge as the means to academic success or a better job. Native people believe that knowledge should be used to serve others; then it becomes wisdom. In his beautiful book about Native American philosophy *No Word for Time,* Algonquin author Evan T. Pritchard says, "Wisdom, *unkeedasee wach'n* in Micmac, means 'the state of thinking big thoughts.' It means you see the greater scope of things, how it all falls together, how we are all linked together in a very wide hoop."[23] The elders teach us to serve community, to do what is necessary to preserve the mental, physical, spiritual, and environmental health of family and neighbors. Service may mean attending a town meeting, writing a letter to a senator, hugging a tree to prevent illegal logging, or getting down on your hands and knees to help an old lady plant her garden.

Service is altruism, free of preoccupation with oneself and thus neither self-serving nor self-sacrificing. The former attitude elevates the ego; the latter all too commonly demeans it. Like a narcissistic child who believes that the world revolves around his personal needs, a self-serving person asks, "What's in it for me?" A self-sacrificing person proclaims, "Let me help you" while inwardly feeling "My own needs are unimportant." What, then, is the proper motivation for service? Compassion. We serve because we realize that our lives and destinies are bound up with others.

Service also means generosity, one of the cardinal virtues in Indian Country. There are two kinds of wealth. First, wealth is having a big family and many relations. The second kind of wealth might sound paradoxical from a non-Native perspective: a wealthy person may have few possessions and little money; wealth is not measured by how much you accumulate but by how much and how often you give. A person who shares resources and helps those in need is a rich and honorable person.

Native Americans often honor a person or an event with a Giveaway Ceremony in which possessions, both previously owned and newly purchased, are given to invited guests. The Giveaway Ceremony is practiced throughout North America, but it is perhaps best known in the Pacific Northwest, where it is known as the *Potlatch,* a word that means "gift" or "to give" in the Chinook language. Occasions for Potlatch may include receiving an Indian name, honoring a dream or dream-spirit, a wedding, a healing, the birth of a child, a good harvest, installing a chief, or passing on an inheritance to a family member. Even a poor family will try their best to cover the floor of a large meeting hall with blankets, household goods, drums, jewelry, money, and other items. I know a cancer patient who remortgaged his home in order to borrow enough money to purchase goods to honor the community that had helped him and prayed for his healing. In one of the largest Potlatches I have attended, items were distributed among approximately three hundred guests by the

Potlatch's sponsor and various ceremonial helpers—including children and elders. Amid a general mood of warm celebration, attendants sang, danced, and engaged in traditional oratory to explain the reason and spirit of the Potlatch.

Generosity strengthens the web of connection and kinship. Goods are constantly circulated or "recycled" when other tribal members have their own Giveaways. People begin to feel that everyone owes a debt of kindness to everyone else. Contrast the Giveaway with the Western idea that the "secure" person has money in the bank and possessions under lock and key, lest they be taken away. Which is the real security: knowing that your community will provide for your needs or fearing that you never have enough possessions to insulate against misfortune? The Potlatch made Euro-Americans uncomfortable because it questioned the morality of ownership. In 1885, the Canadian government outlawed the Potlatch at the behest of missionaries and Indian agents. In 1879, Canadian Indian Commissioner G. M. Sproat wrote, "It is not possible that Indians can acquire property, or become industrious with any good result, while under the influence of this [Potlatch] mania."[24] The ban was not lifted until 1951. The United States instituted similar prohibitions during the same time period.

Generosity may be a necessity for profound healing. A healer who is generous with time and service communicates unconditional love. A patient who is generous to the healer and community honors the Source of healing and symbolically releases attachment to material existence, thus opening his spirit to a deeper reality. A Caribou Inuk (singular form of *Inuit*) from Hudson Bay once told Danish explorer Knud Rasmussen, "If a sick person is to have any hope of being cured, he must own nothing but his breath."[25]

9. LIVING

It is not enough to know and speak the truth; we must put it into action—we must live it. Grandma Twylah says that the meaning of living the truth can be found by asking ourselves four essential questions, which she calls "The Four Guidelines of Self-Development":

1. Am I happy doing what I am doing?
2. What am I doing to add to the confusion?
3. What am I doing to bring about peace?
4. How will I be remembered after I am gone?

To truthfully answer "Am I happy doing what I am doing?" you must think carefully about your priorities and distinguish wants from needs. For example, are you happy if you are working only for money? Are you doing what you need to be doing or what is expected of you by parents or peers? Would you be happier doing something else? Ultimately, you must ask, "Am I happy with myself?" If the answer is no, then inquire how you are adding to the confusion within yourself and perhaps in your environment. Issues related to the second question include "Am I giving mixed messages to the people around me? Is my lifestyle creating stress and worry? Can I have the courage to express my opinion and make my voice heard?" The third question implies that each person is responsible for bringing clarity out of confusion and being an example of peace. Peace is not only up to our political leaders. There will be no peace on earth until each person is at peace within. The fourth question is, unfortunately, one that most people do not think about until late in life: "Will I be remembered as an honorable person?" Innu elder N'Tsukw once told me, "When we die, we are not extinguished. We still exist as memory." What do we need to do, release, or change to ensure that we will leave a good memory?

Living the truth implies deliberate, focused action and balanced use of the mind's power to focus. Set noble goals in your life and then do your best to accomplish them. You should also be wary, however, of the dangers of too much willpower. If you stubbornly insist on staying on a particular path, you may miss a trail that is more beautiful and interesting or a shortcut. A person with a stubborn, willful attitude misses opportunities in life.

The nine o'clock position on the wheel is the autumn season. The earth that receives the decaying autumn leaves is the same earth that brings forth new life in the spring. The earth supports and nurtures all forms and stages of life, and teaches observant people to do the same. She is a role model of unconditional caring and living in balance.

10. WORKING

To Grandfather Moses Shongo, "work" meant far more than earning money or "making a living." It involved the hands, the mind, the heart, and the cooperation of others—the kind of work common in ancient indigenous societies, including healing, craft making, hunting, farming, constructing dwellings, and making clothes. Smohalla (circa 1818–circa 1907), the Wanapum *yantcha,* "spiritual leader," and prophet from Washington State, was critical of how white society seemed more committed to profit than to people: "My young men shall never work," he said. "Men who work cannot dream, and wisdom comes to us in dreams."[26] Even in a free-enterprise society, many people take dream-crushing jobs because of lack of education, apathy, or the unavailability of meaningful work.

The Omaha have a saying: "A man should make his own arrows." This means that good work is creative and self-reliant. Yet self-reliance is not the same thing as individualism. The self-reliant person is ready and willing to work with the group to accomplish community goals. Among Native people, one of the worst insults you can say about someone is "He lives as though he had no relatives." We can turn this around to say that a spiritual person lives as though everyone were a relative. In Micmac ceremonies, just saying *Nogomaq,* "We are all related," creates harmony and blessings.

In the Wolf Clan Teaching Lodge, work is symbolized by the turtle. The turtle does everything slowly and carefully. His pace is dictated by the rhythms of nature. He is on "Indian time." Things get done when they need to get done. No schedules or clocks. No type A personalities. There is a Hasidic story of a man walking quickly and anxiously past his rabbi. The rabbi grabs his shoulder and asks, "Why the rush?" The man replies, "I have to rush to make a living." The rabbi reprimands him, "Maybe if you slow down, your living will catch up to you!"

I feel it is tragic that so few people examine the relationship between hastiness and happiness. Faster computers and commuter trains increase productivity but decrease leisure time and overall satisfaction with life. When I last visited New York City, I saw a middle-aged man wearing a T-shirt that said, "First Place Winner: NYC Rat Race." The problem is that if you win the rat race, you're still a rat. Personally, I would rather be a turtle.

Anthropologists have shown that cultures with the least technology have the slowest pace of life and the most leisure. According to Marshall Sahlins's classic *Stone Age Economics*, people living in subsistence cultures "do not work hard. The average length of time per person per day put into the appropriation and preparation of food was four or five hours. Moreover, they do not work continuously. The subsistence quest was highly intermittent. It would stop for the time being when the people had procured enough . . . which left them plenty of time to spare."[27] Hunters are described as having an "economic confidence" that allowed laughter during times of want. Contrary to the idea that subsistence people toil to survive, Sahlins says that it might be truer if the conventional beliefs were reversed: "[T]he amount of work (per capita) increases with the evolution of culture, and the amount of leisure decreases."[28]

Does this mean that we should reverse the clock and go back to a less complex and more leisurely lifestyle? I recognize that subsistence living is neither an interest nor an option for most people today, whether Native or white. With a population of more than 6 billion, there are simply too many people in the world to survive from hunting and foraging. Additionally, the wilderness, primordial forests, plants, and animals that sustained original peoples have been largely destroyed. We can, however, help to preserve and restore what is left of the earth and of our humanity by adopting the values embodied in traditional Native American work: cooperation, self-reliance, simplicity, and the importance of slowing down.

11. WALKING

In the Cycles of Truth, "walking"—or as Grandma Twylah says, "walking the truth"—means walking a spiritual path through life and remaining in motion; that is, realizing that spirituality is dynamic rather than passive. The spiritual person does not meditate in a cave waiting for enlightenment. Instead, he or she values what Tibetan Buddhists call "meditation in action," a spirituality that is fully engaged with life.

To the early Native Americans, walking was more than recreation or exercise; it was a matter of survival. To walk is to appreciate and learn from the landscape and to discover the location of building and craft materials and edible plants and animals. Walking, sledding, and paddling canoes or kayaks were the major forms of transportation—horses came with the white man. People walked to neighboring communities to trade and participate in ceremonies and festivities. People walked to discover escape or attack routes during times of warfare. Walking was also essential for spiritual survival; a person who walked on pilgrimage to a holy place renewed his or her connection with tribal history and sacred lore.

During healing ceremonies in the Northwest, dancers never dance in one spot for an extended period. The elders say that to stay too long in one place creates a kind of energetic stagnation that may prevent spiritual forces from flowing to and within a person. "Everything flows," said the Greek philosopher Heraclitus. A life in harmony with nature also flows.

To walk a spiritual trail is to walk with courage and commitment. Walk your vision, walk your goals. Even if you don't know what ultimately lies in store, have the courage to step onto and along that path. Once you know that the path exists, no detour can be satisfying.

"Walking" is dynamic spirituality. "The spiritual person is always on the front lines," Rolling Thunder was fond of saying. Holy people like Crazy Horse (Lakota) or Gokhlayeh (the real name of Geronimo, Apache) were the first in battle. Today, medicine people remain active in many important tribal decisions. They advise the chief, testify before the U.S. Congress, and defend their people against social and political injustice.

My favorite example of dynamic spirituality is a true story about the Lakota leader Sitting Bull. On August 14, 1872, four hundred soldiers under Major E. M. Baker were accompanying a surveying party of the Northern Pacific Railroad Company along the south bank of the Yellowstone, in violation of a recent treaty. Sitting Bull rode with his warriors to meet the soldiers, hoping to speak with them and warn them to stay out of Lakota country. They reached the soldiers at daybreak, but before a word could be spoken, the soldiers opened fire. There was no choice but to fight.

The soldiers were on a cutbank, and the Indians were on the prairie about a quarter of a mile away. After fighting all morning and with many warriors wounded, a medicine man named Long Holy convinced one group of warriors to ride toward the soldiers in circles, each time approaching closer in. After the fourth circle, they would charge the soldiers. Long Holy prayed to make the warriors "bulletproof" and taught them his song:

There is nobody holy besides me.
The Sun said so; the Rock said so;
He gave me this medicine, and said so.[29]

Unfortunately, the medicine did not prove adequate protection. As the warriors advanced, they were hit. After the third circle, Sitting Bull galloped across the prairie between the lines of soldiers and warriors, shouting at his men to turn back. Reluctantly, they did so. Long Holy did not appreciate Sitting Bull's interference. Sitting Bull was not a show-off. He was a courageous, wise, and humble leader of his people. Nevertheless, he needed to demonstrate the power of his own visions and muster the loyalty and unity of his people so they might return home without further injury.

Sitting Bull laid down his gun and quiver and took out his sacred pipebag. Stanley Vestal portrays the excitement of the scene in his 1932 biography *Sitting Bull: Champion of the Sioux*. Sitting Bull then walked

coolly out in front of the Indian line, as if he were taking a stroll through the camp at evening. He walked right out in front of the soldiers, and sat down on the grass a hundred yards in front of the Indian line, right on the open prairie, in plain sight of the firing soldiers. Then he got out his flint and steel, struck fire, lighted his pipe, and began to puff away in his usual leisurely fashion. Turning his head toward his own astonished men, he yelled to them, "Any Indians who wish to smoke with me, come on!"[30]

Sitting Bull was joined by his nephew White Bull, another Lakota named Gets-the-Best-of-Them, and two Cheyenne. The warriors' hearts were racing as Sitting Bull calmly proceeded with the Pipe Ceremony, passing the pipe in a circle to each of the men. Bullets whizzed past them, kicking up dust. When the ceremony was over, Sitting Bull carefully cleaned the pipe and returned it to the pipebag. The young warriors ran to the Indian line as Sitting Bull slowly sauntered back. He mounted his horse and led his men back home.

What about battles not between nations but within oneself, between the body's immune system and the invading host of bacteria, viruses, carcinogens, and other pathogenic forces? Does dynamic spirituality play a role in healing? Both indigenous and Western medicine say that a passive attitude is bad for health. Do not wallow in despair or be a victim of disease. Scientific research confirms that feisty people are better at fighting illness.[31]

12. GRATITUDE

The zenith of the wheel is the North, the direction of wisdom and strength. It represents the quality of gratefulness, the gift that takes us closest to the Source of Life. The simplest and profoundest Native American prayer is to say "Thank you" four or seven times. Seneca Indians greet one another with this beautiful phrase: *Nyaweh Skanoh,* "I am thankful [*nyaweh*] you are healthy." Haudenosaunee ceremonies, like those of most Native Americans, begin and end with a prayer of gratitude to the Great Spirit. Author Paul A. W. Wallace discusses the importance of "the prayer of thanksgiving" in his 1946 classic *The White Roots of Peace,* the story of the Peacemaker, who established the Haudenosaunee Confederacy in the distant past. The Peacemaker said that to open an assembly of the Confederacy, a statesman from the Onondaga Nation shall

> *return thanks to the earth where men dwell, to the streams of water, the pools, the springs, and the lakes, to the maize and the fruits, to the medicinal herbs and trees, to the forest trees for their usefulness, to the animals that serve as food and give their pelts for clothing, to the great winds and the lesser winds, to the Thunderers, to the Sun, the mighty warrior, to the Moon, to the messengers of the Creator who reveal his wishes, and to the Great Creator who dwells in the heavens above, who gives all things useful to man, and who is the source and the ruler of health and life.*[32]

When Native people pray, they do not say, "I want . . . Give me . . ." but "I offer . . . I am grateful. . . ." Gratefulness is a free expression of the heart. It is offered without demanding or expecting something in return. "Thank you" is such a sacred expression that in some Native cultures, the term is reserved for prayer. This is a difficult concept for some non-Indians to grasp. In white culture, when you perform a service or give something to someone, you expect an obvious and timely expression of gratitude, both verbally and perhaps with a thank-you note. It is considered polite to demonstrate gratitude with emotion and enthusiasm. For Lakota and other Native people, such behavior could be insulting. According to Dorothy Mack, writing in the Native newsletter *Red Cedar Bark,* "overt expression of thanks is a sign of currying favor or begging."[33] If someone does something that should be done by any caring person, to thank him may imply that he was acting out of character. Native people do express their thanks, but more subtly than whites— perhaps with a gift, a gentle word, or by helping out with a task.

Gratitude is healing. Some diseases cannot be cured. However, we can improve quality of life by changing our attitude toward a disease or disability. The easiest way to do this is by shifting attention away from our weaknesses and toward the things for which we are grateful. Healing spirits prefer people who are grateful to those who are thankless, unappreciative, or resentful. When you are thankful for your blessings, you attract more of them. People who are grateful to the Great Spirit are also more likely to change unhealthy, disease-promoting behavior. Instead of being depressed about their condition, they do something about it!

THE PATHWAY OF PEACE MEDITATION

We need to develop our twelve gifts in order to have a happy, beautiful, and meaningful life. According to Moses Shongo, the Cycles of Truth helps people "restore the peace where it belongs," which I interpret as a reference to the human heart. Peace can never be achieved through political action unless it is accompanied by a change of heart and a commitment to peaceful values.

How do you develop your gifts? I wish there were an easy answer to this question, or to any of the truly important questions in life. A poor question has one simple answer; a good question has many answers, and sometimes, no answer at all. Grandma Twylah had the advantage of a loving grandfather who explained and modeled spiritual gifts from the time she was an infant. Most of us are not so fortunate. If you are asking yourself the question "How can I understand and more fully live according to the ancient teachings?" then you are well on your way to the answer. The question itself attests to your dedication to the Great Spirit. He will answer your heart's prayer.

The most important way to cultivate the twelve gifts is by reflecting on them, thinking about how and whether you are using them in your life. For example, if you discover that you are very good at speaking, the six o'clock position on the wheel, but not very good at listening, the five o'clock position, then you can begin to hold back from volunteering opinions until you have carefully and silently considered whether your words are necessary and whether you are expressing them in a way that can be heard. Or if you discover that you have a problem expressing gratitude, even in subtle indigenous ways, you may need to examine what has hardened your heart. The gifts in the Cycles of Truth are twelve doorways into different aspects of yourself.

The Wolf Clan Teaching Lodge has a specific meditation called the "Pathway of Peace" to help people open their spirits to the healing power of the Cycles of Truth. Like the Four Winds, the gifts in the Cycles of Truth are both principles and powers. We can think about the East Wind, or we can invite the blessing of the East Wind. We can contemplate the meaning of "love," or we can make ourselves receptive to the power of love.

The Pathway of Peace meditation is based on gifts six through twelve, the seven gifts that comprise the left-hand portion of the Cycles of Truth, and opens our spirits to their power and blessing. Why practice a meditation with only seven parts and not with all twelve? We cannot be certain why Grandfather Moses Shongo taught this particular meditation. Native teachers do not always reveal the sources of their information, as the importance and authority of information lie in its truthfulness, not in its origin. The Pathway of Peace probably appeared to Grandfather in a dream or vision. It is not surprising that spirits would teach a meditation based on the holy number seven, which creates efficacy in ceremonial procedures.

First read the meditation to familiarize yourself with it. Then either try it on your own or ask someone to read it to you.

Sit on the ground or in a chair with your eyes closed. Rest your hands comfortably in your lap.

Imagine seven stepping-stones to the heavens, leading gradually up toward your source in the Great Mystery. As you step on each stone, you will receive a blessing from the gift that stone represents. Maintain the image of each stone for about thirty seconds to one minute, according to your comfort and ability to concentrate.

You step onto the first stone, beautiful red in color. It glows like a ruby. This is the stone of speaking the truth. You have the courage to speak what is in your heart, directly and honestly. This is also the stone of faith: faith in yourself and in the Creator. The red energy of speaking and faith enters every cell of your being. Stand in stillness and receive this blessing.

You step up to the second stone. It is a bright solar yellow, the power of love. You have the ability to give and receive love. Your mind and heart are nourished and healed by love. The yellow warmth of love fills and permeates you. You are grateful as you receive this gift.

You step up to the third stone, of service. It is deep ocean blue. The blue color washes through you, gently cleansing you like a calm sea. The blue energy brings the power to serve and nourish both yourself and others. It makes your mind deep and intuitive, so you can sense what is needed. You serve because you are in harmony with all your relations.

You take another step upward and stand on the bright green stone of life. You are a warrior for peace and a warrior for the Earth, willing to do what it takes to protect the harmony of the Earth and all who dwell upon her. The green of nature flows through you. This is also the stone of balanced willpower and balanced decision making. You receive these gifts from the green stone of Mother Earth.

You step still higher, onto the fifth stone, glowing pink like sunset skies. It is the stone of working in harmony. You receive the pink energy of this stone. It teaches you the importance of being self-reliant yet connected to others. It teaches you to work slowly, carefully, patiently, and creatively and not to settle for anything less than what you know is the best way to live. With a quiet mind, receive the blessings.

You step confidently onto the sixth stone, a clear crystalline stone of walking the truth. You have the mental clarity of the crystal and the strength to walk your talk. You are committed to releasing limitations and obstructions and making the changes necessary to live in a balanced way. The clear light of this stone rises into you.

With humility, you step onto the seventh and highest stone, the one closest to the light of the Creator. It is the purple stone of gratitude. Here at the top of the trail, your being is filled with the purple light of gratitude. All of the gifts in the Cycles of Truth are included in this one feeling of "I am grateful." You receive the healing power of gratitude, and you send it out with an inner prayer that it reach all who need it.

Now let the images go. With your eyes still closed, be aware of your body and surroundings. Focus on your breath, noticing its calm, quiet pace. Open your eyes whenever you wish.

4

— THE VISION AND VISION QUEST —
Messages from the Spirit

A vision is a mystical experience of seeing or knowing. Native Americans believe that it is a gift from Spirit, a source of wisdom and guidance beyond the individual self. In the previous two chapters I discussed spiritual powers and gifts. It is through visions that we connect with these powers and find out what our unique gifts are and how to use them. Visions can point out a meaningful life path and provide answers to important life questions, such as where to live or what kind of career would be most fulfilling. Knowledge of healing songs and methods, spiritual dances, the design of medicine bundles, or the location and properties of herbs may come to a healer during a vision. We can all have access to visionary realms at times of deep intuition, during powerful dreams, and in expanded states of consciousness, when the boundary between waking and dreaming becomes fluid and tenuous. In *The Varieties of Religious Experience,* author William James describes this potential as follows:

> [O]ur normal waking consciousness, rational consciousness as we call it, is but one special type of consciousness, whilst all about it, parted from it by the filmiest of screens, there lie potential forms of consciousness entirely different. We may go through life without suspecting their existence; but apply the requisite stimulus, and at a touch they are there in all their completeness. . . . [1]

The most powerful visions come during the Vision Quest, an important activity in all Native American cultures.

WHAT IS A VISION QUEST?

The Native American Vision Quest is typically a one- to four-day period of isolation, fasting, and prayer in pursuit of guidance from the Great Creator. The "vision" may be a waking or sleeping dream, a meaningful encounter with an animal or a helping spirit, or it may arrive when the spirit of a natural phenomenon, such as wind or thunder, visits the quester. The vision guides us as we try to live our truth and during times of crisis. It may reveal a person's life purpose and gifts and bestow on the quester the power to achieve them and to overcome adversity. The Odawa, an Algonquian-speaking people from the Great Lakes, say that the Vision Quest helps a person achieve the Good Life, or *Pimadaziwin,* defined by anthropologist A. Irving Hallowell in his *Culture and Experience* as "a long life and a life free from illness and other misfortune."[2]

The Vision Quest is a purposeful undertaking and, as such, is often considered a ceremony. The "dreamer" does not wait passively for a vision; he or she seeks it. Although the first Vision Quest is commonly a ritual of puberty, which helps the young person to find a spiritual center during this period of shifting hormones and emotions, one is never too old to seek the Great Spirit's guidance or to walk in a new or better direction. The Lakota word for the Vision Quest is *Hanblecheyapi,* "crying (*cheya*) for a vision (*hanble*)," implying that the vision comes in response to the deep longing of the soul.

The Vision Quest generally occurs in a remote place in nature: on a hill, mountain, or butte, in the forest or desert, near rocky outcroppings ("dreaming rocks," as the Cree call them), by sacred lakes or other bodies of water, or in a kind of earth-womb such as an L-shaped pit in the ground. The Tsistsistas (Cheyenne)—originally from the upper Minnesota River Valley and southern Canada and, later, the Dakotas, Montana, and Oklahoma—sometimes go to natural caves, *maheonoxsz,* to receive guidance or to be granted knowledge of ceremonies by powerful spirits. The most famous of these sacred caves is inside *Nowah'wus* ("The Sacred Mountain Where People Are Taught"), commonly known as Bear Butte, in the Black Hills of South Dakota.[3] In 1931, anthropologist A. L. Kroeber described in his paper "The Seri" how Seri healers (*ko'te*) from Tiburon Island in the Gulf of California seek power in caves that only appear to the eye of spirit, mystical openings in solid rock.[4] Vision Quests may also be held in man-made structures: a tipi, cabin (sometimes called a "medicine house"), or other lodge that is only used for sacred purposes. The Western Woods Cree sometimes erect a wooden platform between trees, generally at least ten feet off the ground. This "bird's nest," the *waciston,* is used specifically for fasting and vision- and dream-seeking. Wherever they are, such sites are holy and only used for Vision Quests or other sacred ceremonies.

The Vision Quest is not a one-time event. Many Native Americans return every year to particular sites to fulfill sacred vows and to renew their connection to the Great Mystery. Dreams and life experiences also corroborate and expand one's understanding of the vision.

VARIETY OF CUSTOMS

Typically, during a vigil, the dreamer stays within the well-defined perimeter of the sacred ground, fasting and praying, exposed to the elements, with only a blanket or an animal hide for a cover. In the Pacific Northwest, the quest may be a sacred pilgrimage—similar to the Walkabout of the Australian aborigines—that includes praying at and bathing in each body of water that one passes. Some Native California healers return each winter evening to a spring or other body of water until the inhabiting spirit teaches them directly or appears in a dream. Most dreamers seek the advice, support, and prayers of an elder "sponsor," who helps them prepare for the quest and later interpret their vision. However, some people are spontaneously called to vision. They leave on their quest "when the time is right" and return after an indefinite period of time.[5]

The Cree, like other Native Americans, say that the dreamer and the vision site must be pure, clean, and holy (*pikistowin,* in the Cree language), so that negative energies cannot block the revelations of Spirit. The dreamer purifies himself or herself physically and spiritually by ritual bathing or sweating, by fasting and chastity, and most important, by removing himself or herself from what the Cree call the *widipiswin,* "unclean and polluted" influences of civilization. Only when the "cup" of the mind is empty of everything unnatural can it be replenished from the Source. The wilderness outside leads one to the wilderness within, a place where the human mind is in touch with its original, God-given wisdom.

THE DREAM IMAGE

The Omaha call the Vision Quest *Nózhinzhon,* "to stand sleeping," because during the Vision Quest, waking and dreaming reality seem to merge. The dreamer becomes aware of a realm of spirituality and meaning that underlies our everyday reality. The Cree say that the dreamer encounters the *pawakan,* or "dream image," meaning the soul, spirit, or sacred presence of an animal, a bird, an object, or a place. Although the English words *Vision Quest* imply visual perception, spiritual messages can also be received through sound, intuition, feeling, smell, taste, touch, or any combination of the senses. The vision may take several forms; it might be a numinous image or presence in your mind or the actual, physical appearance of an animal, a bird, a fish, or an insect. It might be more accurate to call a vision "a listening," as it implies the ability to listen and receive the spiritual message with your whole being.

A few weeks after the tragic events of September 11, 2001, a mountain spirit urged me to visit it on a particular mountain within view of my home, a few miles to the west. I heard the voice of the mountain and felt it through every cell of my being. I was uncertain why I was suddenly called to make the journey, though I suspected that it had something to do with America's new war on terrorism.

One afternoon in late September, I hiked to the mountain and up the trail on its east slope. It was twenty degrees outside, and three inches of fresh snow covered the ground. Although I had not consulted an elder, nor prepared myself with ritual purifications, such as the Sweat Lodge Ceremony, in the face of the world's problems, I felt that it would be selfish and perhaps even dangerous to hesitate to follow the call of Spirit. I knew that "the time was right."

Three hours later, just before sunset, I stopped three-quarters of the way up the mountainside, in a small clearing surrounded by a ring of leafless aspen trees at an elevation of about ten thousand feet. I offered a pinch of tobacco on the ground, in gratitude to the spirit of the place, then made a small shelter of pine and aspen saplings, covered with dry yellow leaves and the tarp I had carried in my backpack. I spread my sleeping bag on a thin blue plastic pad and then sat on a rock to watch the shadows lengthen and the stars brighten in the clear, freezing sky. That night, the rocky ground pressed through my sleeping pad and kept me in a half-awake state. Nevertheless, the mountain spirit visited me in a dream and spoke these words:

> *The wars will not cease until human beings learn the lesson of simplicity. Two-leggeds are removing the bones of their ancestors, the plant people whose ancient bodies are coal, oil, and gas ["fossil fuels," created when carbon in vegetation is compressed underground for millions of years]. These bones are sacred. When you mine coal, oil, or gas, you rob the graves of your ancestors.*

> *When you stand on the ground, you stand on your plant elders. They support you, and their energy is the source of feeling centered, rooted, and in touch with nature. As two-leggeds pull up their own roots, they become incapable of making wise decisions, whether in the Middle East, the United States, or elsewhere. If they hoard resources or continue to disrespectfully excavate, burn, and consume my body, conflict will continue or get worse.*

I got the message. I returned home the next morning.

A DEEPER REALITY

A vision is not a daydream, a flight of fancy, nor a beautiful thought or image, experiences common to our ordinary waking reality. Yet the division between a vision received during the Vision Quest and one that occurs in everyday life, sometimes as a grace, unbidden and unasked for, is not rigid. A vision may be a special kind of waking or sleeping dream. A vision can be distinguished from an ordinary dream because both the dreamer and the community and elders with whom he or she shares it recognize that it is a direct communication from a spiritual realm. The vision feels more "real" than ordinary waking "reality," and it teaches truths that are too deep to be adequately conveyed in words. The great Lakota holy man Black Elk realized this ineffable quality of vision when, as an old man, he reflected on the great vision he had as a child:

> I am sure now that I was then too young to understand it all, and that I only felt it. It was the pictures I remembered and the words that went with them; for nothing I have ever seen with my eyes was so clear and bright as what my vision showed me; and no words that I have ever heard with my ears were like the words I heard. I did not have to remember these things; they have remembered themselves all these years. It was as I grew older that the meanings came clearer and clearer out of the pictures and the words; and even now I know that more was shown to me than I can tell.[6]

Visions often occur during times of transition or crisis, *if* we can surrender to a higher and deeper source of guidance. We cannot hear the voice of Spirit if we are wrapped up in personal concerns and worries. When the ego-barrier is gone, Spirit can be heard. Vision, in other words, requires entering the silence.

The appreciation of silence is not unique to Native American spirituality. Every major world religion has dreamers and prophets who hear the voice of God during times of deepest quietude. The Prophets of the Old Testament were visionaries. The Hebrew word for Prophet, *Navie,* is related to the roots *navuv,* "hollow," and *nava,* "to flow through, to gush forth," suggesting that the Prophet empties himself or herself of ego and selfishness so that the divine message can be received and communicated to others.[7] Moses is the archetypal dreamer in the Judeo-Christian tradition. He climbs the holy mountain and sees God in a Holy Fire, a burning bush.[8] Interestingly, Rabbi Lawrence Kushner believes that we can uncover hidden depths in the Bible by interpreting each person and story in it as part of a personal dream or by seeing how the stories are enacted during waking life.[9] If you are dedicated, persevering, and seeking truth for a noble purpose—such as the good of your nation—you can also see God on a mountaintop.

VISIONS THAT SERVE THE COMMON GOOD

The Vision Quest is not always a personal matter. Many people seek or spontaneously receive visions specifically for the good of their communities. These visions are generally considered the most noble. Today, a Native American might seek a vision to help solve his or her tribe's social, economic, or legal problems. In the past, tribes commonly relied on visionaries to locate animals' migration routes; determine the best places for fishing, foraging, hunting, or farming; and warn people of natural or supernatural danger. Native American spiritual leaders such as Handsome Lake, Wovoka, and Smohalla had visions that shaped new religions and helped Indian nations survive in the face of persecution and oppression.[10]

The great vision of Chief Plenty Coups, recounted in Frank Linderman's 1930 classic *Plenty-Coups: Chief of the Crows,* changed the destiny of his entire tribe. In 1857, the nine-year-old future chief dreamed that the buffalo would disappear from the Northern Plains and be replaced by strange spotted buffalo. He also saw a terrible storm destroying a forest of beautiful trees and birds, leaving only one tree standing. This tree was the lodge of the sensitive and wise Chickadee. Plenty Coups told his vision to the medicine man Yellow-Bear, and the entire tribe agreed with Yellow-Bear's interpretation. A storm of white people would soon sweep across the plains and attempt to uproot the Absarokee people. The Indian way of life, represented by the buffalo, would be destroyed and replaced by white ways, represented by the "strange buffalo," which Yellow-Bear recognized as cattle. The Chickadee is a good listener and learns from experience. Even in the midst of a storm, the small Chickadee avoids disaster by pitching her lodge in a safe tree. The Absarokee could learn from her example. As a result of Plenty Coups's vision, the Absarokee were one of the first plains nations to sign treaties with the whites and were able to preserve much of their beautiful, original lands.

Before he died, Plenty Coups asked that his personal home—a simple wooden house on the reservation—and the surrounding land with its cottonwood trees and stream be preserved as a place of peace and friendship for all peoples, nations, and cultures. I have visited the Chief Plenty Coups Peace Park (Crow, or *Absarokee,* Nation, Montana) with my family and experienced there a palpable presence of peace, serenity, and wisdom. It was easy to feel the warmth and hospitality of the people in the friendly *Kahee,* "Welcome," offered by Absarokee park volunteers.[11]

SPIRITUAL SACRIFICE

Sacrifice is an important element of Native American spirituality. To sacrifice means to offer something special to a spirit or deity as a symbol of gratitude or as an act of worship. During the Vision Quest, to attract the attention and compassion of spirits, Native Americans sacrifice the comforts of home, food, and water. Just as a wealthy Native American gives possessions to one who is poor, so powerful spirits may give the relatively weak quester a gift of vision, knowledge, and power. According to Cree tradition, fasting (*kowahkatahow*) increases sensitivity and receptivity to the spiritual beings or forces, a concept that is fundamental to vision questing in all indigenous cultures.

Fasting usually means fasting from food and water. If the Vision Quest takes place in a covered pit, a cave, or a darkened room, the seeker also "fasts" from light. In addition, the seeker abstains from sex for at least a few days prior to and, of course, during a quest. Yet a fast is more than a deliberate surrender of normal comforts; it is an attempt to face life directly and nakedly. Among many tribes, the dreamer may have no more than a buffalo robe to protect him from the evening cold. Professor Rodney Frey, scholar and student of Absarokee culture, says that the Absarokee faster is destitute like an orphan, *akéeleete,* a word that means "one with no possessions, one who has nothing."[12] An orphan is likely to be "adopted" by a protecting and helping spirit. In *Grateful Prey: Rock Cree Human-Animal Relationships,* anthropologist Robert Brightman writes, "In more social terms, the act of fasting evokes the 'pity' of potential guardians, conveying to them the seriousness of the novice's intentions."[13] A vision is the reward for sacrifice; you have put your life and soul in the hands of Creator.

When my Leni-Lenape friend Tom Laughing Bear Heidlebaugh was studying the flute with the great Comanche musician Doc Tate Nevaguaya, he was instructed to fast and pray in the woods until he was in such a deep communion with Spirit that he couldn't help crying. Then the spirit of the woods would speak to him and allow him to express its spirit, its breath, through the wooden flute. Dreamers among the Absarokee, Arapaho, Assiniboine, Hidatsa, Kiowa, Lakota, Mandan, and Tsistsistas weep to attract the pity of helping spirits. In the ceremonial longhouses of the Pacific Northwest, dreamers sometimes emit heartrending, otherworldly cries as spiritual forces shatter and reshape the soul. I wrote the following poem in the winter of 1991 after attending a traditional northwest ceremony during which dreamers honored their spirit powers with dance and song.

Shaman's Cry

The cry is an obsidian blade
That pierces this reality.
It cuts open a window
Into the dreamtime.

My suffering is unavoidable;
I must release the pain of separation.
I must release the pain of language;
I must release even my self.
I cry, and the Creator pities me.

I have shed my human form
I have entered the Bear Robe.

I look at you but cannot see you
Unless you have prayed yourself into being.

A Vision Quest is a sacred ceremony not to be undertaken lightly, but neither should it be avoided when it is necessary. Spirits sometimes instruct people to make significant changes in their lives; enacting them may require new levels of discipline and self-control. If you are not ready to try your best to follow such directives, don't even think about pursuing a Vision Quest. Ignoring the advice of Spirit can have serious consequences. A person who dreams of Thunder yet ignores Thunder's advice may be struck by lightning or develop a problem in the body's electrical (nervous) system. An Eagle dreamer who rejects the Eagle's gifts of spiritual insight, healing, or prophecy or who uses them irresponsibly may lose his gifts and become spiritually blind, nonintuitive, and dull-witted.

This does not mean that you have to carry out the instructions of a vision to the letter or that you need fear that it will make demands that are impossible to meet. Modern life is sometimes incompatible with spiritual obligations. Let's imagine that a Chumash Indian from California receives guidance to provide for his family by fishing in a traditional lagoon. Today, it might be impossible to obey that vision. The lagoon may be on private or federally "protected" lands or its waters polluted with mercury. Instead of taking the vision literally, the Indian can honor it by working to protect the environment and by fighting for Indian rights. The key to fulfilling a vision is always commitment, effort, and discipline.

Like dreams, visions often contain symbols, and it is up to the dreamer and his or her spiritual advisers to interpret them correctly. For example, a disabled friend fasted in a cave for two days. He had a vision that he rolled his wheelchair off the edge of a cliff. The chair disappeared, and he turned into an Albatross, a beautiful seabird with a six-foot wingspan, sailing over the ocean. The vision helped him realize that his spirit could still soar and encouraged him to fulfill his childhood dream of sailing to Australia, where the Albatross lives. Visions must be interpreted intuitively and creatively.

You may have the impression that the Vision Quest is always successful. What if you fast and pray and nothing happens? Perhaps your lesson is patience. Perhaps your lesson is to pay closer attention. The world always has something to teach if we are observant. Lakota elders advise that the essence of the Vision Quest is *wacinksapa*, "attentiveness," and *waableza*, "clear understanding." Lee Irwin, assistant professor of religion at the College of Charleston, relates in his landmark book *The Dream Seekers* that the act of fasting may confer fortitude and power whether or not a vision is received.[14] The Vision Quest may be considered successful if it lessens the power of the ego and thus increases the realization of kinship with life.

THE SACRED LAKE: A PERSONAL VISION

I grew up in Queens, one of the five boroughs of urban New York, an environment that was not especially conducive to deep communion with the spirits of nature. Yet I had visionary experiences from age six, when I became occasionally and unpredictably aware of a powerful energy in my body that produced tingling, warmth, and a feeling of greater aliveness. One day, when I was twelve years old, I realized "the energy is who I am." I knew that my experience was unusual and dangerous because it conflicted with the version of reality that most people trusted. I wondered if my awareness made me seem different; perhaps it explained why my elementary school classmates mistrusted, resented, and bullied me. As I was thinking these thoughts, I suddenly saw everything around me become crystalline and luminous, as though light of varying intensities were shining through both people and nature. I felt joyous, even ecstatic, and remained in a state of expanded awareness for the rest of that very special day.

When I was seventeen, I began studying qigong, a Chinese system of exercises and meditations that cultivates awareness of healing energy in the body. It felt very familiar and natural but did not satisfy my longing for a deeper understanding of the energy, light, and hidden power in nature. When I was in my twenties, I began traveling across North America and spent many nights camping under the stars. One night, as I lay asleep in a motel room in Colorado, I was suddenly awakened by a feeling of spiritual presence. I pulled the curtains from the window and looking outside saw two beings in a nearby pine tree: a red shadow and a brilliant black bird, shining like obsidian, with a wingspan of about nine feet. I knew intuitively that the red shadow was sent by the Great Mystery to direct me on a journey. I recognized the bird as Thunderbird, a messenger from the West. The next day, I asked the clerk at a local camping supply store what was due west of the town where I was staying. He described a wilderness region of pine and aspen forests and twelve-thousand-foot peaks. I decided to follow the call of the spirit beings and set up camp in that area.

Some friends drove me out of town: twenty miles up a steep canyon road and another ten miles to the start of the trail. I hiked west for about six or seven hours, gradually ascending into a world of delicate tundra and dwarfed alpine flowers. The cascading river at my side leveled out into a clear, flat brook. I reached the source of the waters and the end of the trail at a half-frozen lake fed by a glacier that covered the nearby peak. From a vantage point just above the lake, I could see snowcapped granite peaks in all directions. I recognized this place as the home of the Thunderbird and of the Red Spirit of the East, the wind of new directions. I didn't really know what that new direction was, but I knew that I had taken the first step. I had found my special, sacred place. I bent down and rested my two palms on the earth in gratitude. I sensed that I would someday return to the sacred lake for a formal Vision Quest.

My travels eventually led me to Berkeley, California, where I attended graduate school and began to study with various Native American teachers. After five years, I was ready to stop learning about nature and to start living in it. The combined stress of poverty, polluted cities, and a disintegrating marriage had caused a flare-up of my childhood problem of chronic bronchitis. I needed to live in a simpler, purer environment. I moved to a small town in the mountains of Colorado and, after a painful and protracted divorce, was in desperate need of the Great Spirit's guidance. Seven years from the time of my first visit to the sacred lake, I was ready to return.

I once again climbed the trails to the glacier-fed alpine lake. This time, I was guided by my elders to fast and pray. As I reached the lake, the clouds, which had been rolling in over the divide, now formed a dark, heavy blanket. A sound of rolling thunder reverberated through the circle formed by the snowcapped granite peaks. Just as I set up my camp, the sacred space of my quest, lightning began to flash, and hailstones the size of golf balls crashed on the roof of my simple lean-to. I took out my sacred Native American pipe, the Canunpa, *and began to pray and ask for direction. As soon as I lit the pipe, the hail stopped; one ray of light broke through the cloud cover and illuminated my dwelling. I stepped outside to blow a puff of smoke, an offering of gratitude, out toward the thunderclouds. Directly in front of me, seated on a tree branch about ten feet away, was a small eagle. This was not merely an Eagle of Vision, an Eagle seen with the mind's eye—it was physically present. The eagle looked at me for a moment, then flew off to the East, down the valley through which I had just passed.*

As I continued to smoke, I heard a voice in and through my mind that said, "Now you are like this small eagle flying to the East, but soon you will be like us. Look up!" I looked up and saw two eagles circling overhead. I heard another spirit voice: "Always remember, there is no virtue in suffering, only follow the Way of the Pipe." The voice repeated itself: "Always remember, there is no virtue in suffering, only follow the Way of the Pipe." I continued to watch the eagles as they circled slowly and gracefully above. The clouds quickly dissipated and left a clear blue, sparkling sky.

I know that part of my mission is to teach the importance of holy joy and that we must avoid suffering for suffering's sake. Suffering is not, of itself, ennobling, yet one must accept suffering as a part of life. It may be a side effect of following a spiritual and an honorable life path. And I know that I must follow the Way of the Pipe, which means dedicating myself to the instructions of the Great Spirit and making every step a prayer. The message of my Vision Quest has stayed with me, strengthened and corroborated by subsequent visions.

Life is indeed punctuated by cycles of the holy number seven. I made a vow to return to my site two more times, a total of four times in twenty-eight years. I have completed my vow.

SHARING THE VISION

Sharing a vision is a sacred act. As a sign of respect for the dream helpers, a vision should only be shared in a sacred setting, when the time is right, and with the right people. One or more medicine people help the dreamer arrive at a meaningful interpretation. Mourning Dove (1888–1936), a member of the Colville Federated Tribes of eastern Washington State, wrote in her autobiography, "While the power and the guidance for a career came from a spirit, it was the elders, learned in these tribal traditions, who provided the fine points of usage and established the social context for approved practice."[15] The telling of a vision is a form of ritual speech, called "dreamtalk" (*hanbloglaka,* in Lakota), that takes place after listeners have purified themselves in a Sweat Lodge or other ceremony. The dreamer allows the vision to speak itself. He or she speaks the images and invokes the power of the dream, allowing the listeners to share in some aspects of the experience. Listening to a vision is always a blessing and a gift.

In indigenous cultures, sharing a vision with others is often more a responsibility than an option. Marilyn Schlitz, director of research for the Institute of Noetic Sciences, reflects on her experience among the Huaorani tribe of the Amazon: "It is in the shared exploration of a reality considered more real than ordinary experience that meaning takes form within the social collective."[16] The vision builds community by affirming common values such as the importance of valuing, trusting, and acting on spiritual guidance. The prevalence of dream images in discourse, art, and ritual draws other tribal members into the dream and creates wider awareness of and access to spiritual realms.

Some visions include directions about how or if they must be shared. Spirits told The-Fringe, a mid-nineteenth-century Absarokee medicine man, to share his vision only after four sweat lodges had been constructed in a row, from east to west. He was to pray in each of them before telling his vision to eleven "Wise Ones" (medicine men).[17] Some visions must be allowed to deepen and mature in the dreamer's mind before they are spoken. If you were to pray in each of the directions regularly for a year, asking that Sacred Wind the meaning of your vision, then you might be ready to speak intelligently about it or perhaps not to speak at all. Visions demand patience and discretion. A Native colleague illustrated this point humorously:

A woman stood up during a healing ceremony and said, "I just received a vision that I would like to share." She explained that she had, during the previous hour of singing and drumming, been visited by what she called "a releasing spirit." She volunteered to sing the song of the releasing spirit. Immediately after the song, several people rushed off to the bathroom. The elder commented, "Before sharing your vision, you should have asked the spirit what kind of releasing spirit it was. I think that you invoked the Poop Spirit!"

AN UNEXPECTED LESSON

Visions can be grand and prophetic, like that of Plenty Coups, or they might seem quite mundane. A Native friend told me a story about how, as a young man, he was disappointed that he had not yet had a vision. One day, after rising from bed, he stood up and glanced about, suddenly shrieking as he saw a hideous image standing in front of him in the pale dawn light. A thought flashed through his mind: "I am learning to see evil spirits; I am on my way to becoming a medicine man!" Just as suddenly, the thought evaporated, and his awe and terror turned to laughter. He was looking at himself in a full-length mirror! A wise elder explained, "How can you have a vision if you are afraid of yourself?" My friend learned an important lesson. A vision cannot arise from the depths if we haven't plumbed the shallows.

A Native American educator told me how she expected to see eagles during her first Vision Quest and instead saw only a row of black worker ants. It was a lesson in humility. Even the smallest creature has something important to teach. Whether a vision is of mighty whales or a simple mouse, its message is always unexpected.

When I was a young man and searching for romance and adventure, like many young men, I once had a dream of an extraordinarily beautiful woman. She seemed to be the embodiment of everything I had ever loved or dreamed of in a woman. She was multiracial and had characteristics that I could identify as African, Asian, and Native American. She moved with quiet grace yet great inner strength. Her eyes were dark and deep, full of wisdom and love. She was both sensual and spiritual, beautiful in body and mind. When I woke up, I was determined to meet her! The dream seemed so real that I actually believed it was prophetic of a woman I would meet in ordinary, nondreaming reality. I decided to practice a method of spirit journeying with the hope that I might discover her location. I wanted an "address" and a phone number.

I prayed to be taken to the dream woman. To my surprise, my body became light as a feather. I floated up like a cloud and began to travel with incredible speed. I crossed the ocean, traveled over Europe, Africa, Asia, Australia, all of the continents. I found that I could mentally control my height and speed, now and again descending close to the earth to observe the people or terrain. But I didn't find her, no matter where I looked.

Eventually, I made a complete circuit of the earth and found myself back at home, at my starting point. Yet I wasn't disappointed. I heard a voice, a sweet, wonderful voice, coming from both the outside and deep within my mind. It said, "I am the Earth. I am your mother. I appear to you in many forms."

This vision was an important lesson. I discovered that the Earth Mother is everywhere, and all women represent her. Since she is everywhere, there is no need to pursue her vigorously, to look far away for what is close at hand. I just needed to be patient and allow life to unfold.

SELLING DREAMS:
THE CONSEQUENCES OF A LIFE WITHOUT VISION

The images we see every day affect who we are and what we become. Native Americans who follow their old traditions place tremendous value on images seen in dreams and visions. The images are shared in storytelling and "dreamtalk," enacted in ritual—for example, in the Pacific Northwest, the portrayal of dream stories in masked dances—and represented in art, including ancient Native American petroglyphs and pictographs. In the Northern Plains, spirits seen during Vision Quests were often painted on tipis, reminding the family who dwelled there of the powers that protected and guided them. Until very recently, dream images were always noncommercial, valued entirely for their spiritual rather than monetary value. (Today's Native Americans are not immune from materialism. There is a controversy raging in Indian Country about whether artwork with sacred images—such as a blanket with a religious symbol or a ritual mask—should be sold.)

In Euro-American culture, secular and commercial images often guide people's lives: violent images in the newspaper, billboards on the highway, a storefront display, or a TV ad for updated Internet software or a new car. In the Hollywood movie *Enemy Mine,* an alien from another planet tells the earthling that he had assumed from intercepted radio and TV broadcasts that Mickey Mouse was the name of the human God. Although religious and artistic images are certainly important in the West, they are not central to everyday experience. An advertising agent once told me, "I am in the business of selling dreams." How sad—when dreams become commodities and when fears, hopes, desires, values, and even reality are shaped by the images projected by television and mass media.

The objects people carry on their bodies, such as a medicine bag, a piece of jewelry, or a wallet, are also images that have more than utilitarian value. When people see them or hold them, they remind them of who they are; they represent personal or cultural dreams. The traditional Native American medicine bag is a small buckskin pouch, generally worn around the neck, which contains objects that represent dream helpers and the power of nature—for example, a piece of turtle shell or a bear's tooth. The modern American "medicine bag"—carried by both Indians and whites—contains symbols of consumerism: credit cards and slips of paper inscribed with pictures of U.S. presidents, many of whom were Indian killers.[18]

Yet there is reason to hope. Westerners are becoming tremendously interested in dreams, and the twentieth century provided the world with great role models of spiritual visionaries: Mahatma Gandhi, Mother Teresa, Nelson Mandela, and Dr. Martin Luther King Jr., who declared, "I have a dream." They are respected by Native Americans as true holy people who bravely gave their visions the priority they deserved.

Life is tragic if we do not follow our dreams. Even if a dream is never fully realized, we are happier if we make the effort to listen to its guidance. When I meet someone who has succumbed to dream-extinguishing pressures, I sense a great loss to humanity. Some people do not realize the importance of their dreams until they are about to return to the mind of the Great Dreamer—the Great Mystery. Are we perhaps but images in his or her mind?

5

— WHERE HEALING DWELLS —
The Importance of Sacred Space

Physicians and holistic healers often work in a geographic vacuum, focusing on the *why* and *how* of disease, but not the *where*. Do herbs or massage work as effectively in the city as at the seashore? Does penicillin destroy bacteria as quickly in a busy hospital as in the comfort of your home? Certainly, many of us have been in places that don't feel right, that make us feel tense, uncomfortable, or even sick, or conversely, that make us feel happy, relaxed, and well. Does the place itself influence healing? Even if scientific proof were lacking—which it is not—common sense tells us that it does.

Native American healers recognize that specific healing powers, as well as the plants and animals that embody them, reside in specific locations. To treat a patient's injured spine, a healer might travel to a desert to fast, pray, and gather snake power, a medicine related to the flow of electrical signals in the nervous system. If he needs star power, perhaps for greater clarity and guidance, he might fast on a mountaintop, to be physically closer to the stars. To deepen introspective power and improve counseling skills, he might seclude himself in a cave. Clues about the healing power of a certain place can often be found in Indian rock art. Near Moab, Utah, there is a boulder with a petroglyph of a woman giving birth. It is likely that pregnant women prayed and made offerings of tobacco or cornmeal there to seek spiritual help for a safe and easy childbirth.[1]

Sometimes, it is the patient who must make a pilgrimage to aid in his or her own healing, perhaps to gather a medicinal plant or commune with a healing power. The very act of traveling to a new landscape helps us release unhealthy habits and opens the mind to unexpected vistas. A pilgrimage into nature can also be powerful *preventive* medicine. Nature strengthens us *directly* by feeding us with the natural "nu-

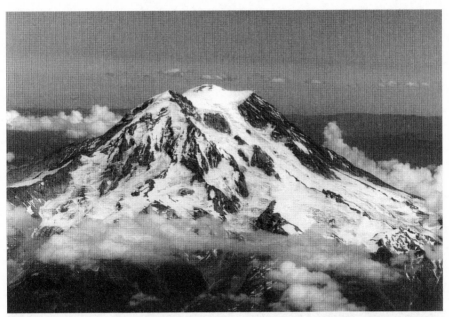

Mount Rainier—known to the Puyallup Tribe as Tahoma, the "Great White Mountain"—rises like a giant breast 14,408 feet above Washington's Puget Sound. Her glacial milk is a source of water and nourishment for the lands below.

trients" of air, earth, sky, mountain, and plant, and *indirectly* by expanding our awareness and awakening our intuition, faculties that can help us create healthful changes in our everyday lives. We can make a pilgrimage more healing and rewarding by *celebrating the landscape,* a custom of indigenous people throughout the world. When passing Mother Earth's beautiful features, compose poems and songs to honor their beauty. The purpose of pilgrimage is beautifully captured in ethnologist Alice C. Fletcher's *The Hako: Song, Pipe, and Unity in a Pawnee Calumet Ceremony,* a description of the Hako, a prayer ceremony for children and for the health, happiness, and peace of the tribe:

> *The journey we are taking is for a sacred purpose, and as we are led by the supernatural power in Mother Corn, we must address with song every object we meet, because Tira'wa [the Great Spirit] is in all things. Everything we come to as we travel can give us help, and send help by us to the Children.*[2]

As we travel, we can listen to the songs that the land is singing: the rushing wind, the rippling stream, ice breaking in the river, rain falling on the lake, the whistling hawks, chirping sparrows, and squirrels scurrying through the undergrowth. These are the songs that we can hear with the physical ears. Our spiritual ears can also hear songs. The Earth is truly alive, and all her beings have the capacity to speak or sing to the human mind. The sagebrush sings; the salmon sing. Sometimes, the songs are in the language of the listener; sometimes, they consist largely of sounds that in themselves have no meaning, such as the *vocables* used in Native American songs— "hey ya, hi ya, ya wey ya hey ya, wey ya hey yo, ya na wa na ya na, ung ung ung ung,"

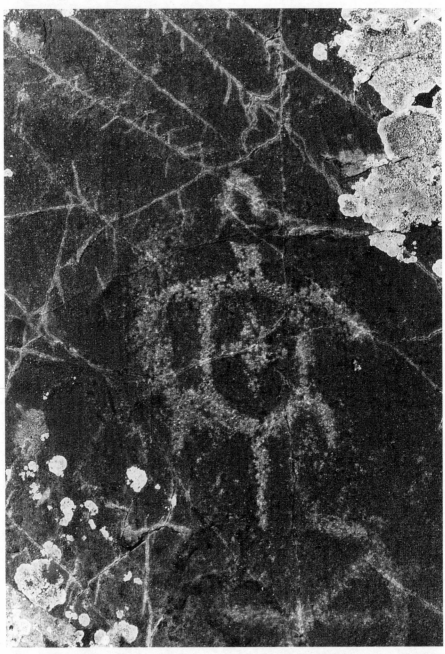

Turtle with Four Winds symbol on back. Rock art from Jeffers Petroglyphs Historic Site, Minnesota.

and so forth—which evoke both moods and spirits and express the pure, rhythmic energy of life.

With permission of the Paiute Tribal Council, I once offered a healing seminar on the banks of a sacred lake within the borders of the Paiute Nation, several hours' drive from Reno, Nevada. One evening after we sang around the campfire, we continued to hear faint drumming and voices carried on the wind. It seemed to be a symphony of chants and songs of old warriors who had once fasted and prayed here, mixed with a shrill background noise, like a ceremonial eagle-bone whistle. Sentrylike boulders behind us echoed these sounds out over the moonlit lake and created the mysterious impression that they were coming from everywhere at once. We felt deeply honored by this ancient presence.

Turtle Island, an ancient Native American name for North America, is filled with places of sacred pilgrimage and healing power. (To learn about them and find out which ones may be visited, see "Indian Country Travel Guides" in the "Native American Resources" section.) Native American spirituality is not a universal religion that can be adopted by people living anywhere. A Catholic person can study and practice his religion in Sri Lanka; indeed, many Christians have tried to spread their religion to other countries. By contrast, Native American songs, stories, and teachings belong to the North American landscape. Creation took place *here*, at *this* cave. The First People lived on *this* desert mesa. For Black Elk, the sacred center of Lakota spirituality was Harney Peak in the Black Hills.[3] Native Americans are bonded historically, culturally, and spiritually to their original lands, which are sources of inspiration, cultural renewal, and healing power.

EUROPEAN SACRED SITES

The power of place was important in ancient European medicine. Professor C. A. Meier, former president of the Carl Jung Institute in Zurich, reminds us of a universal truth: "Marvelous cures have a tendency to occur in particular places, for sanctity is bound up with locality."[4] Ancient Greeks sought healing dreams in temples devoted to Asclepios, the God of Healing. A patient or a person proxying for a patient would prepare for his quest by taking a ritual bath to purify body and soul. Then, if he felt genuinely called to seek healing, he would enter the innermost sanctuary, the *abaton,* a word that means "place not to be entered unbidden." There, the patient would lie down on a *kline,* a couch, and await a dream that revealed the means to recovery. The English word *clinic* is derived from this dream couch. Today, "dream couches" are found in offices rather than temples, and the only Western healers who seek healing clues within dreams are psychotherapists.[5]

Early Christians were also aware of the sacred quality of places. In the Gospel According to Thomas, a text written in Coptic, a language closer to Jesus' own Aramaic than the common Greek in which his words were later recorded, Jesus is asked, "Where is the Kingdom of Heaven?" He says, "The Kingdom of Heaven is already spread upon the earth but people do not see it!" When we perceive clearly, we feel God's presence everywhere, in every place. *Makom*, "Place," is one of the ancient Hebrew words for God. God is, literally, here and now.[6]

Spiritual Christians, like followers of Native American tradition, make healing pilgrimages. The most famous pilgrimage site is the spring at Lourdes, in the French Pyrenees. In February 1848, a fourteen-year-old girl, Bernadette Soubirous, was gathering firewood when she suddenly heard a roaring sound, like the wind. Looking up toward a cavelike depression in the rocky cliff, she saw a beautiful woman dressed in a white garment with a blue sash. The apparition announced that she was the Immaculate Conception and revealed to Bernadette the location of an underground spring. Bernadette dug with her hands until water appeared, and the spring continues to flow to this day. Within a month, four "miracle cures" had occurred at the spring. Today, more than 4 million pilgrims visit Lourdes annually, among whom approximately 65,000 are ill. More than 6,000 individuals have claimed that they were cured at the spring. Sixty-four of these cures have been certified as "miracles" by the Catholic Church.[7]

Two of these miracles were reported during the second half of the twentieth century. In April 1962, a twenty-two-year-old Italian soldier named Vittorio Micheli was admitted to the Verona military hospital because of debilitating hip pain. Extensive testing, including X rays and biopsies, confirmed a diagnosis of sarcoma (cancer) of the left pelvis. His health deteriorated quickly, and within months, the cancer had almost completely destroyed his left pelvic bone. Doctors placed Micheli in a hip-to-toe cast to immobilize that part of his body, enabling limited movement and, hopefully, reducing pain and slowing down deterioration, but the cancer continued to attack his bones. By January 1963, his femur was no longer connected to the pelvis. Then the doctors tried chemotherapy and radiation, but the therapy was ineffective, and treatment was discontinued after several sessions. Micheli was in severe and unremitting pain.

In May 1963, Micheli went to Lourdes hoping against hope for a miracle to ease his suffering. After his first bath, he felt hungry, a characteristic of the Lourdes cures. Several baths later, the pain diminished, and Micheli reported to his doctors that it felt as though his leg were reattaching itself to the pelvis. A month later, still in a cast, he was walking. In August, X rays confirmed that the sarcoma had regressed and that his bones were regenerating. Soon, doctors could find no trace of cancer; his left hip joint returned to normal. Micheli took a job in a factory, standing for eight to ten hours a day. The Medical Bureau of Lourdes followed his case for five years, during which time there was no recurrence of the cancer. In 1976, after review by pathology professors and international medical and canonical commissions showed it to be scientifically inexplicable, the Catholic Church declared Micheli's cure a miracle.

That same year, Delizia Cirolli, a twelve-year-old girl from a village on the slopes of Mount Etna in Sicily, saw her doctor because of a painful and swollen right knee. Her doctor sent her to the Orthopedic Clinic at the University of Catania, where X rays and biopsy showed metastasized bone cancer. The biopsy slides were examined by the most eminent bone tumor specialists in France, who confirmed a diagnosis of Ewing's tumor, a rare and always fatal type of cancer. Delizia's family refused all treatments, including the amputation and radiation advised by her doctors. Instead, they took her to Lourdes, where she spent four days bathing in the sacred waters and praying. However, Delizia's condition did not improve. After the family returned home, her mother gave her Lourdes holy water to drink, and people from her village prayed to Our Lady of Lourdes for a miracle, but the cancer continued to grow. Her family prepared for her funeral.

Then, shortly before Christmas, four months after the pilgrimage to Lourdes, Delizia suddenly declared that she wanted to stand up and walk. Inexplicably, her knee was no longer swollen. She was able to walk briefly without pain, and X rays showed that the cancer was gone. Six years later, in 1982, after consultation with Delizia's doctors and an exhaustive review of her medical records, the church pronounced that her cure, too, was a miracle.

Although the healings at Lourdes are the best known and most rigorously tested, similar pilgrimage sites are found throughout the world. Iceland has its own Lourdes, the holy spring near Snaefellsnes, where the Virgin Mary appeared to an Icelandic bishop a thousand years ago. Drinking from the spring is said to confer a lifelong blessing. The nearby holy mountain, Helgafel, was probably a Vision Quest site for practitioners of *seidr,* ancient Norse shamanism. Icelandic tradition states that anyone who makes a silent pilgrimage to the summit and stands in the center of its circular stone shrine will have three wishes granted, provided the wishes are good and kept secret.

CHRISTIAN CHURCHES ON PAGAN SOIL

European churches were frequently built over Pagan "power places," areas that were said to be inhabited by elves, fairies, or other pagan spirits and had been used for Pagan worship. Church founders were probably intuitively attracted to the power of these places. Unfortunately, they also denied the basis of this power by not accepting the sacredness of the earth and by labeling nature spirits as "devils." In his A.D. 604 letter of instruction to the Abbot Mellitus, Pope Gregory wrote, "I have determined, after mature deliberation on English affairs, that the temples of the idols of that nation ought by no means to be destroyed. . . . Provided the temples are well built, it is requisite that they should be converted from the worship of devils to the service of the True God."

The history of the Pagan and Christian relationship to place is excellently summarized in British scholar Nigel Pennick's *The Ancient Science of Geomancy.* Pennick notes that in Lichfield, England, the Cathedral of Saint Mary and Saint Chad was built on a site that was originally dedicated to Mars, the God of War, or his Celtic counterpart. The feast of Saint Chad is still celebrated on March 2, a day formerly dedicated to the worship of Mars. The land on which the cathedral sits was also once the site of an ancient ceremony called "beating the bounds," in which eight sacred wells, representing the four cardinal directions and four intermediate points bounding the site, were visited in turn.

A similar reinterpretation and blanketing of an indigenous sacred site is found near Española, New Mexico, at *El Sanctuario de Chimayo,* the Chimayo Catholic Church, sometimes called the "Lourdes of America." The energetic center of the church is a small room near the altar that has a hole in the floor filled with the local, natural mud. The nearby Tewa Indians remember this area for its volcanic fires and smoke and for a pool of bubbling hot mud that was used for healing. It was called *Nam Po'uare,* "Earth Blessed," and *Tsimajopokwi,* derived from the words *Tsimajo,* which is believed to mean either "obsidian" (a volcanic stone found in the area) or "place where the big stones stand," and *pokwi,* "pool." Extraordinarily, geologists confirm that the area was volcanic and geothermally active close to a million years ago. The fact that Native people knew of such activity long before it was "discovered" by scientists in the 1940s lends further credence to the great antiquity of their oral history and habitation of North America.

In 1818, a Catholic church was built over the healing soil. Today, Christians rub the earth over their bodies and pray for healing as Indians did for millennia before them. Dr. Stephen F. De Borhegyi, former curator of the University of Oklahoma Museum, writes in an essay about Chimayo, "This earth is supposed to contain great medical powers that can cure pains, rheumatism, sadness, sore throat, paralysis, and is particularly useful during childbirth."[8] The walls in the Chimayo Church are lined with discarded crutches and photos and testimonials of miraculous, though scientifically undocumented, healings. I have no doubt that good-hearted Christians and Indians, however divergent their beliefs, helped to maintain the sanctity of this place by their common emphasis on the healing power of prayer.

ACKNOWLEDGING THE SACRED AWAKENS THE SACRED

Prayers can heal both people and landscapes. Praying for and with the land protects it from destructive influences and helps it stay healthy. In the 1970s, Rolling Thunder purchased 262 acres of flat and sandy desert land a few miles from Carlin, Nevada, to create an intertribal community called Meta Tantay (Shoshone for "Go in Peace"). The previous owner had tried unsuccessfully to find well water. There was a dried streambed on the land that only filled briefly each spring, supplying mud for the magpies' nests. Local ranchers told Rolling Thunder that the land "was worthless" because it could not be cultivated and would always remain arid and barren. No land is worthless. It achieves value when people acknowledge the Creator's power and beauty, which is everywhere present to the eye of spirit.

Meta-Tantay was my home for two or more months each year from 1980 to 1984. The community of approximately forty Native and non-Native residents and guests began each day with a sunrise campfire and prayers of gratitude to the rising sun and the new day. I will never forget the voice of the camp crier early each morning, heard easily through the thin walls of the wickiup, a dome-shaped home made of tree branches and various coverings. "Time to get up. Sunrise in forty minutes." When you start the day by sharing good thoughts with the Great Spirit and with one another, blessings stay with you all day long. Lifelong friendships were made around that prayer circle. We also prayed for the health of the land. If one wondered about the power of prayer, one had only to walk over to the once dried-up riverbed, now flowing year-round, or to drink from one of our gushing wells or to eat one of the giant vegetables growing in the garden. Prayer had turned this "worthless" land into a paradise.

In the 1980s, I experienced a powerful example of the connection between prayer and place while visiting my Cree family in Canada. Around 1985, with the encouragement of Cree elders, my adopted Cree brother Joseph and I made a pilgrimage to the Meewasin Valley Medicine Wheel near the South Saskatchewan River. This is one of the northernmost medicine wheels in North America. It consists of a central cairn surrounded by a ring of stones, with three smaller cairns nearby. Pottery fragments and arrowheads indicate that the wheel had been used since at least A.D. 500. No one is certain, however, *how* it was used. Unlike other wheels, it does not have radiating spokes or any clear astronomical alignments. It does not mark the solstice or equinox nor the position of any known asterism or astronomical event. Yet, like all medicine wheels, it has a powerful, sacred presence.

Because it was rumored that the wheel was going to be disturbed or dug up and analyzed by non-Indian archaeologists, we wanted to do something spiritual to preserve it. We circled the wheel respectfully seven times and then sat near it to smoke the sacred pipe in a traditional Pipe Ceremony. I prayed that the wheel and land

— WHERE IS THE KINGDOM OF HEAVEN? —

Native people like to spice up spiritual teachings with jokes or humorous stories. The following is a personal variation of one of my favorites. It illustrates Western and indigenous perspectives on place:

An elder and chief from Vancouver Island, British Columbia, was invited by the pope to visit the Vatican as a representative of her nation and its religion. Grandmother was pleased with this recognition of First Nation spirituality and political sovereignty. The pope and his attendants took Grandmother on a grand tour of the magnificent buildings, art, and archives. Later, when the pope and the Indian Grandmother were alone in the basement of the great basilica, the pope pointed out a closed red door that was barely visible among the endless rows of sacred texts. He explained in a reverent whisper, "Only a few great religious leaders have seen what lies beyond that door. I escorted the Dalai Lama into that room, and now I am going to show you." The pope opened the door.

The splendor of the Vatican contrasted sharply with the simple view that greeted Grandmother: a fifteen-foot-square chamber in the center of which were a small table and a wooden chair. There was an antique-looking gold-colored telephone on the table. The pope pointed, inquiring, "You wonder how I speak to God? How I get my instructions?" Knowing that Grandmother would welcome the opportunity to speak to the Almighty, he continued, "Of course, the call is long-distance. If you have a credit card, I can let you try the phone for three minutes."

"I am poor," Grandmother explained, with proper regret. "I do not have a credit card and so must decline the honor. But *Ee Heychka,* Thank you so much, for offering."

Most people have only heard that half of the story and are unaware of what happened next. Now let me continue with the rest of the tale:

A year later, while the pope was visiting western Canada, he received an invitation to attend a longhouse welcoming feast in his honor at a small village on Vancouver Island. The pope accepted and was pleased to see the

Grandmother whom he had met earlier. After the nightlong festivities, as dawn was breaking, Grandmother invited the pope for a walk around the village. The pope observed the fishermen pushing out to sea and enjoyed the cool fog drifting among the cedar trees. They stood silently for a few minutes, as the fog lifted to reveal a simple cedarwood shack with a red door.

The pope looked incredulously. "You don't mean . . . ?" "Yes," replied Grandmother, calmly. They went inside. An earthen floor and a room barren but for the red telephone on the ground. The pope reached in his pants pocket, anxiously searching for his wallet. "Oh, no need for a credit card," Grandmother declared. "From here it's a local call."

around it be protected from harm and preserved for the future generations, especially for the future generations of the Cree Nation, to whom it belonged. While there, I received a vision that this wheel was an altar to *Keewaytin,* Cree for "the Wind and Spirit of the North." A few days after the ceremony, Joseph and I visited the Cree spiritual leader, Albert Lightning, who heartily approved of our ceremony and agreed with the information I had received.

This story has a very good ending. In fact, the story is a kind of "medicine circle" that illustrates how things happen in the Indian world. I had first been invited to share healing ways with the Cree by respected elder Smith Atimoyoo in 1984. I worked extensively among them during the following five years. In 1989, the Meewasin Medicine Wheel became part of a three-hundred-acre Cree heritage park called *Wanuskewin,* a Cree word for "seeking peace of mind."[9] I felt certain that the Pipe Ceremony four years earlier along with the prayers and hard work of so many Cree people had helped to bring this about. Smith Atimoyoo was one of the elders who named the park.

I did not have an opportunity to see the new park or to return to the wheel until the summer of 1997, when I was invited to attend a beautiful outdoor blessing ceremony at Wanuskewin. Grandfather Smith was the ceremonial leader. My wife was delighted to round-dance next to Grandfather during the celebration at the end of the ceremony. I felt that life had also moved in a circle and that we were all blessed that day by the spirit of the elder North Wind, Keewaytin.

THE POWER OF PLACE IN MODERN MEDICINE

"Harmony with nature" is more than a figure of speech. Scientists have documented that natural environments enhance health. The human body is literally tuned to the earth. The earth's natural electromagnetic field (EMF) helps regulate and balance the body's biological cycles. When a person is shielded from this field by spending too much time indoors or when the background "noise" of computers and electronic appliances interferes with this signal, sleeping and eating patterns are disrupted, and the mind becomes confused and disoriented. One of the greatest challenges of modern medicine is how to create hospitals that, in spite of technology, do not block nature's healing power.

People have always gone to nature for retreat, comfort, and healing. In the early 1900s, patients with tuberculosis or other serious chronic diseases for which medicine did not provide a cure, commonly went to a sanitorium, to rest and, hopefully, recuperate in a beautiful place in nature. Unfortunately, nature's restorative powers have rarely been brought to the place where patients need it most: the hospital. Scientists know a great deal about the harmful effects of lead paint, radon gas, carbon monoxide, and formaldehyde-treated carpets but very little about the kind of environments that promote health. Research in healthy environments began in earnest only during the last decades of the twentieth century.

A lack of attention to the healing influence of place is most clearly seen in the intensive care unit (ICU). Closed windows, meant to keep drafts and germs out, also keep germs inside and happy to multiply on warm surfaces. Machines that monitor a patient's vital signs are uncomfortably attached to his body with needles or tubes, robbing him of self-reliance, self-control, and self-confidence. His environment is filled with odd-colored lights from monitors; the beeps, clicks, and buzzes of machinery that seem to be sounding an alarm even when they are not; the chatter of nurses and doctors; the moans of other patients; and many unpleasant or disturbing smells. Alice Ware Davidson, Ph.D., R.N., writing in the science newsletter *Bridges,* has documented the adverse effects of this toxic environment.[10] She notes that ICUs "have high levels of sensory interference that can interfere with sleep and impair mental functioning." She discusses how when a group of cardiac ICU patients were allowed to recuperate in an environment of reduced light and noise, their blood pressure and skin temperature were more normal than controls.

Davidson compared a new cancer care center with the previous oncology unit in a major hospital. "Both quantitative and qualitative methods were used to collect data for three months to compare the new Cancer Care Center (CCC) to the previous Oncology Unit (OU) (before it closed)." The CCC was quiet and beautiful and had kitchen facilities where the family could cook meals for or with the patient. As expected, Davidson found that the harmonious environment of the CCC led to a greater sense of well-being, care, and comfort for patients and their families. "In addition *there was no statistically significant difference in cost per patient day* between the OU and the CCC. And patients had a *shorter length of stay* in the CCC than on the OU."

The influence of an aesthetic hospital environment was also reported by Roger S. Ulrich in his article "View through a Window May Influence Recovery from Surgery," published in the journal *Science*.[11] Ulrich examined the records of forty-six patients who, while recovering from gallbladder surgery, had been randomly assigned rooms that faced either trees or brick walls. Patients in both groups were matched by age, gender, and both past and present health status and were cared for by the same nurses. Those whose rooms faced trees required less medication, healed more quickly, and were released earlier.

It makes good scientific sense that the experience of beauty, even in a hospital, can improve health. A beautiful environment creates a positive mood, which stimulates the release of health-enhancing biochemicals called endorphins. It also encourages families to spend more time with patients. Lack of isolation and a feeling of love and support increase patients' expectations of healing ("placebo effect") and create better therapeutic outcomes.[12] Hospitals are beginning to take these facts to heart. Some hospitals, such as the California Pacific Medical Center in San Francisco and Longmont United Hospital in Longmont, Colorado, are trying to create spalike environments, with painted walkways; rooms with earth-tone walls and wooden floors and decorated with natural fibers; areas for meditation; and a variety of complementary therapies. Old ideas about the irrelevance of *place* are slowly dying out.

According to Native American tradition, the most powerful healing environment is nature because nature is not only beautiful but *powerful*.[13] Hospital rooms facing trees, as in the Ulrich experiment cited above, enhance healing because they expose the patient to the power and spirit of trees. When patients are hospitalized, we should bring as much of nature into their rooms as possible, such as flowers, stones, and shells. An Apache healer once told me that she liked to "program" quartz crystals with healing prayers and place them in patients' hospital rooms. Natural healing power can also be transmitted through sound and scent—by playing indigenous musical instruments such as the drum, rattle, or flute or, as we will soon learn, by exposing the patient to the scent of a fragrant healing plant, such as sage.

SMUDGING: INVITING NATURE HOME

Native healers recognize that a sick person cannot always make a pilgrimage to nature, but he or she can always make nature's purifying and healing power more present by *smudging*. *Smudging* means using the smoke and scent of a smoldering aromatic plant to purify a space of toxic energy, feelings, thoughts, or spirits and to create a fragrant atmosphere that attracts healing and helping powers. Many Native people smudge as a daily ritual; it cleanses the home and work-space and makes them more health-promoting. Or smudging may be practiced when the need arises, such as during illness or before a ceremony. Before a healing ceremony or consultation, I always smudge myself, the participants, the physical space, and ceremonial objects such as musical instruments, feathers, and herbs.

I recommend that all health care providers—whether allopathic or alternative—smudge their offices between clients. Pathogenic energy lingers in a space and may infect the next client. This may present a special danger in a psychotherapist's office, where patients are expected to open their minds and reveal deep feelings, leaving them vulnerable to both suggestion and subtle pathogenic energies. The fact that these energies are generally below the threshold of consciousness does not make them any less potent.

Sensing the energy of place is a common human experience. Have you ever been in a home and just *known* that someone was ill or had just had an argument? Young children are especially sensitive to the influence of place and express in words or behavior their reaction to environmental moods and energies. I have introduced smudging and Native American culture to many kindergarten and elementary school classes. I tell the children to "take a shower in the smoke," by waving the smoke around their bodies as I hold the container of burning herbs. I have found over and over again that young children consider smudging to be completely natural and obviously beneficial because "it feels good."

Not all plants can be used for smudging. It seems that the Great Spirit placed only some plants on Mother Earth for purification purposes. The principal smudging plants are sweetgrass, cedar, and sage. Some tribes burn juniper leaves, angelica root, osha root (*Ligusticum porteri*), white spruce pitch, pepperwood leaves (*Umbellularia californica*), yarrow leaves and flowers, Labrador tea (*Ledum*) leaves, cow parsnip roots or seeds (*Heracleum lanatum*), pearly everlasting leaves or flowers (*Anaphalis margaritacea*), or pine needles (in the Northeast, the white pine, *Pinus strobus*). It is best to use the local species because this plant is in tune with, and can have the greatest effect on, the energy of the place. What about incense, such as the popular Asian sandalwood sticks? Asian incense helps to create a serene mood and is appropriate for Hindu or Buddhist meditation or other Asian religious or contemplative practices. But here on Turtle Island, you must use a local plant to heal yourself or your environment. (Interestingly, Tibetan Buddhist pilgrims in India, Nepal, and what remains of Communist-ravaged Tibet carry pouches of local sage, cedar, and juniper during their journeys. They use the smoke of these plants to purify themselves and as an offering to sacred places and their residing deities.)

OTHER USES OF SMOKE

The smoke of the burning plant is its breath. As the plant burns and smolders, it sends its energy and your prayers up to the Creator. Smoke is/was generally used by Native American people in one of four ways:

1. The smoke of an ordinary campfire hides the human scent and helps hunters move closer to their prey. It also has the practical effect of chasing away flies and mosquitoes. Ancient hunters may have discovered smudging when they sensed the effects of wood smoke on physical energy, mental clarity, and spiritual awareness.

2. Smoke of some sacred plants, particularly tobacco, can be used to communicate with the Great Spirit. The plant is placed in a fire, either outdoors or in a lit pipe. Prayers are carried up and out with the smoke. In some Native traditions, to "burn tobacco" means "to pray."

3. Smoke can be therapeutic for a patient who inhales, smells, or smudges in it. Some herbs produce continuous smoke when they are lit directly; others are placed over coals or on hot stones in the Sweat Lodge. In the Plains region, *echinacea* smoke is used for headaches. Cherokee inhale mullein (*jola iyusdi*, "looks like tobacco") root and leaf smoke for asthma and bronchial congestion. Diné people from Arizona and their distantly related cousins, the Dene of the Canadian Northwest, treat headaches by inhaling the smoke from a mix of smoldering yarrow flowers and leaves.

4. Some plants have broad therapeutic properties and are used to purify people, places, or ceremonial objects. As I mentioned earlier, the most common of these sacred plants are sweetgrass, cedar, and sage. Tobacco is also sometimes used for spiritual cleansing, but since it is primarily a ceremonial herb offered with prayer, I will not describe it as a smudging agent. Tobacco is a "prescription medicine" for the spirit; it should be used cautiously and only in certain circumstances. I discuss the characteristics of tobacco in Chapter 13.

THE ORIGIN OF SACRED PLANTS

Anishinabe educator Edward Benton-Banai shares beautiful insight into the origin of sacred plants in *The Mishomis Book*.[14] As the four sons of the First People wandered to the directions, they were each given teachings and gifts. The Doorkeeper of the North lit a braid of sweetgrass and explained that *We-skwu' ma-shko-seh'*, "sweetgrass," is braided like hair because it is the hair of Mother Earth and the first plant to grow upon her. "The smoke of this sweetgrass will keep evil away from your home and will keep you safe on your travels."

The Doorkeeper of the East, the source of all knowledge, gave another son the gift of *Ah-say-ma,* "tobacco." He explained that when tobacco is put in a fire, it makes thoughts visible and carries them to the Spirit World. Tobacco is used to communicate with the Creator.

The third son visited the land of birth and growth in the South. As the Doorkeeper placed a handful of an herb into the fire, he said, "This is *Gi-shee-kan'-dug,* 'cedar.' Use this to purify your body from disease and to protect you from evil."

The fourth son crossed great mountains to reach the home of the West. There, he was given *Mush'-ko-day-wushk',* "sage," an herb that can purify people and their surroundings and help people maintain good health.

SWEETGRASS, CEDAR, AND SAGE

My relationship to the sweet-smelling sweetgrass (*Hierochloe odorata*) changed dramatically the first time I went herb picking with my Cree relatives. There is something deeply satisfying about singing to and then respectfully gathering and braiding the graceful hair of Mother Earth. The flat green blades rise out of reddish stems to a height of three feet or higher. The Cree, like other Northern Plains people, use sweetgrass in most spiritual ceremonies, sometimes burning it continuously on an altar. The sacred pipe is smudged over sweetgrass and lit with a glowing braid. Sweetgrass is often included in the tobacco smoking mixture. Some medicine people follow a subtle scent of sweetgrass to discover healing stones or other natural healing objects.

This beautiful herb is also used for medicinal purposes. Sweetgrass tea is drunk by the Cree and Blackfeet to treat sore throats, coughs, and sexually transmitted diseases. Women drink it to help stop vaginal bleeding after childbirth. Sweetgrass tea is used by men and women as a hairwash to make the hair healthier, stronger, and of course, sweet-smelling. Sometimes, the grasses are braided directly into men's and women's hair. Sweetgrass has also long been woven into beautiful baskets, bags, jewelry, or clothing.

The scent of sweetgrass, variously described as vanilla or haylike, can last as long as a hundred years. When the weather is humid, dried braids come to life and fill a room with their sacred presence.

Bathing in cedar (*Thujus occidentalis*) smoke is so common that many Native people speak of "cedaring" rather than smudging. In the Dakota language, cedar has the distinction of having the holy word *sha,* "red," the symbol of life, as part of its name: *hante sha.* Because the Thunderbird nests in cedar boughs, cedar attached to tipi poles acts as a spiritual lightning rod, protecting the tipi. Cherokee people use cedar to keep moths away from furniture or clothing, as do non-Native people. Native Americans keep feathers and ceremonial objects safe and fragrant in cedar boxes. In the Northwest, cedar is the sacred wood of homes, clothes, canoes, and baskets. At feasts and celebrations in the Northwest, Native peoples bake or smoke salmon on cedarwood planks to give it an incomparable flavor. Cedar is sometimes made into a tea. When the Lakota holy man Red Cloud was a young man, he was cured of cholera by drinking cedar leaf tea and bathing in cedar leaf water. In 1945, Erna Gunther reported in her classic work on western Washington ethnobotany[15] that the Skagit use cedar leaf tea for coughs, and the Klallam boil cedar limbs to make tuberculosis medicine. The Skokomish boil the buds to make a mouthwash. Cedar should not be taken internally during pregnancy or by people suffering from irritable coughs.

The Pawnee and Leni-Lenape both use cedar twig smoke to avert bad dreams. I also recommend cedar as one of the best dreaming incenses, to clear your room of energies that obstruct or inhibit positive and meaningful dreams. When I smell cedar, I am immediately transported to the Northwest. Among the Puget Sound tribes, cedar smoke is a constant presence in healing and ceremony. When I step into a Medicine House in which the cedar smoke is thick as a fog, I know that I can see the world as it really is.

The plant commonly called "cedar" by the Montana Cree is botanically the alpine fir (*Abies lasiocarpa*), the needles of which are burned on a hollowed rock or brick. In the American Southwest, Native people commonly apply the term *cedar* to the plant that is actually juniper (*Juniperus,* various species). Juniper may be used as a smudge or carried in a medicine bag for spiritual protection. The Rocky Mountain juniper (*Juniper scopulorum*) is commonly used by tribes in western Washington State. To purify a home, the leaves may be burned or boiled in water. Juniper root infusions are used to bathe arthritic feet. Juniper leaf tea is added to bathwater or drunk for general health. Interestingly, juniper has a powerful antiviral compound, *deoxypodophtllotoxin,* that may inhibit flu and herpes viruses. Former United States Department of Agriculture researcher James A. Duke, Ph.D., says that he likes to drink juniper tea when he feels a cold coming on.[16] Every part of this versatile plant has medicinal properties. The berries are commonly cooked with wild meat: ten berries per pound of meat.

The cautions for using juniper internally are similar to those for other fragrant herbs. Juniper's volatile oils can irritate the urinary tract and may have a vasodilating effect on the uterine lining. Therefore, juniper tea and berries should be avoided by patients with kidney disease and during pregnancy.[17]

The plants commonly called sage or sagebrush among Native people are not the domesticated, garden sages (*Salvia*) but rather the plants botanists recognize as wormwood or mugwort, or more technically, the various members of the genus *Artemisia*.[18] The word *Artemisia* is linked with the name of the Greek goddess of vegetation, Artemis, and has the root syllable *art,* meaning "bear." The bear is a universal symbol of healing. "Sage" was extremely common in the ancient world, and its scent may evoke deeply imprinted memories, even for Europeans. From thirty-five thousand to eleven thousand years ago, the northern Mediterranean region—including North Africa, Spain, Greece, Italy, Iran, and Syria—was dominated by cool, dry steppes covered with artemisia.[19] The smell of sage is the ancient smell of the earth.

The sages commonly used by Native Americans include fringed sagebrush (*Artemisia frigida,* called "Woman Sage" by the Blackfeet), silver sage (*Artemisia ludoviciana,* called "Man Sage" by the Blackfeet), and big sagebrush (*Artemisia tridentata*). Their wonderful scent is caused by aromatic oils, including camphor. Sage has been a central feature of Native American ceremonial and healing traditions since very ancient times. Native American hunters sometimes place sage in the nose and mouth of their kill as an act of purification and respect. For similar reasons, sage may be placed in the eyes, nose, and mouth of animal skulls used in ceremonial altars.

Sage was found among two-thousand-year-old remains excavated at Jemez Cave, New Mexico, and used as a tea or condiment by the Anasazi of the Southwest.[20] Native people continue to drink various species of sage tea for indigestion, for sore throats and colds, as a purification before athletics or long hikes, and for irregular menstruation. When I lived at Meta Tantay, I loved the scent of sage smoke and sage tea that greeted me each morning when I went to the "cook-shack," the cabin that served as kitchen and dining room. The residents smudged every morning before the sunrise ceremony. People who were feeling ill ladled out some sage tea from a pot always simmering on the woodstove. The sage was always picked fresh in the desert and prepared with prayers and love.

Both wormwood and true sage teas should be avoided by pregnant women. *Plants with volatile oils can be stimulating and irritating, causing reflex actions, and thus must not be taken internally during pregnancy.*

Although any of the purification herbs may be used both to cleanse negativity and to attract healing power, many Plains people believe that there are subtle differences in their effects. Sage and cedar purge a person or space of evil, destructive, or disease-causing forces. Sweetgrass tends to attract positive healing spirits. All three plants protect the user from misfortune. When I travel and conduct ceremonies in areas away from home, I like to burn a mixture of sage, because it grows in my region, with some of the local purification plant. This creates a spiritual bridge of friendship between the two places.

Sage is like a person whose presence is healing. Hanging sage from the rafters spreads a fresh scent through the home. I like to suspend some from my car's rearview mirror. Sage is also used to wrap sacred objects or as a bed on which to rest them. The whole, fresh herb can be waved or rubbed over the body for purification and as preparation for Vision Quest or other ceremonies. When I am hiking, I like to pinch a sage bud occasionally and rub it in my palms. I wipe the scent over my face, as though washing with it. Sage clears my mind and gives me the energy to continue hiking.

HOW TO SMUDGE

It is best to gather sage and cedar in nature. Pick only as much as you need, thanking the plant and being careful not to pull the roots. Never deplete an area of the plant. Always leave enough whole plants and roots for regrowth and reseeding. You can find sweetgrass braids and bundles of smudging plants at powwows and some Native art markets. Unless you are Native American or have special permission from Native people, you should not pick sweetgrass, which is endangered in many areas of North America.

After the plant is dried, place some in an open natural container such as a shell or a stone with a natural hollow (coffee cans or sturdy ashtrays will do in an emergency). Open a window or door slightly, so that unneeded forces can find an exit. *It is essential that there be a way for air to escape to the outside whenever you smudge.* And don't forget to temporarily disable any smoke alarms. I once had a humorous experience leading a ceremony in a building that had high, nearly invisible smoke alarms. We were smudged first by smoke and then by water from the sprinkler system.

Light the herbs with a match, and once they have thoroughly caught, blow them gently out. Some smudging herbs, such as sweetgrass, may be kept burning by placing them on a natural wood coal. Smudge yourself before smudging a space. Wave the smoke over your body, not forgetting the arms and legs. You can use your hands or a feather or wing of a bird from a nonendangered species (such as the turkey or pheasant). If you have a helper, let him or her smudge you as you stand quietly with the palms facing outward. You should also turn to allow the helper to smudge you from the back.

Next, purify the space. As you turn to face each of the Four Winds, hold your smudge container slightly up and away from your body in a humble offering of gratitude. Or you can wave the smoke toward the directions with your hand or feather-fan. At the end, make an offering upward to the Sky and downward to the Earth.

Participants in a healing—patient and helpers—smudge themselves by passing the smudge-shell and waving the smoke over their own bodies, or you can smudge them by playing the role of "helper" as above. Sometimes, in order to create good feeling in a circle, I turn slightly to my left and hold the smudge shell for the person next to me. He smudges, then takes the shell and holds it for the person to his left. In this method of smudging, we all help one another and feel connected. Everyone must be purified before a traditional healing or ceremony. If the smudge starts to go out, gently blow on the herbs. The smudge may be relit as necessary.

Smudging is an example of ritual purification of space common to all indigenous cultures. The exact methods may vary. In the Northwest, candles often accompany the herbal smudge. Both cedar smoke and candlelight are waved over a person and through a space. The Zulu of South Africa also use candlelight in purification ceremonies. What if you must purify a hospital room, where neither flames nor smoke are permitted? Many cultures use water, sound, or the power of the mind to cleanse a person or space. In Hawai'i, a space is purified by dipping a *ti* leaf in ocean water and sprinkling it to the directions (*pi kai*). Chinese Taoists use a nearly identical technique (a willow branch in spring water) to cleanse a temple before ceremonies. The sound of sacred instruments is also cleansing: the beat of a drum, the clear note of a flute, the human voice. A person with strong powers of concentration can imagine a healing power such as sunlight bathing the space. If your mind is clear and strong, a simple prayer may be highly effective. Remember, however, that in North America, the most traditional and common way to cleanse is with sacred smoke.

THE NOSE KNOWS

The primary reason why smudging has such profound effects on consciousness is the spirit and power of the plants, their gift from the Great Spirit. However, modern science also offers an interesting interpretation of the power of smudging. Smells induce altered states of awareness because of their connection with specific parts of the brain.

Think of the different words used to describe the visual, auditory, or kinesthetic senses. Visual terms include *bright, dark, shining, brilliant, transparent, translucent, opaque, sparkling,* and of course, the myriad shades of color. Musicians and dancers have a similar range of descriptive and analytic terms. Chefs have no difficulty describing the subtle tastes and textures of their craft. What about smells? How many kinds of aromas, odors, fragrances, scents, or stinks can you name? Try doing this without using terms that reference other senses such as *rose scent, bitter fragrance, salty smell.* You may find yourself agreeing with G. K. Chesterton's poem "The Song of the Quoodle":

> They haven't got no noses,
> And goodness only knowses
> The noselessness of man.

There is a simple reason why it is difficult to discuss or analyze smell and why we have a dearth of olfactory descriptors. Among all the senses, the sense of smell has the most direct connection with the noncognitive portions of the brain. Sensory information from the skin and skeleton, from the eyes, ears, and tongue all has pathways leading into the cerebral cortex. Smell has no representation in this thinking portion of the brain. Instead, most olfactory impulses are processed in an ancient structure known as the rhinencephalon (literally, "nose brain"), a part of the limbic system. The limbic system is associated with the regulation of heart rate, respiration, hormone levels, emotions, and sexual behavior. Sights and sounds make us think. Smells make us feel. Because smell is connected with the breath, the life energy that we take into our bodies, it is the most intimate sense.

In polite society, it is proper to ask, "Do you hear? Do you see? Do you taste? Do you feel?" All of these imply acceptable modes of sensitivity. When have you heard someone ask, "Do you smell?" Isn't it interesting that a refined person is called a person of taste, not a person of smell. Smell takes us back to a deeper way of knowing. People who smell the world and one another are likely to do unpredictable or passionate things. Smell is subversive to civilization.

The association between smell and the limbic system explains why smells evoke memories, instinctive reactions, and feelings such as attraction or disgust or why sacred scents—incense in temples, sweetgrass in tipis—can awaken ancient ways of knowing.[21] In 1580, the French essayist Michel de Montaigne astutely observed:

> *I have often noticed that [scents] cause changes in me, and act on my spirits according to their qualities; which make me agree with the theory that the introduction of incense and perfume into churches, so ancient and widespread a practice among all nations and religions, was for the purpose of raising our spirits, and of exciting and purifying our senses, the better to fit us for contemplation.*[22]

Olfactory sensitivity is fundamental to physical and social survival. Inuit people can smell different qualities of sea, ice, and weather. Hunters determine with all of their senses, including smell, the location of prey, or they rely on following their more sensitive relations, such as the wolf, who can smell a caribou from three miles away. Lovers breathe and smell each other to kindle their passion. Wrong choices are made because human scents are masked by perfume and deodorants. Divorces occur because of olfactory incompatibilities.

Creating a proper smellscape is essential for Native American healing and highlights an important difference between allopathic and indigenous methods of diagnosis. Native healers know that a sweet smell, like sweetgrass, often indicates good medicine and health. Bad medicine, disease, and toxic spirits smell bad. Allopathic physicians rely exclusively on the visual sense to determine a patient's condition. At one time—and for only a very brief number of years—physicians tapped a patient's chest or placed their ears directly on the skin to diagnose heart disease, and they took careful note of the smells of different diseases. Today, sensual cues have been replaced by laboratory tests, all of which are read visually. Doctors may be able to practice their *science* with only eyes and cortex, but the *art* of treating the whole person requires all of the senses and both sides of the brain.

6

— ASKING FOR HELP —
Finding and Paying a Healer

Native American healers are forbidden by traditional ethics to commercialize or "missionize" healing—that is, to charge exorbitant fees or attempt to coerce people into using their services. If you find a listing for "Medicine Man" in the Yellow Pages, you can safely assume that he is, as Native people say, "made of plastic," not the genuine article. A traditional healer does not display a MEDICINE WOMAN shingle outside her door. Native Americans believe that for healing to be effective, healer and patient must find each other. If life circumstances bring them together and the connection is right, it's synchronicity. In Indian Country, the "moccasin telegraph" helps the process along. Word of mouth is the only acceptable form of advertising for a medicine person.

When you find a healer, it is important to approach him or her in the proper way. The patient makes a sincere verbal request for help and offers a gift that symbolizes gratitude and counts as a kind of "consultation fee." In many tribes, this offering is a pouch of tobacco. If the patient is following the Way of the Pipe, he or she may perform a ritual gesture of holding the pipe in both hands while extending and withdrawing it four times, symbolically asking the medicine person to smoke the pipe and pray for healing. Or the patient may give a pipe to the medicine person. It is also common to offer a woolen blanket, several yards of cloth, and/or a personal gift. Groceries, homemade food, wild game or fish, and fresh-picked berries are also highly appreciated gifts. Although healers rarely charge a set fee, many will accept and very much appreciate a monetary gift. Acceptance of the "consultation fee" does not necessarily mean that the healer has decided to take the case.

If the patient asks for healing, it means that he is either ready to receive healing or at least believes that he is. The healer must also ask for help. A medicine woman asks herself and her sources of spiritual guidance, "What is the patient really asking for? How can I help? Do I have the ability to help?" Today, healers might also ask if the patient needs to see a medical doctor or other therapist as well. For some Native healers, accepting the patient's initial gift seals a contract between them. Other healers may take longer—for example, a ritual period of four days—to consider whether they should or can help.

When Native healing is given without the patient's clear request or against his better judgment, not only is it ineffective, but it can be harmful. For example, a Plains Indian medicine man convinced "Jeremy," a fifty-year-old cancer patient, to travel nearly two thousand miles to take part in a *Yuwipi* ceremony, in which the healer, while sitting in a pitch-black room, calls on spirits to communicate with him and to convey information to the participants. Jeremy was a personal friend, and when he first told me of his travel plans, I felt that he was allowing the healer's persuasive abilities to override his own intuition, which was telling him that he needed to stay home and rest. After this trip, Jeremy's lung cancer, which had been in remission for two years, came back with a vengeance, and he passed on within six months of the ceremony. I have no doubt that the Yuwipi could have helped Jeremy if he had participated *at the right time*. But at that stage in his recovery, the combination of an exhausting journey, intensive ceremonial preparations, and the nightlong ceremony was just too much for his limited resources.

Coercive healing—the attitude that "I know what's best for you; I will fix you whether you like it or not"—is antithetical to the spirit of Native healing. The healer should never assume that his "expertise" entitles him to dismiss or override the patient's wishes. That kind of arrogance disempowers the patient and implies that the healer is himself the source of the healing power. Coercive healing may cause symptoms to worsen or to shift to other parts of the body or into a state of dormacy in which they are hidden and less accessible to healing power. At the very least, it is an invasion of privacy.

Another friend, "Howard," a physician who broke his spine in a car accident, was attending an alternative medicine conference. At various times during the program, people who called themselves healers approached his wheelchair and, without asking permission, placed a palm on his upper spine or waved their hands near his body. One even gave him her business card, saying "I can cure you," a good example of practicing medicine with *license* yet without a license! Howard also noticed other conference attendees staring at him. Such attention is not unusual for people in wheelchairs. What bothered him was his intuitive feeling that people were praying for him or in other ways trying to manipulate him with their intent or energy. At least if someone touched him, he knew when to protest and protect himself, but having to keep up a defense against psychic intrusion was exhausting. He had come to the conference to hone his medical skills, not to be healed.

Uninvited healing efforts can also be bad for the healer. If the patient is energetically and spiritually closed, healing power, unable to enter the patient, is reflected back to the healer, tainted by the patient's illness. The healer becomes ill. I learned this truth many years ago, when I had just begun to practice Native American medicine. A middle-aged non-Native woman named "Mary" requested a healing. Mary worked in a department store as a cashier. She was quite overweight, with a cigarette habit, and was suffering from a serious case of warts. There were dozens of warts all along her arms. She had tried every remedy imaginable, from burning them off with caustic over-the-counter and prescription compounds to herbal lotions and meditation. As she spoke to me of her previous attempts at healing, I began to realize that she was determined to attend every sort of self-improvement workshop but was unwilling to make the changes in lifestyle and outlook that would give her the best chances at healing.

Mary's somewhat challenging tone of voice and brusque manner as she dropped a pouch of tobacco in my palm suggested to me that her request was insincere. She wanted to test Indian healing, to see what it or I could do, but did not really expect that there would be any results. Not that a person needs to believe in Native American medicine for it to work, but he or she must at least be open to the possibility. Instead of admitting my inability to help or discussing lifestyle issues that I perceived as the true problem, my analytic mind got the better of me. I knew that warts, even ones caused by a skin virus, are extremely vulnerable to suggestion and have often been cured by hypnosis, relaxation, or other mind-body interventions. Her case interested me, and I agreed to treat her.

Mary lay on a blanket as I smudged her with sage smoke and prayed. The session lasted approximately thirty minutes. When Mary sat up, to our mutual astonishment, some of her warts had already disappeared. The rest cleared up by the next morning. I, however, had a problem. A painful wart had appeared on my left index finger, and no amount of smudging, praying, or washing would remove it. Two days after the treatment, Mary's warts returned. Mine lasted another few days. Upon later reflection, I felt that there was a lesson in this experience for both of us. I learned to listen more carefully to my intuitive response to the patient. And Mary, hopefully, learned that miracles do happen. Perhaps the spirit powers were testing a skeptic! Unfortunately, in those days, I rarely followed my "cases" and did not learn about any long-term effects of the healing, if it can be called one.

The only time that the rule of "asking" does not apply is with children or anyone who is physically or mentally incapable of asking, such as a patient who is in a coma or has Alzheimer's. In such cases, a friend or family member will ask the healer for help. Synchronistically, as I was writing this chapter, a Cree friend called from a Canadian hospital to request prayers and healing for an elderly chief who had just been admitted for diabetic heart failure. Because the chief had fluid in her lungs and extreme difficulty breathing, she had been put on an artificial respirator, and she had lapsed into a coma. (She came out of the coma later that evening and fell into a peaceful sleep. In the morning, she was moved out of the intensive care unit. Although the various interventions—both allopathic and traditional—did not cure the elder's diabetic heart, they did give her a gift of continued life and breath, keeping her off the respirator.)

When the patient is incapacitated, it is also possible for a friend, relative, or anyone who feels a close personal connection with the patient to act as his proxy—that is, as the healer works on this person, the patient receives the benefits. The proxy must know or intuitively and clearly sense that he has the patient's permission to act on his behalf.

HELP ONE ANOTHER: THE IMPORTANCE OF THE GROUP

Stiwhen stent netsah semken. Pray for one another.
Naelae stent netsah semken. Love one another.
Klishkwas netsah semken. Forgive one another.
Sqowl netsah semken. Help one another.

—A northwest prayer-song

In my healing practice, I follow a tradition common to many Native American healers. Both healer and patient may ask friends, family, and members of their tribe or community to participate in the healing by praying, singing, or performing ceremonial actions that are delegated to them. In many northwest ceremonies, the participants are the healers, and the medicine person may be no more than an "orchestra leader," leading songs and making sure that everyone works in harmony. For example, in the intertribal *Si.Si.Wiss* ("Sacred Breath") healing tradition from the Puget Sound region of Washington State, any number of participants may simultaneously or in succession doctor a patient with songs, prayers, cedar smoke, candlelight, laying on of hands, or noncontact therapy in which the hands move in the air ("energy field") a few inches above the patient's body. I often whisper prayers and good words directly in the patient's ear. I find that a direct expression more powerfully creates the trust and love necessary for healing, although there is ample evidence that nonverbalized intent can heal, even at a distance.[1]

Group participation is also a common feature of Native American counseling and mediation. The medicine person is the primary counselor, but as in Western group therapy, he or she also welcomes ideas and guidance from others. This process is especially potent in bereavement counseling, in which friends offer sympathy and love, helping affirm the bereaved person's worth as an important member of the group. In Diné "peacemaking," a traditional method of therapy used to resolve criminal offenses, a community leader or "peacemaker" meets with the offender, the victim, family members, and any others affected by the offense to talk things out and decide on an acceptable plan of restitution.

As a practical matter, the patient is more likely to follow advice received with others present. This is one reason Western physicians like to advise a patient with the spouse present. If your cholesterol level is high, you are much less likely to indulge in ice cream if your wife has heard the doctor's proscriptions. Involved third parties can make sure the patient stays with a healing regimen. A resistant patient cannot easily retreat to a safe haven of ignorance or denial. Not only does he know what he is supposed to do, but so does everyone else!

The mere presence of community combats the isolation and demoralization that accompany illness. In his book *The Medicine Men,* psychiatrist and medical anthropologist Lewis H. Thomas, M.D., discusses the importance of community in Lakota ritual. "The rituals facilitate a benevolent community participation in the individual's pain and problem and concomitantly encourage the individual's involvement in community concerns, with a therapeutic influence on his or her alienation and narcissism."[2] In a closely knit group of people sharing similar values, the communal experience can be long-lasting. As Drs. Jerome and Julia Frank note in their book *Persuasion and Healing,* a classic overview of modern and cross-cultural methods of psychotherapy, "The more cohesive a group is, the stronger the morale of its members will be, and the more its standards will influence members, both during and between group sessions."[3] Bonds of friendship are created and reinforced by group ceremonies, and participants tend to stay concerned and in touch, offering help to one another when it is needed.

THE SCIENCE OF SOCIAL SUPPORT

Numerous scientific studies confirm the power of social support.[4] One of the best known of these was conducted by David Spiegel, M.D., professor of psychiatry at Stanford University School of Medicine, who in the course of many years of research, went from being a skeptic of alternative medicine to a convert. In the late 1970s, Dr. Spiegel and his colleagues wanted to test the effect of social support on the coping skills of cancer patients. They recruited eighty-six metastatic breast cancer patients and assigned them randomly to either a control group, which received standard cancer therapy, or an experimental group. In addition to standard therapy, the experimental group, led by a psychiatrist or social worker and a therapist who had breast cancer in remission, met once a week for a year. Participants were encouraged to share their grief about their illness, fears of dying, hopes, and coping strategies. They were also taught self-hypnosis techniques to reduce pain. At the end of the study, patients' moods and pain levels were evaluated, and not surprisingly, the experimental group showed significantly less anxiety, depression, and pain. After the results were published in various psychiatric journals in the early 1980s, Dr. Spiegel moved on to other research topics.

As a psychiatrist, Dr. Spiegel expected group therapy to improve cancer patients' psychological health and reduce psychosomatic pain, but he doubted that it could affect their survival. Five years after completing his initial research, he decided that he could easily disprove what he regarded as alternative healers' groundless claims for the influence of consciousness on health by looking at the survival rates of the women who had participated in his earlier study. The results of a new analysis surprised him and many others in the conventional medical community. In his article "Effect of Psychosocial Treatment on Survival of Patients with Metastatic Breast Cancer," published in 1989 in the prestigious British medical journal *The Lancet,* Dr. Spiegel reported that the women in the experimental group had lived an average of twice as long as the controls. He was forced to conclude that social support increased both quality and length of life.[5]

Mortality rates, including suicide, are higher for people who are single than for those who are married. Dr. James P. Lynch, author of the classic *The Broken Heart: The Medical Consequences of Loneliness,* shows that loneliness can literally kill you.[6] Cirrhosis of the liver is seven times more common and tuberculosis ten times more common among divorced men than married men. Widows aged twenty-five to thirty-four are five times as likely to die of a heart attack as married women of the same age. Researchers at Case Western Reserve University in Cleveland studied the incidence of angina (chest pain) among men with high cardiovascular risk factors such as abnormal electrocardiogram, elevated cholesterol levels, and high blood pressure. Those who answered "Yes" to the question "Does your wife show you her love?" had significantly less angina than other patients with the same risk factors.[7]

The damaging effects of social isolation have been documented in many cultures. Researchers at the University of Arizona studied the effect of social support on pregnant, unmarried Diné teenagers. Those who had relatively low levels of social support had four times the number of postpartum complications.[8] In Sweden, researcher Dr. Kristina Orth-Gomér of the National Institute for Psychosocial Factors and Health in Stockholm conducted a six-year study to analyze the effects of loneliness on more than seventeen thousand randomly selected men and women, aged twenty-nine to seventy-four. Those who were the most lonely were four times as likely to die prematurely.[9]

We see these numbers again and again: *twice as likely to die, three times as likely to have a heart attack* . . . In *Love and Survival,* Dr. Ornish summarizes the wealth of scientific data generated by studies conducted between 1979 and 1994: *"Those who were socially isolated had at least two to five times the risk of premature death from all causes when compared to those who had a strong sense of connection and commu-*

nity"[10] (emphasis in original). As Native Americans have been saying for millennia, lack of connection is one of the most significant risk factors for disease, and health is the state of "We are all related."

It is important to remember that the scientific studies cited above point to the negative consequences of *loneliness,* not "aloneness." Loneliness is a feeling of desolation and being cut off from others. Aloneness can be a time of quiet solitude and contemplation, as in the Vision Quest. It is only in solitude that we can fully experience the deep part of ourselves that is intimately connected with all of nature and life. To live wisely and contentedly, we need a balance of solitude and community. I treasure the wise words once spoken to me by a Kanien'kehaka (Mohawk) friend: "Look at the eagles. When they mate, they dance in the sky, swooping down together, then looping up along separate paths. They know the value of aloneness *and* togetherness."

Our human need for connection is universal, yet our lack of connection today is greater than at any time in the past. Young people do not think twice about leaving their families, homes, communities, or land, often because of educational or employment opportunities, but sometimes for no other reason than to demonstrate their independence. Today's communities are more likely to be virtual than actual. But instant access is no substitute for meaningful communication. A hand cannot reach out across a computer screen to offer comfort. It is ironic that psychologists recognize the dangers of pathological codependence and dependent personality disorders, but not the most common disease of our times: *independent personality disorder.*[11] Our insistence on individualism and self-sufficiency has cost us our contentment and happiness. Independence is an illusion; we need one another and nature to survive.

The differences in health between people who are lonely and people who feel connected to others can be partially explained by a variety of factors, including the stress-buffering effect of groups; the power of hopefulness, sense of belonging, and positive expectations of help from others; healthful behavioral changes recommended by associates; and the proliferation of immune-enhancing endorphins, the body's good-mood chemicals. We cannot rule out the possibility, however, that supportive and caring groups create subtle energetic networks or invoke powers that protect participants from harm. Religious affiliation, attitudes, and behavior have been proved to exert a positive influence on health.[12] Isn't it possible that the Great Spirit blesses people whose minds are open to his or her guidance?

PAYMENT FOR SERVICES

In Western medicine, the quality of care that a patient receives is dependent on his or her ability to pay. Sometimes financial resources determine *if* the patient will receive care. From the Native American perspective, exorbitant medical fees are a sign of contemptible professional ethics. Native American healers never charge fixed or unreasonably high fees, because this would take advantage of the patient at precisely the time when he or she is weak and most in need of help. When people are ill, we should be generous and help them be appreciative of their riches rather than disheartened by their poverty.

Winona, a nineteen-year-old Native American, had suffered from suicidal thoughts and inexplicable bouts of depression for many years. Her family had paid for a succession of psychiatrists, who prescribed medications that brought some relief but offered no cure. I counseled Winona and her family and asked her family to be present during a smudging and prayer ceremony, in which each person had a chance to pray in his or her own way or just to speak from the heart. In this sacred space, Winona's family was able to clearly and powerfully articulate their love and hopes for her recovery.

Within a few weeks, Winona's therapist was able to reduce the level of medication. Winona was feeling more secure and happy than she had felt in many years. Winona explained, "The most powerful part of the whole process was when I asked you what your fee was and you said, 'There is no fee. People give whatever they wish. A gift for a gift.' It was the first time I ever felt that a therapist was offering me help without ulterior motives, simply because he cared. I think this helped me to really hear not only your words but what my parents felt about me. I felt loved and appreciated."

Because healing is always a gift and grace from the Great Spirit, we cannot put a price on it. As armed as he or she might be with the weapons to wage war on disease, no physician has yet fully explained what ultimately causes healing. Whether an individual patient will respond to treatment is unknown. Many diseases are self-limiting—that is, the body heals itself with or without the healer's intervention. In Richard Katz's compelling work *Boiling Energy,* the African Kung-San healer Gau expresses thoughts common to all indigenous healers: "Maybe our num [healing power] and European medicine are similar, because sometimes people who get European medicine die, and sometimes they live. That is the same with ours."[13] In the last analysis, the most any healer can do is create the most favorable conditions for healing to occur.

Yet the fact that healing is a mystery and a grace does not quite mean that it should be free. We must give something in order to receive. It is an act that honors the Great Spirit, the spirit powers, and the healer, through which these powers work. If a patient is capable of giving yet gives nothing, or if he gives something that has little personal value, it means that he places little value on the healing. A stingy, self-centered person is not open to healing. There is also the practical matter of providing for the healer. In the past, Native American patients gave healers blankets, furs, weapons, or horses. Today, weapons do not put food on the table, and horses do not pay the rent or electric bills. Determining appropriate reimbursement for healing is a delicate balancing act between one's belief in traditional values and accepting the needs of modern life.

How, then, does a patient pay a traditional healer? This can vary from tribe to tribe, and the customary offerings have also changed over time. In the 1930s, Morris Edward Opler, professor of anthropology at the University of Oklahoma, wrote that an Apache healer required four ceremonial offerings: typically, a pouch of pollen, an unblemished buckskin, an eagle feather, and a piece of turquoise.[14] The patient could also give other gifts as tokens of respect and gratitude. In 1964, L. Bryce Boyer, M.D., a researcher at the University of New Mexico Department of Anthropology, noted that Apache medicine men required the following gifts as payment in advance of a healing: tobacco, a black-handled knife, material for clothing, money, and sometimes a piece of turquoise.[15]

A few hundred years ago, Cherokee patients commonly offered their healers a deerskin or pair of moccasins. In the 1880s, ethnologist James Mooney observed that Cherokee healers were generally given a quantity of cloth, a garment, or a handkerchief, all of which were used in healing ceremonies.[16] Today, patients may offer similar practical gifts—cloth, groceries, money—that may help the healer to survive or other personal gifts to express gratitude. In the Cherokee language, payment for services is called ugista'ti, probably derived from the verb tsi'giû, "I take" or "I eat." The Cherokee, however, like other Indian people, consider healing a spiritual matter beyond price. As Mooney says, the ugista'ti is not "payment" in the usual sense of the word but rather a necessity for "the removal and banishment of the disease spirit."[17] Helping spirits reward generous people.

Today, a pouch of tobacco is probably the most common gift for requesting a healing or consultation. The pouch should be beautiful, perhaps handmade. If it is plastic and store-bought, it should be wrapped in "Indian wrapping paper": red flannel, a piece of buckskin, or other natural material, to add a personal touch. Giving tobacco is equivalent to saying, "I respect your spirituality and request prayers for help and healing."

The Comanche medicine woman Sanapia (b. 1895) required dark green cloth, a bag of Bull Durham tobacco, and four corn-shuck "cigarette papers" to consider healing a patient of physical deformities caused by ghosts.[18] The patient rolled tobacco into a corn husk, lit the "cigarette," and took four puffs. He or she then offered the cigarette to Sanapia. Her acceptance signified a pledge to accept the person as a patient. After the healing, Sanapia received whatever gifts the patient offered. During the late 1960s, Sanapia treated an average of twenty to thirty patients per year, with each patient offering about thirty dollars, some groceries, and enough cloth to make several dresses. Like other Indian healers, Sanapia was not a millionaire.

The patient should ask a healer's family or associates how much money or other offerings are customary. Some healers, in spite of great personal hardships and poverty, will not accept money or will not specify amounts, being unwilling to quantify the sacred. They may, however, be willing to accept a financial gift. Be as generous as possible; don't insult a healer by handing him a ten-dollar bill. But don't flaunt your wealth either, as though money entitles you to enter the Kingdom of Heaven. A street person once gave me a dollar with a very sincere request for help. It felt to me like a million dollars. On the other hand, if someone tries to buy my services or treats Spirit as a commodity, no amount of money is adequate.

At the Seminole Green Corn Ceremony, a speaker cries out, *Malatka tagis!* "Get your donations ready." According to James H. Howard and Willie Lena's *Oklahoma Seminoles,* "One gives the medicine man *malatka* in the firm belief that doing so will make the treatment more efficacious, and that without gifts the treatment will probably be of little value. The *malatka* can be money, yard goods, whatever one wishes. Usually the doctor doesn't ask for a specific sum, but simply leaves it up to the patient and his or her family."[19] Sometimes, the greatest financial demand on the patient is providing transportation, food, and accommodations for the healer and his or her singers and helpers, and a feast for everyone who helps in the healing.

"Not commercializing the medicine" is one of many spiritual laws that a student or practitioner of Native American healing or spirituality must learn.[20]

Part II

METHODS

— OF —

HEALING

7

━ WHAT IS INVOLVED IN A NATIVE ━ AMERICAN HEALING?
Traditions, Protocols, and Moontime Power

It is important to understand that Native American healing methods are not practiced separately from one another. In this chapter, I will discuss how they fit together to form a holistic system as well as the traditional etiquette and protocol one must know to receive or practice Native American healing. I will also describe "moontime power," the special medicine power of women, and how Native American elders advise women to honor this power.

DIVERSITY AND UNITY IN NATIVE AMERICAN HEALING

Although Native American healing is based on widely shared principles and values, in its practical application, there is an enormous diversity of techniques and ceremonies based on differences in tribal cultures as well as in the talents of individual healers. It is well beyond the scope of this or any book to discuss them all. Nevertheless, several broad categories of intervention are considered important among virtually all Native American healers, including vision-seeking, smudging, prayer, music, counseling, massage, ceremony, and herbs. The names and purposes of these healing therapies are outlined in the accompanying table.

Vision-seeking and smudging have been introduced in earlier chapters because the principles and values they embody, the importance of life purpose and sacred space, are central to any understanding of Native American healing. Prayer and music, recurrent themes throughout this book, are also components of all indigenous healing interventions.

COMMON THERAPEUTIC METHODS

METHOD	PURPOSE
Vision-seeking, dreaming, and fasting	Healer and/or patient retrieve information, guidance, or solution to problems or illness; attract and commune with helping spirits and spiritual power.
Smudging: • Wormwood • Sage • Cedar • Sweetgrass • Juniper • Pine needles	Purify the healing space, the healer, patient, helpers, and ritual objects; induce spiritual state of mind; increase awareness of both helpful and disease-causing forces; invite and offer respect to helping spirits.
Prayer and chant: • Sacred expression • Communion • Invocation • Petition	Focus the mind on healing; engender positive, health-promoting values such as love, peace, acceptance, and trust; induce expanded and receptive state of consciousness in healer, patient, and helpers; commune with, invoke, empower, and express gratitude to sacred healing forces; increase patient self-esteem by helping him or her to feel worthy of divine help; attend gathering and administration of herbs or other medicines.
Music: • Voice • Drum • Rattle • Flute • Whistle • Rasp • Clacker • Violin[1] • Bull roarer	Same as prayer; also entrain consciousness and induce harmony and unity among healer, patient, and helpers; accompaniment to any healing intervention, especially dance and ceremony.
Counseling: • Talking things out • Advice of elder/adviser	Explore or clarify disease etiology and pathogenesis, including physical, behavioral, and spiritual components of disease;

• Dream and vision interpretation • Seeking guidance from nature • Healing imagery • Humor	discover new sources of inner strength, confidence, and self-understanding; encourage positive behavioral changes, including strategies for coping with disease; strengthen family and community relations.
Energy therapies: • Conventional massage methods • Laying on of hands • Pressing or puncturing therapeutic points • "Psychic surgery": scooping out harmful intrusive objects or forces • Noncontact treatment • Placing stones, feathers, earth on or near the body	Aid healing of body, mind, and spirit; relieve pain; transmit healing intent, healing energy, and spiritual power.
Ceremony: • Sweat Lodge • Sacred Pipe • Other tribal healing ceremonies (for example, Diné Sand Painting, Salish Winter Spirit Dances) • Ceremonies that belong to individual healers	Enact visions or instructions received from Spirit. Empower and provide a formal structure for healing methods; commune with natural and spiritual forces, the Great Spirit, and/or the spirit of the disease; induce positive and health-enhancing state of consciousness; affirm shared cultural identity and values.
Herbs	Establish physical, mental, and spiritual balance; combat specific physical or spiritual pathogens.

— MULTIFACETED HEALING —

In Native American healing, there is no clear division between therapies used to help others and those used to help oneself. It may sometimes be difficult to tell if healing methods are meant for the patient, are empowering practices for the healer, or are methods of enhancing wellness that may be practiced by anyone. For example, either the healer or the patient may go on a Vision Quest to contact healing powers and receive information leading to a cure. Native American counseling, although primarily a way for a healer to help a patient understand the psychological component of illness, includes many self-help methods—for example, how to seek guidance from nature or dreams. To practice massage, a Native American healer must learn how to sense and project energy through the hands. In the process of learning or practicing massage, he or she learns as much about the inner workings of his or her own body as about the patient. As I discuss in Chapter 11, "The Paleolithic Posture," humanity's physically fit hunter-gatherer ancestors had postural habits that encouraged good personal health and also made them effective healers, aware of the physical and spiritual aspects of the body.

Treatment, even by a healer who has a "specialty," is always a combination of modalities. A Native massage therapist, for instance, may also be a counselor and a singer. For clarity's sake, I generally discuss healing methods separately; in practice any or all of them can work together. The term *holistic* in Native American medicine implies not only treating the whole person but also using multifaceted treatments that address all dimensions of the disease.

For example, let's imagine that a patient named "Tom" goes to a Native healer because his doctor has diagnosed a benign liver tumor. The first stage of treatment is a counseling session. During this session, the healer first smudges himself, his healing tools, the patient, and the space with sage smoke. He offers a prayer or an invocation and invites Tom to pray out loud and in his own way. The healer then talks with Tom to try to understand him as a person, not just a disease: he may ask questions about his family and work and how he feels about his own problem, including any information about it he may have received in dreams. Tom may describe his difficult childhood relationship with his father, who never understood or appreciated him, and who, even now, years after his death, Tom describes as "a thorn in my side."

If a patient's illness is rooted in the emotions, a counseling session may provide all the therapy that he needs. As the patient releases bound-up emotions and makes healthy behavioral changes based on the healer's recommendations, the physical problem disappears. Tom, however, requires additional therapy. As they continue to talk, the healer begins to see with his spiritual eyes that there is indeed a "thorn" in Tom's side. It is an intrusive and toxic energy actually shaped like a thorn. It must be released emotionally *and* physically if Tom is to heal. The healer encourages Tom to talk more about his feelings, and slowly, the emotional knots start to loosen. Now the healer will practice "hand doctoring," a Native American form of massage.

Placing his palms a few inches above Tom's body, the healer moves his hands slowly, with great sensitivity, along the contours of the subtle energy field that surrounds Tom, sensing physical and psychic aberrations. He projects energy into depleted areas, brushes away pain, and pulls out invisible toxic threads from the tumor. The healer picks up his drum and begins to sing a healing song, while imagining that a badger is burrowing into Tom's liver to dig out the toxic "thorn" and the tumor itself. He adds more sage to the smudge, as an offering of respect and to feed the badger spirit power with the smoke. When the session is over, the healer gives Tom a mixture of sassafras root, dandelion leaves, and other healing herbs. "Drink this herbal tea every day for the next seven days. Don't forget to doctor up the tea with prayer and good thoughts before you drink it."

Two weeks later, Tom's physician tells him that the tumor is gone. Tom arranges a Giveaway and a feast to thank the healer and the many friends and family members who had been praying for him.

— THE BENEFITS OF SEEING THE WHOLE ELEPHANT —

It makes sense that combined therapies should be more effective than a single approach to disease, even though this goes against the increasing trend in modern medicine toward more specialization. A Native healer looks at the whole person and flexibly matches the therapy or therapies to the needs of the patient.

The problem with specialists is that by examining the patient through the microscopic lens of their discipline, they miss the larger picture, illustrated in this famous story from India: Four men are in a pitch-black room with a sleeping elephant. One touches the ear and says it is a fan. Another touches a leg and says it is a pillar. One leaps back in fear as he touches the tail, believing it is a snake. The fourth tells the others that they are all mistaken. The object in question is certainly a water hose.

Many patients in the United States see both alternative healers and conventional physicians. This is good because it may give the patients a better chance at finding a cure that works. But it is also confusing because patients sometimes feel that their providers are groping in the dark, like the men in the story. A general practitioner sees a patient who has a hacking cough, diagnoses "bronchitis," and prescribes an antibiotic. An acupuncturist determines that the cough is caused by "toxic heat in the large intestine" and recommends a diet of "cooling foods," like cucumber. Finally, the patient decides to see a massage therapist, who says, "Of course you are coughing. Your back muscles are tight, your shoulders are raised, and your chest muscles are spasming." Each person sees the patient differently and believes that he or she has correctly diagnosed him. Who is right?

It's not that each type of therapy isn't important or doesn't have its place. A cancer patient needs the oncologist to treat cancer and the counselor to help confront the fear of death. But patients also long for someone who understands them beyond the narrow confines of their discipline and can appreciate the physical, emotional, and spiritual sides of their disease. Native American healers are able to see the whole "elephant." The four men in the dark room had forgotten that there is a light switch. The light is the eye of spirit. Members of the Swinomish Tribal Mental Health Project from the state of Washington write in their excellent textbook *A Gathering of Wisdoms,* "[S]pirituality is understood [by Native Americans] to be a fundamental reality of all life and all people, inseparable, connected to physical reality, bodily events, interpersonal relations, individual destiny, mental processes, and emotional well-being."[2] Native American healers are intimate with the spiritual realm. *Their "stew" of combined therapies draws the patient into this reality, which, because it is the source of the physical, is one of almost infinite possibility. Treating a disease effectively in the Spirit World often cures it in the physical.*

Modern science has examined and to a large extent confirmed the effectiveness of the Native American multifaceted approach to healing. It may seem hard to believe that an empirical discipline could have anything positive to say about spiritual realities, but it does. Remember, however, that science can detect only quantifiable aspects of Native American healing—those that register on its instruments. The spirit powers leave a much stronger imprint on the human mind than on a computer screen. Measuring their true power is beyond the capability of science.

One of the best examples of how Native American healing combines therapies is the "Winter Spirit Dances," a ceremonial tradition practiced among the Coast Salish tribes in the Pacific Northwest. Beginning in late October, tribal members gather periodically—in some cases, every weekend—throughout the winter in "smokehouses," cedarwood buildings slightly larger than gymnasiums, to honor their *syowen* ("spirit powers") with dance and song. The ceremonies begin in the late afternoon and may continue past midnight. Performing or observing the dance (considered a form of support and participation) has powerful cleansing and healing effects, due, in part, to the sheer intensity of the experience. A participant is stimulated *visually* by the vibrant, colorful imagery of the dance masks and regalia; *auditorily* because of the intense drumming, singing, foot-stomping, and perhaps bell-ringing (the music is sometimes of such volume that a singer cannot hear herself singing); *kinesthetically* and *tactually* by dancing or moving about; *olfactorily* by clouds of cedar smoke used in smudging; and *mentally/spiritually* by hearing the words and rhythms of song and prayer. In technical terms, the participant is immersed in "multiple sensory saturation."

The powerful drumming and dancing rhythms have an *entraining* effect on listeners, whose minds, bodies, and spirits start to resonate at the same rhythmic frequency, as when one tuning fork causes another to vibrate with it. Since the 1940s, scientists have documented that drumming produces a synchronous firing of the brain's neurons, known as *auditory driving,*[3] and a profound shift in the *frequency* and *amplitude* of the brain waves. The frequency of a brain wave is measured in waves per second, like counting the number of ocean waves that hit the shore per second, while the amplitude of a brain wave is measured in voltage, the height and power of the wave. Drumming rhythms, such as those that accompany Northwest spirit dancing, cause the frequency of participants' brain waves to slow down, indicating a relaxed and intuitive state, while the amplitude increases dramatically, signifying that large areas of the brain are working in powerful unison. Unified minds can produce, invoke, and concentrate strong healing energies. Interestingly, Tewa Indian educator Gregory Cajete, Ph.D., writes in *A People's Ecology* that in the Tewa language of the Southwest, psychological illness is sometimes called *pingeh heh*, "split thought or thinking, or doing things with only half of one's mind."[4] A divided mind is weak and incapable of healing oneself or others.

Spirit dancers may be especially receptive to the effects of such sensory stimulation because they prepare themselves for the winter ceremonials by undergoing periods of fasting, silence, and darkness. *From a scientific perspective, we could say that sensory quietude followed by sensory saturation in a supportive community setting causes a dramatic change in reality, including the reality of disease.*[5] The human mind and body are a complex system, with so many interdependent parts and functions that if only one aspect of a disease is treated, it is unlikely to be eradicated. The deepest healing can only result from a global rather than partial or incremental transformation.

TRADITIONAL ETIQUETTE AND PROTOCOL

Several years ago, I met a young white woman, "Deborah," who leads women's pilgrimages to Native American power places. She told me about a recent pilgrimage. When her group arrived at the Hopi Nation, they decided not to participate in the traditional ceremonies on the mesa and went instead to an adjacent part of the reservation where they donned handmade papier-mâché masks and performed their own "kachina dance." As she recounted the story, it was clear to me that Deborah had not been invited to Hopi land in the first place and that she certainly had not received permission from the Hopi elders to perform her own dance. Deborah seemed blithely unaware that she had violated an important protocol. I explained that *it requires permission to enter someone else's home and that, once there, one is expected to abide by the rules of the house.* Deborah answered in a haughty tone, "I was exercising my freedom of religion." It is useless to argue with someone who exercises freedom so irresponsibly. Freedom of religion does not include the freedom to trespass or to act disrespectfully.

Many American spiritual seekers are attracted to a form of spirituality grounded in the American landscape and, having found conventional religion rigid and unfulfilling, have embraced Native American culture out of genuine interest and desire to learn. This is a good thing, but a problem arises when the nonhierarchical, nondogmatic Native American spirituality is confused with a philosophy of

— MS. MEDICINE MANNERS —

Here are some general rules of ceremonial and social etiquette, including suggested behavior at cultural events such as powwows or feasts:

- Do not consume alcohol or drugs before, during, or, hopefully, long after a cultural event. Be pure and peaceful in body, mind, and spirit.
- Treat all people with respect and courtesy.
- Offer elders a chair and a cup of coffee whenever appropriate. At a meal, serve them food first. Elders deserve and receive special attention.
- Use kinship terms when addressing elders. For instance, the Innu call a male elder *nimushum,* "my grandfather," and a female elder *nukum,* "my grandmother." Among many tribes, it is disrespectful to address an elder or a spiritual leader by his or her personal name.
- Don't ask too many questions or interrupt when someone—especially an elder—is speaking. Remember that silence is the mark of respect.
- Maintain the confidentiality of sacred and personal information whether shared during a ceremony or at other times.
- Do not take notes, record, or photograph without permission.
- In many tribes, when a storyteller or other speaker is talking, it is polite to periodically exclaim a specific word such as *Ho, Aho, To,* or *Hau,* to indicate that you are listening and to show support and encouragement. Storytellers in the Northwest occasionally pause at the end of a sentence and wait for the listeners to say "I am listening" before continuing.
- Dress comfortably and modestly: slacks for men and ankle-length skirts for women; no shorts or miniskirts.
- Never instigate or accept sexual advances during a ceremony or while in the role of a ceremonial leader or teacher.[6]
- Before attending a ceremony, ask the ceremonial leader or knowledgeable participants about specific rules that may apply as well as any purifications or preparations you will need to make in advance.
- Do not step or pass things over an altar or a ceremonial object.
- Do not point with your finger; it is considered impolite. Instead, "point" by looking or by pursing your lips and inclining your head in the direction.

- Be mindful that ceremonial actions will be performed in either a clockwise or counterclockwise direction, depending on the ceremony or tribe.
- Use your eyes in a manner that communicates respect. Some tribes have traditions regarding where people should focus or not focus their eyes. For example, among many Plains tribes, to look directly in a speaker's eyes is considered challenging and a sign that one is only listening to the words rather than "seeing" the meaning and spirit behind them. Instead, listeners avert their eyes to the side or downward and remain attentive. As another example, to stare at a beautiful piece of jewelry may communicate envy and greed rather than admiration, or it may imply that you are so poor that it should be given to you.
- Help out by observing what experienced participants are doing and which activities are gender- or age-specific. People often arrive before a ceremony to help prepare for it, perhaps by chopping wood or cooking food, and stay afterward to help clean up. There is generally no need to ask, "Can I help you?" or "What should I do?" Just go into the kitchen and get to work. Or if necessary, put on your thinking cap for ten minutes as you decide if the mess on the floor should be mopped up, and then wait around for someone to compliment you on your unusual thoughtfulness.
- Don't imitate. Be yourself. Be humble but do not shy away from full participation in group songs, prayers, or dances. When called to speak, do not mutter to yourself. Speak strongly so that other participants and the Great Spirit know that you stand by your words.
- Be patient and attentive but not solemn. Lighten up!

"anything goes." In fact, there are clear rules concerning how traditions are practiced and standards of conduct that are expected of anyone, Native or not, who participates in a ceremony or other cultural activity.

Actions that are considered courteous or respectful in one culture may be interpreted as disrespectful in another. For example, when I was first married, my wife had a hard time getting used to my Indian way of doing things. A southerner by birth, she expected a gentleman to hold a door for a lady and allow her to enter a room first. Yet I always did the opposite. In Native culture, the man goes first because he wants to protect the woman, exposing himself to any harm. When my wife found out my reasoning, she decided that Native Americans had even better etiquette than southerners!

I am not trying to scare you away from participating in Native American culture when appropriate. Some ceremonies are only for members of particular Native nations or medicine societies and are simply forbidden to outsiders. But many activities—such as Indian art and culture fairs, Indian-run reservation tours, and powwows—are open to everyone. At powwows, even non-Indians may dance when invited by the master of ceremonies: "Let's have an intertribal dance—everybody come out to the dance floor!" That includes the white "tribe."

When you visit a foreign country, you are bound to encounter unfamiliar customs. Even if it is your first time with Native people, if you are open-minded, nonjudgmental, and patient with yourself, you will be treated with fairness. People will explain things to you, and God will not strike you down with a lightning bolt if you make a mistake. (Of course, the Great Spirit might! Just kidding.)

— PERMISSION OF THE ELDERS AND LAND —

To attend a ceremony, including a healing, a participant such as the medicine person, patient, or previously invited guest—perhaps a member of the patient's family—must invite you. You may not just show up. Native American ceremonial leaders and healers must also, in a sense, be invited. The healer must have proper training and the consent of the elders and the land. How can "the land" give you permission? When you intuitively listen to the voice of the earth in waking and sleeping dreams, you will know if your work is in harmony with the local spirits, or you may receive a natural omen, such as the call of a bird or the appearance of an animal at an auspicious moment.

My first experience with such an omen occurred when I was on the way to a Cherokee spring planting festival at which I had been invited to sing. I was just beginning my healing work, and I felt insecure about this responsibility because I had not yet gotten over the idea that my ability to lead an indigenous ceremony might be hindered by my ethnicity. Also, I did not know whether the song or songs I would be asked to sing would be within my repertoire. Although an elder had invited me, I was hoping for an additional sign of encouragement from the Spirit World. Driving to the ceremonial site, I felt a tingling sensation in my hands, which is frequently my personal indication of the call of a helping spirit. Although I was unfamiliar with the area, I turned off the main highway onto a dirt road. I continued following my spiritual sense of direction and made other detours. The road ended at a serene and beautiful lake.

I parked the car and walked over to a giant oak tree at the edge of the lake. Sitting cross-legged on the ground under the tree, I spread out a red-and-white woolen altar blanket that I had brought with me. I removed my sacred pipe from its smoked moose-hide bag and placed it on the blanket along with the tobacco, special stones, shells, seeds, and other items that symbolize my spiritual ideals. As soon as I was ready to begin the Pipe Ceremony, a water moccasin swam to the edge of the lake and slithered to a halt about five feet from me. I had no doubt that this poisonous snake was there to bless, not to harm. She watched intensely as I smoked the pipe and seemed to accept the smoke I blew toward her. "Thank you, little sister, for joining me this morning. I ask for your guidance. Help me to have a clear mind and pure heart so I can perform my duties in a good way." The moment I separated the pipe-bowl from the stem, signifying the end of the ceremony, the snake slid back into the water.

My encounter with the snake reminded me of a snake song that I had learned several years earlier. During the next two hours, as I continued driving, I practiced the song. When I arrived in the late afternoon at the festival grounds, the ceremonial leader asked me if I would sing a snake song. I felt well prepared.

Frequently, omens also appear *after* a healing ceremony, as a kind of affirmation that the ceremony was performed in a good way. For example, Rolling Thunder often accurately predicted that rain would fall soon after a ceremony. Rain is a natural symbol of blessing and new growth.

A snake appeared in more subtle yet dramatic guise a few years after the Cherokee festival, at the close of another event. I had been conducting a weeklong seminar about how exercises and meditations modeled on the snake teach people to be supple, sensitive, and adept at self-healing. Although the workshop took place at an alpine retreat, where snakes are rare, I had informed the group of twenty students that they would *all* see a snake by the week's end.

One stormy morning, I sensed that the snake would arrive. I donned my finest Indian jewelry and ceremonial attire to greet an honored guest. A few minutes after the participants had gathered in their customary circle, lightning crashed outside the open doorway and rolled into the center of the room as a ball of blinding light. Fortunately, no one was sitting or standing in the lightning's path. Although we were all briefly blinded and deafened by the "ball lightning," as this phenomenon is called, no one was hurt. I explained a commonly held Native American belief that the electricity of life may appear as a snake on the earth and as lightning in the heavens.

The snake had also left a physical mark. On a lodgepole pine tree to the side of the retreat entrance, a charred black line was clearly visible winding from the top of the tree to the bottom, where the lightning had first struck the tree before entering the hall. The tree had not been split or otherwise damaged. Twenty years later, the tree was still alive and healthy and a visible testament to the Great Spirit's power.

— A TIME AND PLACE FOR EVERYTHING —

Among different peoples, some ceremonies can only be performed at certain times or in specific locations. It may be appropriate only at a particular time of day, such as sunrise for a sunrise ceremony, or during certain seasons. Some ceremonies must be timed with natural events, such as the solstices and equinoxes, the phases of the moon, the ripening of crops, or the appearance of particular constellations in the night sky. Winter, for example, is the storytelling season for many Native Americans, and they will not share sacred stories at any other time of year. Northwest spirit dances take place in the winter, which is also an important season for vision questing. By contrast, most Northern Plains tribes begin "crying for a vision" only after the first thunderstorm of spring. Similarly, some songs may only be sung as part of the ceremony to which they belong. If a spring bear song is sung during the winter, the bears might awaken in an angry mood. It is as inappropriate to practice a seasonal ceremony out of season as it would be to plant seeds in the fall.

If you are given permission to share a medicine teaching, whether in the form of storytelling or ceremony, you will also learn and be required to respect the rules that govern it. To disobey those rules is to upset the natural harmony and balance among people, time, and place, which may have dangerous consequences to personal and community health.

— CARETAKING MEDICINE OBJECTS —

Medicine bags, jewelry, and ceremonial objects are considered private and sacred. It is considered a serious breach to touch one without permission. In fact, unless you are a close friend, even asking may be offensive.

My wife once went to a salon for a haircut, wearing her special copper bracelet and turquoise rings in honor of our wedding anniversary. As Rebecca settled into the chair, the stylist complimented her and couldn't resist touching the bracelet. Rebecca gently moved her arm away. Then the stylist picked up Rebecca's hand to get a closer look at the rings. Rebecca moved her hand under the sheet that covered her shoulders and arms. When the stylist tried to move the sheet aside, Rebecca said, "That's rude. Do not touch!" The stylist was insulted at being prevented from invading another person's privacy.

Such experiences are common. I have learned to wear my medicine pouch, bear claw, or whatever Indian jewelry hangs on my neck under my shirt to avoid these perhaps well-meaning but ignorant transgressions. My elders are not always as subtle in their response. I once saw Rolling Thunder put an overly zealous television reporter firmly in his place. The reporter, seeking out Rolling Thunder for a prearranged interview, approached a group of people surrounding the elder and blurted out, "Which one of you is Rolling Thunder?," an odd question considering that the elder was the only one in the group carrying an eighteen-inch-long wolverine-skin medicine bag and wearing a traditional Cherokee "turban," a gray cloth wrapped around his head, with eagle and hawk feathers suspended from it. Rolling Thunder replied, "I am Rolling Thunder," whereupon the reporter, instead of reaching out to shake hands, immediately grabbed Rolling Thunder's medicine bag with one hand and tried to put his other hand inside as he asked, "What's this?" Rolling Thunder cut through the man with his eyes. "It's my medicine bag," he replied. "I keep two live rattlers inside it. Now why don't you just put your hand all the way inside there and check it out!" Although there was humor in Rolling Thunder's handling of this uncomfortable situation, it did not belie his serious intent. The reporter kept a more respectful distance through the rest of the meeting.

Because medicine objects are powerful, proper care and storage are essential. In fact, the stronger the power, the greater the danger from neglect or misuse. Sacred objects must be ceremonially blessed—"awakened"—during their first use, then periodically reawakened, renewed, or purified by exposing them to the sun, moon, wind, water, or other natural powers. Sacred pipes are stored in special pipe bags, with bowl and stem separated. Drums, rattles, stones, and masks may need to be stored with sage or other plants or facing specific directions. According to ethnologist William N. Fenton's *The False Faces of the Iroquois,* if the sacred wooden medicine "faces" (masks) are neglected, stored facing the wrong direction, or wrapped improperly, they may cause their owners to become fearful, possessed by spirits, ill, or deformed.[7] Fenton tells the story of a woman from the Onondaga Nation in New York State whose "mouth had commenced to grow crooked because of a neglected mask . . . but her cure commenced when the mask was used in a dance following a proper tobacco invocation."[8] In his nineteenth-century classic *Myths of the Cherokee,* anthropologist James Mooney describes a sacred Cherokee quartz crystal that was once part of the forehead of the Uktena, a dragonlike creature that lived in lakes in the Cherokee homeland. It must be kept "wrapped in a whole deerskin, inside an earthen jar hidden away in a secret cave in the mountains"[9] and periodically fed with a ritual offering of the blood of small game. "Should he [the caretaker] forget to feed it at the proper time it would come out from its cave at night in a shape of fire and fly through the air to slake its thirst with the lifeblood of the conjurer [medicine man] or some one of his people."[10]

Since medicine objects amplify mental and spiritual energies, they should not be used by anyone who is under the influence of alcohol, recreational drugs, or negative thinking. For example, if an angry person uses a feather in a rainmaking ceremony to end a drought, it may instead bring on a flood. During healings, weddings, warrior training, and other traditional ceremonies, participants sometimes paint their faces with red ocher, a natural earth pigment, to attract blessings. But if a drunken person paints his own or another person's face with red ocher, he offends the spirits, all of whom value sobriety, and may attract a curse. The Taoists of ancient China had a saying that is relevant here: "If the wrong person uses the right means, the right means work in the wrong way."

— RECLAIMING CULTURAL TREASURES —

Many Euro-American museums and homes display "artifacts"—Indian shields, pipes, pottery, regalia, effigies, medicine bags, or masks—that have cultural or historical value to Native Americans. Some of these are sacred objects that should only be kept by authorized Indian people. Native nations are seeking their return. For example, the Grand Council of Chiefs of the Hodenosaunee (alternate spelling for Haudenosaunee) heads an effort to restore their confederacy's sacred objects to their proper caretakers. In an undated policy statement, the council wrote:

> *All wooden and corn husk masks of the Hodenosaunee are sacred regardless of size or age. . . . There are no masks that can be made for commercial purposes. . . . Each Hodenosaunee reservation has a medicine mask society that has authority over the use of masks for individual and community needs. . . . The public exhibition [or reproduction, photographing, or illustration] of all medicine masks is forbidden. Medicine masks are not intended for everyone to see and such exhibition does not recognize the sacred duties and special functions of the masks.*

The Grand Council asks that all people help in this effort; the return of sacred objects by museums—though, unfortunately, not by private individuals—is a federal law.

Revered ceremonial objects do not belong in museums but rather in the hands of the people who know how to use them. I have seen and experienced the pride and joy that Native Americans feel when their cultural treasures return "home." I will always feel blessed that I was invited to smoke the *Canunpa,* "Sacred Pipe," of the holy man Sitting Bull with Lakota people shortly after the Smithsonian Institution returned it to the tribe.

— RECORDING AND PHOTOGRAPHING —

Native American healing techniques, ceremonies, and sacred songs are still largely passed on orally, from elder to student, from grandparent, uncle, or other relative to the younger generation in an unbroken chain of transmission. For this and many other reasons already covered in this book—such as preventing dilution and commercialization of spiritual power; protecting people who, with access to power, could be harmed or cause harm to others; and obeying the wishes of the spirits themselves—Indian communities do not, except in the rarest of circumstances, allow sacred ceremonies and events to be taped, photographed, or otherwise recorded. At some Cherokee ceremonies, the medicine man "doctors up" old men to give them the power to sniff out and scare away uninvited anthropologists. During the ceremony, that frail old man may look to such intruders like a menacing giant!

Yet the distinction between sacred or private and social or public is sometimes subtle or even blurry. Native American songs are considered sacred or social, but some fall between the two categories, and the decision whether or not to record them may be up to the song group or individual artist. Social songs include "pow-wow" dance songs as well as new and popular genres of music that combine traditional and modern instruments and singing styles, exemplified in the exquisite music of Joanne Shenandoah. Although these are widely available in music shops, the recording of sacred songs is discouraged even for educational purposes. Ceremonial songs should be learned experientially, by hearing them performed during a ceremony. Among many tribes, you are allowed to sing a sacred song only if it is deliberately "given" (taught) to you by a previous owner.

Songs recorded on audiocassettes are stored on a shelf and easily forgotten; they become *inert information,* removed from life experiences. If, however, every time you perform a buffalo dance or ritual, an elder coaches you on the words to the buffalo song, you never forget that song, never take it for granted, and it is always full of meaning and power. Through dedication and effort, you have earned the song and deserve the gifts it evokes. When you have memorized a traditional song, you may feel "I climbed the mountain, so I'm entitled to the view."[11]

Ceremonies are not for spectators, and this is another reason that photography, film, and note taking are forbidden. They remove us from the experience and limit understanding to fixed images and concepts. Ethnographers can seriously distort information by filtering it through their cultural screens and intellectual or moral standards or by selectively editing whatever statements or images might offend or confuse their audience. Historical ethnographers such as Edward Curtis advertised their own versions of Indian culture by staging their photographs or by asking their subjects to pose. Their works may thus communicate false, decontextualized, and partial information. As anthropologist Felicitas Goodman, Ph.D., once commented to me, "You could fill the Library of Congress twice over with what the anthropologists have *not* documented!"

MOONTIME POWER

Sacred information must be shared with discretion. Yet I believe that *the most sacred of all Native American ceremonies,* the Moontime Ceremony, should be understood by everyone. It is the way that women, the givers of life, honor and renew their power.

Among virtually all indigenous peoples, menstruation is a time when women isolate themselves in a sacred dwelling for prayer and meditation, taking a welcome break from family and community responsibilities. This Moontime Ceremony was created by women to honor their feminine power and their roles as mothers, caretakers, and providers. It is an example of neither patriarchal oppression nor men's fear of shifting hormones. Moontime separation is based on an understanding of the differences between men's and women's power and how honoring that power influences harmony, creativity, and health. The Moontime Ceremony is central to the understanding and practice of Native American healing. Although I describe traditional moontime customs in the present tense, readers should be aware that some practices—particularly separate dwelling—are rarely followed today. Tragically, moontime rituals, in spite of their importance, are practiced less than other rituals described in this book.

According to Anishinabe elders, men are caretakers of fire, women of water.[12] These associations are also widely accepted by other tribes.[13] Fire is an agent of change and transformation; it is a spiritual power that underlies the intellect and toolmaking, including modern technology. Men must learn to control this power with wisdom and compassion, or it can become destructive. Women have the gentle strength of water and the subtle power of intuition. They were instructed by the Creator to do everything in their power to protect the purity of streams, lakes, and oceans. Our waters are polluted because the politically dominant men of Western society have rarely listened to the counsel of women and never to the counsel of indigenous women.[14]

Water is life. It nourishes the seeds on earth as well as the seeds of life in a woman's body. Once a month, women purge their old water and fluids during menstruation. It is called "moontime" because the moon controls the tides of water on the earth and in the bodies of women. Women tend to ovulate, conceive, and begin menstruation during particular phases of the moon. In preindustrial times, many women ovulated during the full moon or the day before and began menstrual bleeding during the moon's waning. Today, electric lights have interfered with the activity of the light-sensitive hormone melatonin, with a resulting disruption in normal biological cycles.

Women are fortunate that their bodies are so tuned to the Earth Mother and Grandmother Moon that they go through cyclic purifications, waxings and wanings. As a Mexican *curandera* ("folk healer") once told me, "Most women are cleaner after their periods than any man will be during his lifetime." Women gain power as they honor their ability to cleanse and grow fresh "seeds," recognizing their moontime as the sacred way that Creator prepares their bodies for birth, whether this be the birth of a child or the birth of new ideas and intuitive insight. As Keepers of the Water, women have the power to nourish, nurture, counsel, and create life and life-giving values.

Traditional indigenous women treat moontime as a natural sacred ceremony. In order not to mix their power with that of men, they isolate themselves in separate beds or, whenever possible, in a separate dwelling called a "moon lodge." The moon lodge may be a private moontime retreat hut or a communal lodge where women can join in sisterhood with other women who are in their moontime.[15] For several days each month, women shift their focus away from their day-to-day work and responsibilities toward a broader and less personal reality linked to nature's cycles. I believe that by honoring this time, they help maintain not only family health but the health and balance of life on Earth.

The sanctity of moontime is part of the Creator's original instructions. The Moontime Ceremony and the custom of moontime retreat were created by women for women and are a natural outcome of their cyclic need for aloneness, quiet, and introspection. Women normally teach other women about moontime; men learn about it from other men and from their spouses. Before I was married, I was sometimes in the awkward position of explaining the Moontime Ceremony to my female students. To make sure that I knew the respectful way to describe moontime proscriptions, a Lakota female elder taught me about moontime medicine and allowed me to attend what would have been an all-women's teaching circle. I will never forget Grandmother's reaction when a young white woman asked if her husband could still hug her during her moontime. Shaking her fist in the air, the elder replied, "When I still had periods, my husband never dared lay a hand on me. If he ever did, I would wallop him for such disrespect." The effect of her statement was especially dramatic for those of us who knew her husband, a brawny full-blood Lakota man who towered more than a foot above her. According to Theda Perdue, noted historian and scholar of Cherokee women's culture, "Women secluded themselves; men did not force restrictions of them. Men, in fact, often observed similar restrictions before and after warfare, and they, like women, regarded seclusion as a practical precaution and a demonstration of the elevated plane they had achieved."[16]

Cree elder George Kehewin shares his insights about moontime with Cree journalist Dianne Meili, in her *Those Who Know: Profiles of Alberta's Native Elders:* "Women are far, far ahead of men. It's quite hard to understand, but when you start living the Native culture, you will. You are like Mother Earth, who once a year in the spring, washes herself down the river to the ocean. Everything . . . all debris is washed away. Same thing with a woman, except it's every month. It's the power you have."[17]

Women stay in the moon lodge from the first spot of blood until the last. During their respite from work, they meditate, pray, read, converse with other moontime women, and work on crafts or other personal projects. Food is brought to them by women attendants, or they prepare the food themselves.[18] When moontime women leave the moon lodge, they close their ceremony by smudging and bathing. I have lived among traditional Native Americans who adhere to these traditions. My personal impression is that after dwelling in the moon lodge, women return to their community with renewed clarity, radiance, and beauty.[19]

It is interesting to note that for most of human history, menstruation was *not* a monthly occurrence, and Native American women may have visited the moon lodge only twenty to thirty times during their lifetimes. Nursing mothers produce the hormone prolactin, which suppresses ovulation and acts as a natural contraceptive, preventing menstruation. In indigenous societies, a woman generally conceived soon after puberty, bore a child, nursed for three years, had a few menstrual cycles, and became pregnant again. This pattern was repeated until menopause. In *Why Zebras Don't Get Ulcers,* Robert M. Sapolsky, professor of biological sciences and neuroscience at Stanford University, writes:

> [O]ver the course of her life span, she [the indigenous woman] has perhaps two dozen periods. Contrast that with modern Western women, who average perhaps 500 periods over their lifetime. . . . Perhaps some of the gynecological diseases that plague modern Westernized women have something to do with this activation of a major piece of physiological machinery 500 times when it may have evolved to be used only 20 times; an example of this is probably endometriosis, which is more common among women with fewer pregnancies and who start [childbearing] at a later age.[20]

Moontime separation is practiced for both physical and spiritual reasons. It is a ritual of purification and renewal that, from the Native American viewpoint, fosters well-being, health (especially reproductive health), and healthier children. When author James H. Howard conducted research for his classic book *The Ponca Tribe* during the early 1950s, his Northern Ponca consultants in Nebraska and Southern Ponca consultants in Oklahoma "attributed much of the disease of present-day Indians to the fact that the menstrual taboo is no longer strictly observed."[21]

Cleansing the body of unneeded blood and cells also creates vulnerabilities. Sanapia, a well-known medicine woman, felt that menstruating women could be easily harmed if they either performed or observed traditional doctoring. As author David E. Jones writes in *Sanapia: Comanche Medicine Woman,* "loss of blood means weakness, and weakness makes an individual more susceptible to illness caused by supernatural or natural means."[22]

While cleansing, women keep physically distant from medicine objects, ceremonial areas, and people who are not in moontime. As I said earlier, women's moontime medicine does not mix with men's medicine. Their powerful "water" can put out men's fire and overwhelm the medicine of their sisters, like a flooded river inundating a nearby stream. Sex is forbidden to prevent an imbalanced exchange of energy and because of the possibility that a man might absorb the discharge of unneeded energies through his most sensitive organ. Additionally, in the old days, women protected their men from the scent of blood, lest it prevent hunters and warriors from moving invisibly through the woods. All forms of prey—including fish—are sensitive to the energies and scents of moontime.

Spiritually, moontime is a time of introspection, prayer, and creative dreaming. While in the moon lodge, women may receive important guidance for themselves, their families, communities, or nation. Rebecca D. Cohen, Ph.D., investigated the effects of indigenous menstrual customs on dreaming, intuition, and other factors in her pioneering dissertation "Empowering Women through Sacred Menstrual Customs."[23] Eight non-Native female subjects in committed heterosexual relationships were asked to sleep separately from their husbands during menses in an area that they considered sacred and private. Throughout the seven months of the study, each woman kept a journal of her feelings, dreams, insights, and meaningful experiences. After interviewing the women and analyzing their reports, Dr. Cohen found that:

- Creativity increased during menses for some women.
- The number and meaningfulness of dreams increased for all women.
- Dreams gave more meaningful guidance for daily life during menses compared to dreams that occurred at other times for some women.
- Intuitive insights increased during menses and continued throughout the month for most women.
- Marital relationships improved for all eight women, from the perspective of all the women and all but one of their partners.

Although this initial study needs to be replicated, it is highly suggestive that moontime customs can lead to positive changes for even non-Native women in contemporary Western society.

In an earlier study, Robert L. Van de Castle, Ph.D., former director of the Sleep and Dream Laboratory at the University of Virginia Medical School, examined more than 450 dreams from approximately fifty female nursing students over a three-month period. He found significant differences between the content of dreams during menstruation compared to the content during other phases of the women's cycle. During menstruation, the women tended to initiate more social contacts with male and female dream figures yet were the recipients of less attention or social interaction from them. In his book *Our Dreaming Mind,* Van de Castle comments, "This suggests that the average menstruating woman perceives herself as being more socially isolated at that time than at other phases of her cycle."[24] From the perspective of Native American tradition, I can venture an additional interpretation: women *need* more isolation during moontime than at other phases. Unfortunately, Western society does not provide a way for women to honor and learn from their cyclic need for retreat.

Van de Castle found that as women's hormones shift, their dream images move between polarities such as assertiveness and receptivity, birth and death, independence and dependence, and isolation and relationship. Menstruating women frequently dreamed of engagements and weddings. Their dreams of "being wed to mysterious strangers or receiving engagement rings from boyfriends may represent an attempt to incorporate masculine elements at this time of heightened femininity; a fusion of feminine and masculine energy may be seen as enabling the woman to achieve increased psychic vitality and power."[25] Van de Castle writes that women's cycles give them unique insight into the "bipolarities of being" and an ability to have a balanced perspective on "the realms of the intrapersonal, interpersonal, and transpersonal."

Many Native women do not feel the same need as men to participate in the Sweat Lodge, Vision Quest, or other ceremonies. After all, they are already attuned to the rhythms and energies of life and have their own monthly ceremony brought on by nature. This does not mean that they are less capable of becoming powerful healers and ceremonial leaders, only that there is less urgency to seek these roles. Why quest for a power that is inherent to one's biology? In *Women and Power in Native North America,* Alice B. Kehoe writes about men's and women's roles in Blackfoot society:

> *Women are believed to have more innate power than men, because they are born with power to reproduce both the human and the material components of the social world. Fewer women than men feel the need to go out crying to be pitied and favored with power. . . . Men's inability to bear children was a sign of lesser reproductive power, carrying over to an inability to make—reproduce—tipis, clothing, or well-prepared meals. Men provided raw materials, from semen to slaughtered bison, and women processed raw materials into the components of civilized society.*[26]

In the 1930s, anthropologist Ruth Underhill asked a Tohono O'Odham (Papago) grandmother, Maria Chona, why she and other Indian women did not take part in ceremonies. Chona said that men have dreams, make up stories, and perform ceremonies. "You see, we *have* power. Men have to dream to get power from the spirits and they think of everything they can—songs and speeches and marching around, hoping that the spirits will notice them and give them some power. But we *have* power."[27] Chona then asked the anthropologist if any man can make a child "no matter how brave and wonderful he is." The elder explained that there is no reason for women to envy men, since they made the men!

In general, neither male nor female Native healers doctor a woman during her moontime. This rule is not, however, written in stone, and some healers may doctor

— TRADITIONAL INTERTRIBAL RULES
FOR MOONTIME —

Applicable to women of any ethnicity who are following Native American spirituality.

- Create a sacred space for prayer, retreat, and renewal, even if it is only a room or section of a room in your house.
- Sleep in this space throughout your moontime, separate from your spouse.
- Do not have sex during moontime.
- Do not conduct or participate in indigenous ceremonies, unless they are specifically designed for or include moontime women.
- Do not attempt to heal others, unless the need is urgent and clearly has priority over your need for separation. Do not touch or prepare herbal medicines.
- Do not enter a ceremonial lodge, visit sacred sites, or bathe in lakes, rivers, the ocean, or other natural bodies of water unless they are traditionally recognized places for moontime purification.
- Do not touch or approach ceremonial objects or hunting weapons.
- Do not touch or prepare food that will be consumed by people not in moontime.
- Enjoy your special time and the grace and beauty of Grandmother Moon.

moontime women if the illness is serious and they feel intuitively certain of the appropriateness and timing of the therapy. Some healers may also hesitate to doctor the spouse of a moontime woman. In the past, writes Theda Perdue, Cherokee men whose wives were menstruating "marched and danced behind the others on ceremonial occasions."[28] Cherokee healer Hawk Littlejohn told me that the sacred bond of marriage required him to completely avoid ceremony during his wife's moontime. In 1929, a California Wintu named Syke Mitchell explained, "The perceived dangers of menstruation affected not only the 'moon-sick' woman, but other people to whom she was linked. A husband, for example, would not go hunting during his wife's menstrual period because her condition would affect his prowess and luck: after all, they were of the same family and thus connected as a unit."[29]

I find it odd that many anthropologists and non-Indian women believe that moontime isolation is demeaning. If there is anything demeaning or patriarchal in moontime customs, it is not the isolation or emphasis on ritual purity but rather the denial of moontime's sacred dimension by male writers. Moontime traditions, like other "old ways," were designed by the Great Spirit to ensure the harmony and happiness of *all* of his children.

8

— THE PRINCIPLES OF —
NATIVE AMERICAN COUNSELING

Native American counselors help people find meaning and direction in life and guidance for relief from emotional distress, such as fear, anger, frustration, and sorrow. In this role, the healer is part priest or rabbi, part psychotherapist. The counselor may also be a spirit whom the patient contacts directly or with the help of a medicine person. Because Native American philosophy recognizes the interdependence of body, mind, and spirit, counseling can positively affect physical disease, and some healers always include it in a healing session.

Counseling is one of the least discussed aspects of Native American healing, perhaps because Native people take it almost for granted, and non-Natives are too entranced by exotic rituals to even notice its existence.[1] The Comanche medicine woman Sanapia encouraged her patients to explain their troubles in a monologue that could continue for several hours, arriving at her diagnosis as they spoke.[2] Cherokee scholars Jack and Anna Kilpatrick say that the Cherokee medicine man "is traditionally, among other things, a marriage counselor and an advisor to the forlorn."[3] In his book *Fools Crow: Wisdom and Power*, Thomas Mails explains that the Lakota holy man Fools Crow talked to his patients at great length, describing his method of doctoring; the possible emotional, spiritual, and social causes of the patients' diseases; and how the diseases might be affecting their families. He would also get a complete "history," encouraging the patients to tell him about previous experiences with other healers or therapies. Mails writes, "The purpose of this lengthy discussion was to draw the people completely into the curing process, to engage their total persons, to get them communing fully with *Wakan-Tanka* and the Helpers, and to enhance their own curing abilities and those of the 'hollow bones' [receptive healers] who treated them."[4]

Native American counselors are always on call in the service of their communities. A frightened woman calls Grandmother late at night wanting to know what to do about her abusive husband. A distraught young man hopes that a healer will help him understand why he can't find suitable work. A grieving widower needs advice about how to find inner peace after the death of his wife. Native counselors treat the same range of human problems as psychotherapists, with a strong emphasis on the primary tools of the trade: intuition, insight, and compassion.

A counseling session may help a healer determine whether other healing methods are required. For example, if a patient discusses a dream that seems suggestive or even prophetic of a developing cancer, the healer may prescribe an herbal tea or perform a ceremony to invite or increase the power of protective and disease-preventive spirits. Although traditional Native counseling is based on spiritual wisdom rather than book learning, more and more Native Americans are studying Western psychotherapy and counseling and creating new methodologies that integrate them with traditional values and spirituality.[5] There is no conflict in being a licensed clinical psychologist, social worker, or counselor *and* a traditional healer.

Native counseling, however, is in some respects closer to pastoral counseling than to psychotherapy. The healer embodies spiritual values and prays with and for the patient. He or she is expected to be a model of health and centeredness and thus to effect some degree of healing by example and presence. The Native healer works to instill confidence in a patient by focusing on the patient's strengths, avoiding negative-sounding diagnoses, disease labels, and descriptions.

HAPPINESS IS THE BEST MEDICINE

Because Native healers recognize that patients' chances of survival are much greater when they feel good about themselves, they focus on the "dos" rather than the "don'ts" in treating the disease. For example, a patient with a genetic susceptibility to heart disease should certainly avoid fatty foods, but if he feels deprived, or if he becomes preoccupied with proscriptions, he may develop high levels of stress that might contribute to his problem. Native healers advise the patient to pay attention to positive things in his life, such as the joy of taking walks in nature and the healing power of family love. He should think about what he can do rather than dwelling on what he can't. Speaking personally, when illness or worry has seemed like an inescapable abyss, I am always redeemed when I remember that the earth is beautiful and that I, like the earth, am a child of the Great Spirit.

To put it simply, focusing on the limitations imposed by disease may promote disease or, at the very least, does not encourage healing, a principle illustrated by the following joke:

A man who has been diagnosed with advanced heart disease is presented with an extensive list of "don'ts" by his physician, including many of life's pleasures. Because his blood cholesterol levels are elevated, he must avoid all saturated fats and rich pastas. To prevent strain on his heart, his doctor advises him to quit practicing carpentry and to curtail sexual activity. Since he could drop dead at any time, he can no longer risk long drives in the country by himself, and smoking cigarettes is certainly out. The list goes on and on. The distraught patient asks his doctor, "If I follow your advice and deny myself the things I love, will I live longer?" The doctor replies, "No, but it will certainly seem that way."

We laugh at this joke despite its grim truth: even if we do everything right, there is no guarantee that we will beat a life-threatening disease or that we will necessarily buy ourselves more time. Native healers realize that joy of life is the best medicine, and they do all they can to help patients find or recover it. By "joy of life," I don't mean a hedonistic search for pleasure but rather appreciation and gratitude for the gift of being alive. The dietary restrictions and other lifestyle changes physicians recommend to their patients are generally based on statistical averages, which do not take into account the exceptional healing potential of individuals. In fact, statisticians consider data that falls substantially outside the normal range of expectations to be statistically insignificant. If, for example, most patients with a particular type of cancer survive six months, the small percentage who survive twenty years or more will not even be figured into the average. A physician may consider these survivors irrelevant to his prognosis.

Yet patients routinely defy statistics. As Mark Twain said (quoting Benjamin Disraeli), "There are three kinds of lies: lies, damned lies, and statistics." Counseling is often an essential component of Native American healing because it puts the healer in touch with the patient's uniqueness. A healer must understand a patient's mind and emotions to determine what kind of therapy will really work and how to tailor the therapy to the patient's needs.

THE STORY OF DISEASE

Native American healers realize that an illness is a *story* that expresses a patient's life experiences. Neither a patient's complaints nor the physical signs of disease can give a comprehensive picture of his or her illness. In an article in the journal *Advances in Mind-Body Medicine*, Dr. Brian Campbell Broom, physician and psychotherapist at the Institute for Integrative Health Studies in Christchurch, New Zealand, defines story as "that tapestry of elements relating to the patient's past, present, and future experience as a subject."[6] He explains how modern medicine's lack of attention to the story of disease is a consequence the "biomedical model," in which mind and body are compartmentalized, with the body considered fundamental and subjective experience devalued.

The Native American counselor is an interpreter of the patient's story. He or she wonders, How and why did the illness develop when it did? What does it symbolize or mean to the patient? Is the illness a symbolic message from the Creator or a spirit? Is the patient looking for a painkiller, an escape, or a cure? Will the patient make a commitment to change disease-promoting attitudes or an unhealthy lifestyle? Native healers must also ask themselves the difficult question, "Is the therapy good and meant to be?"—that is, is it necessary or is it necessary *now*? Native healers are guided by their innate sense of whether or not offering a therapy is in harmony with all that is and will truly contribute to a patient's happiness and quality of life. In some situations, timing is everything. A medicine offered at the wrong time may only serve to deepen or shift symptoms.

Bob was a thirty-nine-year-old Vietnam vet who had been homeless and living on the streets for the past ten years, strung out on cocaine. He looked like a burned-out hippie from the sixties. His face was barely visible behind a wide, uneven beard and a mane of curly black hair that fell past his shoulders. Bob could not hold his gaze steady, and he would drift into a wordless stupor after a few minutes of conversation. During the two or three months that he attended a free exercise class I was teaching, I never heard him speak a complete sentence. He tended to utter broken phrases. He was clearly someone who needed healing, but I did not offer him an intensive, personalized healing session because I didn't feel that the timing was right. Frankly, I wasn't certain that he really wanted to change, and without that motivation, there was little I or any other healer could do to help him.

So Bob really took me by surprise one day when he approached me after class and said, "You know. Change. I want to change. Can't. No willpower. Drugs. Dope. It's everywhere." Pleased, I suggested he come for a private counseling session.

At our meeting, Bob slowly and painfully told me the story of his life—an abusive childhood, a brief marriage that ended just before the Vietnam War, then the shady drug deals and the game of street survival, the few hopes and many disappointments he had had about his life. One of the strangest parts of his story concerned a man he met at a homeless shelter shortly after his discharge from the army. He was convinced that this man was "an evil witch who was constantly trying to cast spells on me" and explained that his life had spiraled quickly downward after he had moved into that shelter. I could not yet tell whether the witch was a symbol of Bob's fears and paranoia, a way of rationalizing his tragic circumstances, or whether, indeed, malevolent outside forces were at work. But at this point, the diagnosis was not all that important. Bob was ready to make a change, and the fact that he recognized a problem existed would make a positive outcome possible.

I agreed to do a healing ceremony for Bob on two conditions: (1) that he refrain from using any drugs for four days and (2) that he take a bath, clean his clothes, and cut his hair, even if only a few inches. Bob readily agreed to all of the conditions except the last. He said, "I can't cut my hair. That would be identifying with the Establishment." (Coined by hippies in the social foment of the 1960s, the term refers to government, law enforcement, big business, and education—the traditional holders of power and authority in society.) I replied, "Not cutting your hair is identifying with the 'Establishment.' The Establishment says you are the way you look. Do you believe that?" Bob was still reluctant, so I said to him, "OK, don't cut your hair, but let me ask you, how do you plan to pay me for my services?" He replied that I knew he was broke. "Exactly, but you must give something. I would like you to consider giving something to Creator. You were born naked, without possessions. We really own nothing. So give part of your body. Cut two inches from your beard and hair, and burn it in a small campfire outside. As it burns, offer thanks to the Creator and say, 'I humble myself before you. I know that I own nothing. All I have to give is part of my body. Please help me to heal.' "

I gave Bob a small quartz crystal and asked him to keep it in his shirt pocket until we met again for the healing. I explained that it was a special crystal and that it had the power to make drug dealers think that Bob had become a narcotics agent. "If you don't make the first move and ask for drugs, I guarantee that nobody is going to offer you any."

Four days later, Bob met me and about a dozen ceremonial helpers at a cabin in the mountains. Sober, wearing clean clothes, with hair neatly trimmed and combed, he already looked like a new man. I asked Bob to lie on his back in the center of the room. While the support group sang traditional healing songs, I fanned and smudged Bob with sage. I then placed special healing stones on his body and began to pray out loud. When I finished my prayers and opened my eyes, I saw an eagle hovering a few feet above Bob's head. Instead of an eagle's visage, the bird had the face of a rather sinister-looking man. I knew that this was the face of the "witch" Bob had mentioned. Bob had indeed been hexed. His former housemate had removed, forcibly, Bob's spirit power—the eagle—from his heart (the place where I usually see the helping spirit) in order to make him pessimistic and vulnerable to misfortune, the essence of a hex.

Fanning the eagle with a mixture of sage and tobacco smoke, I prayed to the Great Mystery to lift the human face from the eagle and restore Bob's spirit to wholeness. I asked the Great Mystery to take the human face and do with it whatever might be best, whether it be releasing it into the Light of Love or giving a lesson to the one who sent it. I waved and twirled a feather fan over the human face, as though lifting a mask.

Underneath, the eagle's face was normal and healthy. I shook my feather fan toward the sky to help discharge the human face. I prayed for Bob's welfare, asking that he be forgiven for any misdeeds, that he be given the willpower to resist drugs, and that he find a way to get off the streets and take better care of himself. I asked for a whirlwind to come in and clean out his mind and body, blowing away poisons and negative thinking. As I prayed, an actual whirlwind came up suddenly, shaking the house.

Finally, I gently supported the eagle in my hands and took it to Bob's crown. I then blew it vigorously into his fontanel and visualized it lodged in his heart. I led the group in a closing song.

Bob's healing was nothing short of miraculous. He never went back to hard drugs and over the next several months was able to wean himself off marijuana completely. Immediately after the healing, his gaze became steady and focused, and he could speak normally and coherently. These effects lasted for the next two years that I knew him. He began to study Tai Chi Ch'uan with me and became an outstanding student, well coordinated and healthy. Within two weeks of the healing ceremony, Bob found a sales job in a garden supply store and used his first paycheck to make a deposit on an apartment. He never went back to living on the streets. To my surprise, I received a phone call about a month after the healing from a social worker with the county Department of Social Services who was familiar with Bob's case. She told me that she had never seen an individual go through such a radical transformation in such a short time. "I don't understand what you're doing, but it works." She expressed her hope that I would continue to offer my services to other homeless people.

In 1997, the last time I heard from Bob, he was working as a fitness instructor at a resort in California.

HEALING AND CURING

Sometimes, a healer will know that no healing intervention will cure a chronic, deadly disease. In such cases, the only way to preserve quality of life is to help a patient to accept his or her condition by seeing it in a new light. The healer may need to resolve, "I will not try to fix him." This is a very difficult statement for most allopathic physicians to make; their training focuses almost exclusively on curing disease and saving life. If the body or mind break down, you *must* try to fix them. Native American healers are often more concerned with *healing* than fixing or curing. The word *healing* comes from the Old English *haelan,* "to make whole." It implies helping the patient to discover meaning, harmony, and the highest degree of contentment possible. Wholeness is a feeling of integrity. "I can be true to who I am." A whole person is not shattered by disease or adversity. Wholeness maximizes our healing potentials, but it does not always cure.

When you think of people who have lived with apparently incurable conditions such as diabetes, AIDS, or cancer, it is fairly easy to understand the distinction between "healing" and "curing." As strange as it sounds, I have known AIDS patients who said, "AIDS was the best thing that ever happened to me. I learned how to take care of myself. I learned about who I am and who God is." This certainly does not mean that science should stop pursuing every possible avenue to relieve a patient's suffering or to find a cure. However, finding a cure is not the only measure of success for a healer. Helping a patient find that sense of fulfillment and peace can be equally important.

Allopathic medicine is sometimes considered "heroic medicine." Typically, a physician combats disease at almost any cost—literally and figuratively—to the patient and her family. Healing is seen as an endless series of battles; patients are winners or losers in a "war" against cancer or drug abuse. By comparison, Native American healing is *compassionate healing*. Native healers view life as a series of endless opportunities for growth and change. They believe that every time you see a healer, you should feel better after the encounter than before, or at least be aware of a way to improve your own health and quality of life.

How wonderful it would be for themselves and their patients if Western physicians could adopt this same ethical stance. Heroic medicine tends to pathologize many entirely normal conditions such as childbirth, menopause, and death. Swiss psychiatrist Carl G. Jung once said life itself is a disease with a very poor prognosis. It lingers on for years and invariably ends with death. From the Native perspective, childbirth and menopause are sacred times of transition that should be celebrated rather than treated or anesthetized. Death is natural rather than tragic, and it is sad only to the living, not to those who have died! The healer models a way for the patient to shift her focus away from the specific condition to the "larger picture." During severe pain or incurable disease, relief of symptoms is certainly important. A patient's relationship with her own soul, with her family, and with the Creator, however, are sometimes even more important to her. She may be seeking compassion as much as cure. I have known numerous cancer patients who experienced more relief from a healing song than from any amount of morphine.

THE SEARCH FOR MEANING

Janet is a twenty-five-year-old Native American living in the Southeast. She had been in and out of psychiatric institutions and on psychiatric medications since she was ten years old. A Native American social worker brought her to see me and was present during the consultation. He told me that Janet had been diagnosed as schizophrenic and that no one had been able to help her. Janet was intelligent and articulate and did not seem to have suffered any cognitive impairment from her psychiatric drugs. I asked her, "What do you feel is your basic problem? I don't want any psychiatric labels.

I want to know why you believe that you have been hospitalized so frequently." Janet immediately replied, matter-of-factly, "I'm crazy." "In what way?" I asked. She explained that when she was a young child, the trees, flowers, mountains, and other aspects of nature spoke to her mind, and she felt that she could understand them. When she told her parents, who were fundamentalist Christians, they took her to a psychiatrist. I realized that Janet had been analyzed and drugged during what should have been a very meaningful time of her life. The voice of nature, which could have been for her a source of deep spiritual inspiration, was pathologized, invalidated, and denied.

"What do you need most in your life for true healing?" I asked Janet. "If you could ask God for whatever you need in order to be happy and healthy, what would that be?" "Meaning," she said quietly. "Meaning. I would ask for meaning." I felt that Janet had hit the nail on the head. I gave her a small bag of Indian tobacco, the raw, wild tobacco that is reserved for ceremonial use, and explained how to make a tobacco offering. I suggested that every day at dawn she go to the park at the edge of town and stand on the bank of the river that runs through it. "Hold the tobacco on your open palm and ask the Creator for meaning. Ask and pray in your own way. When your prayer is finished, toss the tobacco into the river. Close your eyes and imagine the river joined by other streams and rivers, the current growing stronger and stronger. It is joined by still other rivers, until the river unites with the sea. Grandmother Ocean receives your tobacco and responds to your prayer. Do this for the next ninety days, then contact me and let me know how you are."

Three months later, both Janet and her social worker reported that Janet was healthier and happier than at any time in her memory. With her psychiatrist's consent, she had begun taking a lower dosage of medication. Janet was no longer in an existential vacuum; she wrote to me that she had found the most important "meaning" of all: "I have a direction, like the river. I am also on a journey toward my source, and whether psychiatrists realize it or not, nature is alive!" Janet's daily tobacco ritual had connected her with the wisdom of her Native ancestors and validated the reality and importance of nature's guidance, the very thing that had been denied during her childhood. Janet soon took up watercolor painting as a hobby and remained in good psychological health throughout the two years that I followed her case.

In the book *Wisdom Keepers: Meetings with Native American Spiritual Elders*, Haudenosaunee Chief Leon Shenandoah says, "Everything is laid out for you. Your path is straight ahead of you. Sometimes it's invisible but it's there. You may not know where it's going, but still you have to follow that path. It's the path to the Creator. That's the only path there is."[7]

The purpose of Native American counseling is to find meaning, both the meaning of the disease, trying to understand if the illness has symbolic meaning in the patient's life; and life meaning, helping the patient find a path through life that has purpose and beauty. The deepest and most satisfying purpose includes, yet moves beyond, the personal, because it creates spiritual unfolding and a closer relationship with the Creator.

In this respect, Native American counseling shares many principles with *logotherapy,* a method of psychotherapy founded by Viennese psychiatrist Viktor E. Frankl. Logotherapy regards meaningfulness (*logos* in Greek) as the key to psychological health. Happiness cannot be found through a mere adjustment and adaptation to society or resolution of internal conflicts. Rather, it requires finding meaning and purpose in life. When we can find meaning in past or present suffering, it ceases to be as painful, or at the very least, we are better able to cope with it. Dr. Frankl discovered the principles of logotherapy while a prisoner for three years in Nazi concentration camps. Even in the most horrific conditions, prisoners who found meaning in their lives were protected from despair, suicide, and death.

Sigmund Freud thought that people are primarily motivated by the desire to find pleasure and to avoid the unpleasurable. Frankl discovered that the "will to meaning" is a far stronger power in people's lives. People will choose a path with meaning over a path that is pleasurable or one that has mere survival value. The will to meaning explains why people have always been willing to fight for a noble cause even at risk to their own lives or why people with integrity choose justice over self-gratification. "Creator, whether the path be easy or difficult, pleasurable or painful, I will fear not," says a Dakota friend when he prays.

In his best-selling book *Man's Search for Meaning,* Dr. Frankl explores deep existential questions that are rarely asked in other works on psychology. How does a psychologist respond to a patient who is ready to consider not only the meaning of his or her own life but the meaning of life itself? Dr. Frankl writes:

> *We needed to stop asking about the meaning of life, and instead to think of ourselves as those who were being questioned by life—daily and hourly. Our answer must consist, not in talk and meditation, but in right action and in right conduct. Life ultimately means taking the responsibility to find the right answer to its problems and to fulfill the tasks which it constantly sets for each individual.*[8]

Dr. Frankl coincidentally repeats the indigenous philosophy that life assigns every person his or her own specific mission to fulfill. And although he says that we need to stop asking about "the meaning of life," he, paradoxically, also supports the idea that an "ultimate meaning" exists. This greater meaning, however, is not one that can be understood with words. Like Native elders, Dr. Frankl says that it exceeds human intellectual capacity and is far deeper than logic. *Logos,* for the Greeks, meant not only "meaning" but "mystery."

WHAT MAKES LIFE SEEM MEANINGLESS?

— NEGATIVE THINKING —

The chief reason that people lose a sense of meaning and purpose is that they succumb to negative thinking. "No evil sorcerer can do as much harm to you as you can do to yourself," says Nu-chah-nulth healer Johnny Moses. In Rolling Thunder's lectures, his constant refrain to the audience was "Pollution begins in the mind. If you don't change your thinking, you're not going to change yourself or the world." In camp, if a turkey buzzard passed overhead, Rolling Thunder was quick to warn us, "Watch what you're thinking!" A buzzard could empower negative thoughts and make them more likely to come true. When someone speaks in a negative way, the Diné say, *Doo'ájíniidah,* "Don't talk that way!" Instead, people should encourage healing by *Hózhooji Nitsihakees* and *Hózhooji Saad,* thinking and talking in a positive way, or, more literally, "in the Beauty Way." The expectation of negative events can create those events. Our beliefs may become self-fulfilling prophecies.[9]

Negative expectations, called *nocebos* in medicine, can affect physical health, creating illness in one's own body or someone else's. Robert A. Hahn, Ph.D., M.P.H., an epidemiologist at the Centers for Disease Control and Prevention in Atlanta, Georgia, writes in the *Journal of the American Medical Association*, "Nocebos are causal in the same way that commonly recognized pathogens are—cigarette smoke of lung cancer and the tubercle bacillus of tuberculosis. They increase the likelihood that sickness . . . will come true."[10] Hahn cites a study in which surgical patients were randomly divided into two groups. In the control group, anesthetists visited the patients briefly the night before surgery; they were cool and "professional," performing their duties without displaying emotion. In the experimental group, the anesthetists were warm and compassionate. "Patients in the experimental group required half as much pain medication and were released 2–6 days earlier than controls."[11]

A healer's negative thoughts, words, or actions can have dire health consequences. Poor prognoses pronounced by an authoritative figure may hex a patient into believing and fulfilling them. Even nonverbal suggestions of negative outcomes can adversely affect treatment. An extraordinary example of the power of nocebo is illustrated by an article published in 1936 in the Indian medical journal *Archives of Neurology and Psychiatry.*[12] Indian prison authorities gave a Hindu physician permission to conduct a gruesome experiment. He asked a healthy young man, who had been sentenced to death by hanging, if he would instead allow himself to be painlessly bled to death. The prisoner agreed. He was strapped to a bed and blindfolded. Unknown to him, a vessel of water was placed on each of the four bedposts and set to drip into basins on the floor. The doctor then scratched him superficially on his arms and legs. Everything was set up to convey the impression that the man was dying. The water began to drip, quickly at first, and then more and more slowly, accompanied by the doctor's gradually lowering tone of voice. The prisoner grew progressively weaker. When the last drop of water fell into the basin, the room became cold and silent. The prisoner was dead, killed by the power of imagination and expectation.

Our thoughts affect more than our physical health. They can influence our quality of life, the kinds of experiences we have, or the people around us. When you are mistrusting, people are more likely to act untrustworthy. Conversely, even scoundrels may demonstrate a shred of goodness if you look through their shells and expect decent behavior. I am not suggesting that you let down your defenses in situations that are potentially dangerous. A mugger is not likely to be transformed by your kind intent. However, the mugger may be less likely to pick you out as a victim if you are not expecting to be one!

From the Native American viewpoint, even positive expectations can have undesirable consequences, not only because they become unrealistic fantasies but because thinking too much about the future may actually change it. Time does not exist in the Spirit World. Destructive or confounding spirits may wait in the future to foil planned-for events. Have you ever noticed that the more carefully you plan, the more likely it is that something will go wrong? No need to be paranoid; the world is not against you. The spirits are simply upholding Murphy's law: whatever can go wrong will go wrong (for example, your line at the supermarket is slowest when you are in a hurry). This does not mean that you should give up goals. Have noble goals, but devote your attention to the here and now. A goal must be realized now, step by step, or it will not be realized at all.

— DENIAL AND FALSE POSITIVE THINKING —

The subtlest form of negative thinking is what might be called "false positive thinking," when we hide our problems from others, and sometimes from ourselves, behind a smile. Though we may hate to admit it, human beings have an extraordinary ability to delude themselves. Sad people can convince themselves that they are happy and drop the pretense only during their most private moments or in their dreams. Additionally, if a person has repressed his problems, he can influence others negatively even if his words and actions seem positive. I am reminded of a story about Carl G. Jung that I heard from mythologist Joseph Campbell. Jung was once astonished to discover a patient in *perfect* psychological health. Though Campbell did not mention it, I imagine that the patient had entered therapy for personal insight rather than to solve a problem. He seemed to be a fully aware and balanced individual, with no worries or difficulties: a man without a *shadow,* Jung's term for the hidden, repressed, or "dark" side of the personality. But then Jung met the man's wife, a woman who seemed anxious and deeply troubled. He realized that the two fit together like two sides of one consciousness, each unaware that the other existed. Jung's task was to teach each of them how to be whole in themselves.

A basic principle of Native American philosophy is that a spiritual person understands and acknowledges the light and the dark, both sides of human nature. On the Si.Si.Wiss altar, these two sides are represented by two candles. When both candles are lit and thus symbolically honored, they make a whole and brighter human being.

A person who fears his shadow is likely to blame others for faults he is unwilling to face in himself. Or he avoids difficult inner work by developing an inflated self-image and seeking the adulation of students who affirm his grandeur.[13] Native medicine people have little tolerance for this kind of cowardice. Get off your high horse and join the rest of us mortals. "We do not like guruizing," Rolling Thunder used to say.

— NOT EXPRESSING YOUR TRUTH —

The Great Spirit endows each person with special gifts and a mission in life that can be used to promote harmony, beauty, peace, and personal fulfillment. For example, my gifts are being a good parent and a good educator, but my mission is to follow the sacred Way of the Pipe—that is, to honor nature, the spirit powers, and the Great Spirit by living with integrity, courage, and prayer. My former car mechanic, a Christian, used his gifts—impeccable honesty, caring, and attention to detail—to make cars and customers safer, doing work he loved to do. He made the world a better place. No gift from Creator is better or more lofty than any other.

We aren't all born knowing our gifts and mission, however. We must discover them. Native Americans seek to learn theirs through the Vision Quest, dreams, meditation, or other spiritual practices. Hearing the Creator's instructions is sometimes the easy part. Our more difficult task is finding the courage to express and live the truth. The original instructions are too easily crushed, buried, or forgotten under the influence of conventional, authoritarian religion and society's "headucational" systems. Many people embrace values that they know in their hearts are meaningless or false; they prize conformity and put money, prestige, and power over integrity. How tragic when, at the end of life, they realize that they have never really lived. Perhaps we need to ask ourselves periodically, "If I live in this way, will I have regrets when I die? How will my children remember me after I am gone?"[14]

A commitment to follow a spiritual path is not to be undertaken lightly. It carries the responsibility to act in accordance with received spiritual guidance. If we ignore that guidance—if we do not make the offerings, perform the ceremonies, or sing the songs—we can become ill. Spiritual powers, like people, do not like to be taken for granted. If we deliberately turn away from spiritual powers that were previously invited, they may depart, temporarily or permanently, leaving us bereft of their protection, auspiciousness, and life-enhancing gifts. From another equally valid viewpoint, it is possible that these powers or medicines do not so much leave as they become hidden. A medicine that is not honored and expressed rots inside and causes sickness. Indian medicine is not a pill you ingest but a gift you receive, embrace, and then offer back to the Creator.

— SOUL FRAGMENTATION —

A meaningful life can only be realized by someone who has achieved inner stability, centeredness, and wholeness. If you feel inwardly divided by repressed, unresolved, or conflicting feelings or pulled apart by the divergent needs of self, family, and work, then personal satisfaction can be an illusive feeling indeed. Sometimes, the job of the counselor is to mend a fragmented or shattered soul.

From the perspective of Western psychology, painful feelings or memories are repressed and lodged in the unconscious, a hidden aspect of the mind. The goal of the psychotherapist is to bring these submerged and sometimes well-defended areas of the psyche back to consciousness by talking about them with the patient. In her book *Soul Retrieval,* Sandra Ingerman, a practitioner of cross-cultural shamanism, explores a contrasting theory of repression.[15] Ingerman writes that indigenous healers commonly believe that fragmented parts of the self exist not in the mind but in another dimension of reality. The healer's work is to journey to other realities, find the soul-part, and bring it back home. Without this "soul retrieval," other counseling methods such as talk therapy may be ineffective, since the counselor would only be talking to a fragment of the whole person and not to the part that needs to be understood, integrated, and healed.

The healer may bring the soul back using a dream- or vision-inspired method, which will generally include prayer, visualization, special breathing techniques (for example, blowing power into the patient's crown), or physical gestures (laying on of hands). Or a specific tribal ceremony may include elements of soul retrieval, such as the Lushootseed Salish (from the Puget Sound region of Washington State) *Sptadaq,* "Spirit Canoe Healing Ceremony," in which a healer and other tribal members travel to the other reality in a spiritual canoe, to retrieve a patient's guardian powers (*sqlalitut*). Although the healer may not seek or retrieve soul fragments, wholeness and healing are achieved nevertheless, because the guardian powers mend the patient's soul.[16]

Ingerman writes that while in an alternate reality, it is possible to perceive the cause of a patient's fragmentation, and I have also found this to be true. For example, a healer might encounter an adult patient as a five-year-old, the age of the patient's split, and ask him why he is there. Or the healer might notice the symbols of past trauma, such as a room where abuse occurred or an object that was used to inflict harm. It is also possible for a healer to discover positive images during a soul retrieval. The fragment may be a symbol of a person's hopes and dreams or a spiritual power that fled in response to negative thinking.

Louise had suffered from muscular weakness, fatigue, and migraines for most of her life. Shortly after she turned fifty, she also began having sporadic rheumatoidlike inflammation of the joints, accompanied by dyslexia and depression. Her physician diagnosed "chronic fatigue syndrome"[17] and could offer only palliative therapy. Neither anti-inflammatories nor antidepressants afforded her much relief.

Even before I started taking her health history, I sensed that there was a major psychological and spiritual component to her illness. Louise was a strikingly beautiful woman, with penetrating blue eyes and an impish smile. I had the impression that she was a playful child trapped in a seriously diseased adult body. She spoke matter-of-factly of her disease. Yet it was obvious that a lifetime of pain had taken a toll on her self-esteem and self-confidence.

I asked Louise about her childhood. She had been born in France, two years after her mother, a devout Catholic, had given birth to a child out of wedlock. The child, a boy, died at birth. Full of grief and guilt, her mother then decided that if she ever married and had another son, it would be a sign that God had forgiven her. But if her second child was a daughter, she believed this would show that God had not forgiven her sin. She would spend eternity in hell.

As Louise finished telling me the story, I looked into the ever-present spiritual reality and saw that Louise's soul had been rejected from the beginning and had never fully incorporated, as if part of it was still in the before-life. I also saw a deer and knew that it was one of her helping spirits. The deer, who symbolizes flexibility of spirit and recognition of inner beauty, moves gracefully between the ordinary and spiritual realities. She was a significant representation of the power Louise had lost.

I asked Louise to lie on a deer hide to honor and invoke her spirit helper. Then I smudged, prayed, and sang an ancestor-honoring song, a deer-honoring song, and two healing songs. As I sang, her soul appeared to me as a sphere of light trapped in a dark cave. It was completely still and unmoving, in a kind of limbo state. I visualized her soul returning to her body and physically blew the sphere of light into the crown of her head. After the ceremony, I taught her the deer-honoring song and advised that she think of and express gratitude to this helper on a regular basis. During the weeks following the healing, Louise's migraines became less frequent and intense. She began to have more and more energy and stamina. All symptoms of chronic fatigue syndrome were completely gone within a few months and never returned.

Physical trauma may also cause splitting of the self. For several years, I worked extensively with physician-referred head injury patients. Health care providers who know such patients before their accidents commonly say that after the injury, patients are not simply disoriented—they seem no longer "present." Patients themselves may remark, "I am not myself. I don't know who I am." As one of my patients astutely observed, "When the car hit, I think I left my body and still haven't returned." A Native healer might return spiritually to the scene of the accident to trace the lost soul-part to an incorporeal realm and then bring it back with a soul retrieval.

The practice of recovering or freeing lost souls is also found in Taoism, Judaism, and other spiritual traditions throughout the world. Taoism, a Chinese religion that began in the fourth century B.C., incorporates many elements of Chinese shamanism (*wu jiao*), which predates it by thousands of years.[18] Taoists practice rituals called *Chao Hun*, "Calling the Soul," to draw a soul back to the body of a person close to death, and *Pu Du*, "Crossing the Physical Realm to Free Souls," to help the spirits of the dead to move into higher realms. Similarly, some Jewish mystics can heal people close to death by retrieving their souls, either by using their own spiritual power, actually grasping the soul and carrying it back, or by pleading their case in the court of the Almighty. The great eighteenth-century Russian rabbi Israel Baal Shem, the founder of Hasidic Judaism, once healed a young bride who suddenly "died" just before her wedding—falling, perhaps, into a coma. As described in Meyer Levin's *Classic Hassidic Tales,* as the rabbi attempted to heal her, onlookers "saw that he had gone into another world. . . . They knew that the Power was come over him, and that he was no longer among them." The rabbi found the woman's soul in the clutches of the spirit of the groom's dead and jealous ex-wife. When he wrenched her soul away, the bride was immediately restored to health. She recognized Rabbi Israel as the one who had brought her back from "over there."[19]

— SORCERY: THE DARK SIDE OF THE FORCE —

Sorcery, the use of supernatural power with evil or malevolent intent or in socially disapproved ways, has always existed in Native societies. Indeed, all indigenous cultures acknowledge the existence of evil spirits. Native Americans commonly call those who wield dark powers "sorcerers" or "witches" and categorize all of their activities as hexes, curses, or black magic. Native counselors take sorcery very seriously because it can sometimes cause illness, emotional problems, or misfortune.

Medicine people are motivated by "the Good Mind" and gain power by communing with the Great Spirit. Sorcerers, by contrast, are driven by anger, jealousy, lust, and other negative emotions or thoughts and are influenced by evil spirits. The Cree, for example, say that medicine people have a close relationship with *Kitchi Manitou,* "the Good Spirit," who is the master of life and creator of the universe, while sorcerers are under the influence of *Matchi Manitou,* "the Evil Spirit," who is the master of destruction and death. Medicine people are dedicated to healing and balance. Sorcerers, like the housemate of Bob I described earlier, cause harm, inflict disease, even death, or they manipulate events or people for their own selfish ends. Under their influence, a person may become depressed, lose hope and meaning, or behave self-destructively. The most powerful sorcerers may even steal or trap a victim's soul.

All indigenous languages contain terms for sorcerers. The Cherokee distinguish *didahnvwisgi,* "healers," from *didahnesesgi,* "one who puts in or draws out," a phrase that implies manipulation of a victim's life energy by either putting in intrusive forces or taking out spiritual power. Similarly, among the Tlingit of southeastern Alaska, the medicine person (*íxt'*) is contrasted with the *nukws'aatí,* "master of sickness," or *neekws'aatí,* "master of pain." In Hawai'i, *kahuna ha* use love (*aloha*) and spirit (*ha*) to heal, whereas *kahuna 'ana'ana* pray people to death. In Central and South America, a distinction is made between *curanderos,* "curers," and *brujos,* "sorcerers," who, for a fee, will attempt to manipulate or harm others.

In the *Code of Handsome Lake,* the ethical teachings of the eighteenth-century Seneca holy man, an entire section is devoted to the dangers of sorcery. Sorcery (*góhtgon*) is described as an "evil practice" that cuts short the number of days given to each person by Creator. I have personally seen far too many examples of sorcery among my patients or while living with Native peoples. I know a Native elder who was given a small piece of bone by a man who claimed to be a traditional healer but who turned out to be a sorcerer. The bone mysteriously disappeared from the elder's medicine pouch and, she believes, entered her body. She passed on from bone cancer six months later. A *kahuna 'ana'ana* was jealous of the popularity and prestige of another elder. Four days after sending him an envelope with a match and an unidentifiable herb, the *kahuna*'s home caught fire. The elder's spiritual "protections" were too strong, and the sorcerer's medicine backfired.

In the 1980s, I was working with a Mexican *curandera,* Marta, who was studying my methods of Native American medicine. She frequently brought her Mexican-American clients to my office, and their concerns taught me a great deal about why some people seek sorcerers. One patient, "Guillermo," a sixty-year-old man recently arrived in the United States from Mexico, professed his love for a twenty-year-old Cuban woman. The problem was the young woman's girlfriend, who disliked Guillermo and kept telling her friend to keep away from him. Guillermo pulled out a fifty-dollar bill and said, "I know that your medicine is powerful. Can you give me the power to seduce my girlfriend, and can you hex my girlfriend's friend?" Guillermo was upset when I refused the money and gently reprimanded him, "A *curandero,* unlike a *brujo,* is never allowed to interfere with another person's fate. All I can do is pray for you. I will ask God to give you self-understanding and the wisdom to make the right decisions in your life." Guillermo, and other clients like him, taught me that people seek sorcerers out of greed, envy, jealousy, and a narcissistic belief that people should be molded according to their wishes or punished for disobeying.

Ethical issues aside, there is scientific evidence that suggests that sorcery works. The mind-body connection goes both ways. Some of the most prestigious medical journals have reported examples of death or cure by nonphysical means. The famed physiologist Walter B. Cannon, writing in *Psychosomatic Medicine*,[20] says that "voodoo death" may be real, although he attributes its power to psychological factors, such as terror and expectation, rather than to the intercession of supernatural forces. If the victim believes that he is doomed, and if family members, friends, and associates share this belief, death may occur within a few days of a hex.

In 1981, the *Journal of the American Medical Association* printed an article that described a twenty-eight-year-old Filipino-American woman who had suffered from systemic lupus erythematosus, a serious and incurable immune system disorder that produces weakness, anemia, and inflammation of the internal organs.[21] Her doctors placed her on various medications to control the symptoms, but when they decided to switch her to a high-dosage, more potent medication, she elected instead to return to the Philippine village of her birth. There, the woman met a spiritual healer who removed a curse that had been placed on her by a previous suitor. Three weeks later, she returned to the United States, where skeptical physicians observed a miraculous change in her health: she was "normal." Although she declined any medication, she was no longer weak, the inflammation was gone, and, twenty-three months later, she was able to give birth to a healthy girl. Dr. Larry Dossey, executive editor of *Alternative Therapies in Health and Medicine,* documents considerable scientific evidence for the damaging effects of hexing and negative prayer in his book *Be Careful What You Pray For . . . You Just Might Get It.*[22]

Not only science but courts of law are also starting to look at the evidence. In 1995, a nineteen-year-old Native Canadian man got into a fight with a *bearwalker,* another word for sorcerer, and used a ceremonial walrus bone to bludgeon him to death. Judge Richard Trainor of the Ontario Court accepted testimony that the slain man was believed to be an evil spirit. Indeed, the man had once boasted about learning "bad medicine" from a woman in the Northwest Territories. Based on the evidence, the judge ruled that the killing was an act of self-defense, and the defendant was acquitted. "I accept the evidence of native spirituality as being a sincerely held belief," Judge Trainor said. "The accused was aware of the victim's propensity for violence, including his reputation for having powers as a bearwalker."[23]

Some sorcery techniques may have evolved from hunting rituals. Hunters call upon their animal spirit guides to help them find their prey and to give them speed, strength, and endurance. Sorcerers use the same technique to hunt human prey. Power objects such as bones and seeds that are used to find game can help a sorcerer find, bait, or procure an enemy's spirit.[24] Most indigenous sorcery practices, including Native American, can be divided into what Filipino *Babay-Lan,* tribal shamans, call *barang* and *paktul. Barang* means that a sorcerer uses ritual and incantations to project a harmful spirit or object, such as a thorn or an insect, into a victim's body. In *paktul,* the sorcerer casts a hex over something that derives from or represents the intended victim—commonly, hair, nail clippings, a drawing, or a photograph.[25] The following story is an example of *paktul.*

Betty, a twenty-five-year-old African-American woman, lived for a few years with a Haitian man who practiced voudun *(commonly known as* voodoo), *an indigenous Caribbean religion. While many* voudun *practitioners are authentic healers who use their gifts in an ethical and helpful way, Betty came to believe that this man was using his power for evil. After he moved out, she felt that he was still trying to pursue her sexually. Though he lived at the other end of town, she often saw him passing by her house. Fearful that she was being stalked, she eventually complained to the police.*

The visits to her neighborhood stopped, but he began frequenting the department store where she worked. He would invariably walk up to her with a question about a piece of merchandise and then begin chanting in a language Betty didn't understand, sometimes switching to English. The only words she ever caught were "You want me. You want me." One day, he dropped some hair clippings on the counter. She recognized the hair as her own and suspected that he had collected it when they were living together. She felt even more frightened by this violation of her privacy.

Betty called me for a Native American counseling session. As she began to tell me her story, I "saw" a large black panther. When she was finished, I asked her, "Does the black panther have anything to do with the Haitian man?" She replied, "Yes, I often saw a panther in my dreams while I was living with him. I think it's his spirit guide." Suddenly, I knew the solution to Betty's problem. I "doctored up" some natural tobacco with prayers and asked her to keep a small pouch of it in her back pocket when she was at work. The next time the man came to her store, she was to drop on the floor a pinch of tobacco from her pocket. The doctored tobacco was an aphrodisiac. The panther would jump out of the man's body and follow the scent, which would lead it down to a muddy, sticky mire. The panther would be stuck there for a few days, during which time her former boyfriend would feel weak and impotent. He would get the message that Betty was not good for his health. Not completely convinced, Betty asked, "What if he leans over the counter and begins chanting again in that strange language?" "Chant back," I told her, "under your breath so he can barely hear you. Chant 'May you find compassion and forgiveness.' Slur the words so that he cannot decipher them."

When I saw Betty again, she reported success. The Haitian man had come to her shop one more time; she did as instructed. She was never bothered by him again.

My indigenous colleagues say that feelings of grievance, lust, envy, or jealousy are the usual motivations for sorcery or seeking a sorcerer's services. A person who feels wronged might want revenge; a person who is envious of another person's power, spouse, material possessions, or status or station in life might want to take these things. As much as I dislike generalizations, there may be some truth to the widely held Native American belief that every race has cultural strengths and weaknesses. The strength of the white race is intellect; its fault, greed. The strength of the red race is earth-connection and earth-wisdom; its weakness, jealousy. According to Annemarie Shimony, author of "Eastern Woodlands: Iroquois of Six Nations," in Deward E. Walker Jr.'s text *Witchcraft and Sorcery of the American Native Peoples,* "[w]itchcraft is believed to be motivated primarily by 'jealousy.' . . . consistently the overt responses from *every* informant"[26] (italics in original). Grandfather Fools Crow wisely advised, "Never bad mouth anybody. Never be envious or jealous of anybody; if you are, you won't be on the right road yourself, because all roads are good."[27]

The Buddha also observed that envy is a major cause of human suffering. According to the "Four Noble Truths"[28] that are the foundation of Buddhist teachings, suffering is caused by self-centered desire, defined as not wanting what one has or wanting what one does not have. Contentment and tranquillity bring relief from suffering. Native Americans add to this profound wisdom their philosophy that contentment or meaning depends on connection and relatedness, and relatedness is found by living close to nature and seeking balance and purpose through Vision.

When I was in my thirties, I experienced the power of sorcery firsthand. One day, I received a threatening phone call and letter from an angry young man who claimed to be Native American, though he would not tell me his name, his nation, or the elder or spiritual adviser (I should have said, "sorcerer") who supported his words. He let me know that I was on his "list." "We will put a stop to you," he threatened. "We do not like non-Indians practicing our ways." If I was as ornery then as I am now, I might have said, "Well, you worship the Great Spirit in your way, and I'll worship him in his!" Instead, I called two trusted Native elders, who confirmed that sorcerers were trying to hex me. They "saw" it. "People are jealous," they warned.

Hexes, like conventional antigens, cannot take hold unless a person's immune system is weak and vulnerable, as mine certainly was at the time. I was under unusual emotional stress for several reasons. I had recently moved to a smaller house and had had to put many possessions in storage. I was in an ambivalent romantic relationship, more out of fear of loneliness than a sense of nurturing connection. And I was broke: it is not easy to maintain peace of mind when you are living on poverty income. Just when I needed it most, I was not praying or doing my spiritual practice as regularly as usual.

Yet I did not believe that a curse could affect me unless I let it. I dismissed any nagging concern I may have felt as irrational. Certainly, no sorcerer could cause harm if one didn't fear or believe in their power.

A few weeks later, while on a scheduled lecture tour, I had an unexpected and frightening dream. I dreamed that a spider was inside my body, near my hips and crawling gradually upward. Within days, I began experiencing pain and pressure in my chest, shortness of breath, and extreme fatigue. I had a moderate fever. My hip muscles began to spasm, sending shooting pains through my lower back and legs. I woke each night from my fitful sleep with an ominous feeling. After a week of this, I canceled my other lectures and made reservations on the next flight home.

My doctor placed me on a broad-spectrum antibiotic and ordered an echocardiogram (ultrasound diagnosis) at the hospital. The echocardiogram revealed an enlarged left ventricle, a thickening of the heart valve leaflets, and "mitral regurgitation"—blood leakage into the heart's upper chamber, the atrium, caused when the valve fails to close completely. My blood pressure was also dangerously elevated. I tried to ignore the hip pain, as did my doctor, because it was not life-threatening. My doctor wanted to do further, more invasive, testing to rule out infection or diseased inflammation of the heart valve, which I—probably unwisely—declined. (It was not until several years later that the source of my hip pain was known. Doctors determined that my hip joints had been seriously damaged by bacteria, probably migrating from the heart. I had probably had an infection of the mitral valve and was lucky to be alive.)

The day after I got the echocardiogram results, Joani, a friend and mask maker trained in African spirituality, called me. Even though I was supposed to be on tour, she knew from a dream that I was ill and at home. In her dream, an owl grabbed my heart in its talons, took two bites, and began to fly to the North, the direction of death and rebirth. I understood that unless I took immediate action, my condition could worsen. In my own waking dreams, I saw that the owl would arrive at the North in four days, suggesting I might only have four days left to live.

I called together a group of both Native and non-Native friends and asked them for help. Joani led the ceremony according to my instructions. The group formed a spiritual canoe[29] and traveled on invisible waters to a spiritual world under the ground. There, they found the owl. Joani respectfully asked the owl to spit out the two pieces of my heart and mend it. Then she saw the owl return from the North and place my heart back in my chest. She sealed the wound with tobacco smoke and prayers. The helpers sang healing songs, and we prayed together for healing, spiritual protection, and to express gratitude to the Great Spirit.

Immediately after the healing, I felt relaxed and a bit light-headed. I was so tired that I fell into a deep sleep in the early evening. The next day, my symptoms were gone. I breathed easily, without chest pain or pressure, and my blood pressure had returned to normal. Although I have not returned for an echocardiogram, three physi-

cians have listened carefully to my heart and cannot detect even a click (mitral pro-lapse), let alone any sound of regurgitation. My heart sounds normal: a medical "im-possibility." My hip muscles no longer spasm, although there is still discomfort in the joint. In the decades since these events, my health has continued to improve.

The owl is a common omen of death and transformation, whether naturally oc-curring or invoked by sorcery. Many years after my experience, I found out about an ancient Diné petroglyph near Manuelito on the Arizona–New Mexico border that pictures an owl, representing a hexed person. Lightning, a symbol of spiritual power, is entering the owl's body. Marc Simmons, in *Witchcraft in the Southwest,* speculates that a sorcerer may have used the petroglyph as a malevolent charm—by drawing the lightning, the sorcerer invokes power and projects it to the victim—or as a commemoration of his success.[30] Though the meaning of the owl in Joani's dream was clear, I was still puzzled by the "two bites." Why two? The question was not answered until 1997, when I spoke with Dr. Larry Dossey about my experience. Dossey, who is a brilliant physician, offered an interpretation worthy of any shaman. "The mitral valve is also called the 'bicuspid valve.' Bicuspid means two leaflets. The two bites symbolized and pinpointed the location of your problem."

Not all hexing is conscious or deliberate. People may be hexed by angry, dis-couraging, or unkind thoughts, words, or behavior, especially from those they care about or trust. Native counselors try to undo these common curses by encouraging mutual forgiveness and healing prayer. Michael Harner, Ph.D.—who is an out-standing scholar, practitioner, and teacher of cross-cultural shamanism—says that one of his reasons for teaching shamanism publicly is that many people use shamanic powers unconsciously and irresponsibly. In an interview published in the *American Theosophist,* Harner says, "I submit that not knowing what spiritual dam-age we may do to others in anger is not a good thing; and therefore I think that one of the biggest dangers connected with shamanism is to be ignorant about the un-conscious shamanic abilities we all have."[31] Shamanic knowledge might be danger-ous—it has the potential to heal or to harm—but, says Harner, "ignorance is far more dangerous."

I agree that if people understand the power of the human mind and spirit, they may be more likely to exercise self-control. I do not, however, agree with teaching the details of specific shamanic techniques outside of the context of indigenous cul-ture. After all, the problem is not so much angry thoughts—we can resolve these with the help of a therapist—but rather, the use of spiritual power to project angry thoughts. There are good reasons for keeping certain medicine ways secret.

I am from the old school that believes that powerful techniques should be with-held until a student demonstrates the wisdom and character to use them properly. Explaining to a child the danger of firearms is not the same as giving him a gun to play with. Papa Bray, Hawaiian elder and son of the famed healer David Kaonohiokala Bray, explained to me that students of healing should seek a balance of *mana* and *ike* (pronounced "eekay"). *Mana* means spiritual power; *ike* is spiritual wisdom. If one only has *mana,* it corrupts and does harm. If one only has *ike,* one does not have the power to put one's wisdom to practical use. "If I had to choose one or the other," said Papa Bray, "I would choose *ike.*"

9

— CULTIVATING THE GOOD MIND —
A Counselor's Gardening Tools

The role of the Native American counselor is to offer support (including reassurance and encouragement), meaningful clarification or interpretation of problems, and spiritual advice to help the patient actualize a fuller potential. "Human development (i.e. the actualization of human potential) is optimum human well-being, which is health," wrote the Council of Native American Elders, gathered in 1982 in Alberta, Canada.[1] Traditional counselors have a wide variety of tools to help them accomplish their goals. Spiritual advice may sometimes be very pragmatic and down-to-earth. For example, a counselor may advise an anxious patient to perform a task that requires mental calm and alertness, such as weaving or fishing. Native counselors also use prayer, humor, healing imagery, and talk therapy in their work. Unlike Western psychotherapists, Native counselors do not analyze problems or try to explain behavior in terms of inflexible psychological theories. Although book learning may be helpful—especially when treating serious pathology—the art of counseling, like other Native healing methods, is learned primarily from life experience, visions, and the mentorship of elders.

TALKING FROM THE HEART

On a cold winter evening, a group of people gather at the home of an elder to share songs, prayers, stories, and teachings. The elder greets the guests and asks each one to find a comfortable place to sit in the gradually widening circle. When everyone is settled, the elder smudges the room with sage smoke. Then he says to the woman sitting to his left, "Tell me something about yourself." She states her name and tells whatever part of her life story feels appropriate. No one interrupts her, and when she finishes, the group responds in unison "Aho!," to acknowledge the importance and worth of her words. The process is repeated as each person in the circle speaks in turn.

This "Talking Circle" creates an atmosphere of respect, attentiveness, and intuitive listening that encourages talking from the heart. It is a basic feature of many types of Native American gatherings. It is used in storytelling, healing, and ritual and to welcome and introduce new people to the group, as in the example above. It may be used in any kind of council, including group therapy or problem solving, wherein participants give their opinions about how to solve a personal or community problem.

Depending on the situation, anyone may take a leading role. For example, when I conduct Native American wedding ceremonies, I generally ask the parents to begin the Talking Circle by blessing the bride and groom, followed by each of the guests. The leader of a Talking Circle will usually pass an object—perhaps a stone, a feather, or a piece of driftwood—hand to hand around the circle. Receiving this "sacred microphone" means "Speak your truth." Your speech can be as long as a lengthy prayer or as short as a moment of silence. Each person tries to speak truthfully, directly, and compassionately, in a way that is respectful to other participants. No sermonizing, obsessing, or intellectualizing allowed.

A Native colleague led a beautiful and highly therapeutic variation of the Talking Circle at the start of a ceremony for a young man who was about to receive his first Indian name. A group of approximately fifty Native and non-Native people sat cross-legged on the floor of the young man's house. My colleague spread a small altar cloth in front of him on which he placed various objects, including, strangely, an ordinary ball of string. He picked up the string and, while holding one end of it, let his eyes fall on a man sitting directly across the circle from him. Telling him, "You are a kind and generous man," my colleague then tossed him the ball of string. Then each participant took a turn intuiting and stating something positive about another person in the circle whom they had picked randomly and threw him or her the string. Soon the room was crisscrossed by a spiderweb of good energy. There was no need to lecture on the idea that "We are all related." In that room, the meaning and truth of this statement were obvious. Once we had thus become a caring family, the leader simply said to the young man, "Your name is . . ." Then the string was collected, and the leader performed other ceremonial actions to bless the man.

Native American counselors aim to help people feel good about themselves and to feel comfortable expressing feelings in a positive way. From the standpoint of the Four Winds, these are gifts of the South. The Council of Native American Elders defined the most valuable gift of the South as "the capacity to express feelings openly and freely in ways that do not hurt other beings. . . . To hold in feelings of hurt or anger without being able to release them can be extremely damaging to our physical, emotional, mental and spiritual well-being."[2] The Swinomish Tribal Mental Health Project, a group that provides "culturally enhanced" mental health services to the Swinomish and Upper Skagit tribes of Washington State, holds a similar point of view: one of the qualities associated with mental health is "being able to express a full range of emotions, including sadness, anger, joy and contentment."[3] Blocked, repressed emotions can poison us. Releasing them, we are purified, as surely as when we attend a Sweat Lodge. Tears wash us clean, like bathing in holy water.

Thus, the first "tool" in the Native counselor's medicine bag is encouraging patients to talk from the heart. Often, the simple act of expressing oneself breaks obsessive thinking and behavior patterns. Sometimes, our problems continue to plague us not because we haven't thought about them enough but because we think about them entirely too much, getting stuck in a fixed way of perceiving and understanding.

CONFESSION AND PRAYER

Confession and prayer are closely related. A person who confesses misdeeds to himself or others has an easier time praying: the words flow effortlessly. Creator is also more likely to listen to a person who is humble enough to admit frailties.

Although Native Americans are very hesitant to criticize one another, because to do so implies moral superiority, self-criticism in the form of personal confession and "owning up" to one's faults or misdeeds is considered cleansing for the soul. It releases guilt and shame, two of the most poisonous emotions to hold inside, and prevents misdeeds from having further negative consequences. Confessing to a medicine person and to those offended is the first step in healing oneself and one's relationship with the community.

In *Boundaries and Passages: Rule and Ritual in Yup'ik Eskimo Oral Tradition,* anthropologist Ann Fienup-Riordan describes how the *angalkut,* or Yup'ik medicine person, begins a healing ceremony by encouraging confession. When a person breaks one of the moral "rules for living," it creates a spiritual opening through which disease can enter the body.

Public confession of misdeeds provided a framework for the social reintegration of the patient into the human community while it cleared away the ritual obstacles that might block recovery. . . . At the same time, the other participants continually expressed their sympathy toward the patient and urged that the consequences of the transgression be mild. Here the power of their minds was believed to affect positively the patient's condition. At the same time, the patient was to think only good thoughts and confess bad ones. Wrong thoughts were as damaging as wrong deeds.[4]

Here, again, we see the importance of "good thoughts." Good thoughts promote ethical behavior, health, and harmony. Native counselors pray for and with the patient, because prayer is the most powerful way of encouraging good thoughts. In *A Good Medicine Collection: Life in Harmony with Nature,* the wise and inspirational author Adolf Hungry Wolf writes:

> *If you make a regular effort at praying—by thinking good thoughts—and you live in an environment that makes you happy, then You will soon find that many of the things you do in your daily life give you good thoughts and can, thus, add strength to your prayers. Your prayers can involve more and more of daily life—by spending more and more of your time doing those things that are good enough to pray about . . . and then all the goodness will make Your Life a Prayer.*[5]

Prayer, for the Native American, is much more than supplication, petitioning, or praising, although it may include these elements. Micmac author Evan T. Pritchard writes in his *No Word for Time: The Way of the Algonquin People* that the Micmac word for prayer, *ahl-soo-tu-my,* means "speaking as one with."[6] It may seem that a Native counselor encourages his patient to pray *to* the Creator or that he prays *to* the Creator *for* the patient's healing. But this is not really correct. A counselor prays and helps the patient pray in communion with the Creator, a process of both speaking and inner listening. Prayer and a prayerful atmosphere help the patient to be honest and direct. A patient is less likely to dodge, hide, or play games with the truth if he or she knows that Creator is listening.

In contrast to the lowered head and soft voice typical of Christian prayer,[7] Native American prayers are recited, chanted, or sung, generally from a proud, upright stance, in a strong and clear voice. Rolling Thunder used to admonish his patients, "Don't whisper when you pray. Are you afraid that God might hear you?" Anishinabe medicine man Kanucas Littlefish's prayer-song "Song to Heal the Body and Spirit," in Pat Moffitt Cook's *Shaman, Jahankri and Néle: Music Healers of Indigenous Cultures,* is typical of the structure and spirit of Native American prayers:

> *Kishi Manitou manshuwan indouwhen*
> *Muquay Manitou manshuwan inniniiquey ininiimish*
> Great Spirit take pity on my relatives
> Bear Spirit take pity on these good women, these good men.[8]

This is more than a simple call for help. The medicine man attracts blessings from the Great Spirit and the healing Bear Spirit by demonstrating humility before them. He also affirms the goodness of his patient and helpers, thereby increasing their happiness and confidence.

One of my favorite prayers comes from Leni-Lenape medicine man Yellow Lark:

Oh Great Spirit, whose voice I hear in the winds and whose breath gives life to all the world, hear me. I am small and weak. I need your strength and wisdom. Let me walk in the beauty of your sunset. Make my hands respectful of the things you have made and my ears sharp to hear your voice. Make me wise so I may understand the things you have taught my people. Let me learn the lessons you have hidden in every leaf and rock. I seek not to be greater than my brothers but to fight my greatest enemy—myself. Make me always ready to come to you with clean hands and straight eyes so when life fades, as the sun sets, may my spirit come to you without shame.

I first learned this prayer from my friend Tom Laughing Bear Heidlebaugh, who learned it from Yellow Lark, his great-grandfather. It has become very popular among Native Americans today and is often attributed to people from other tribes. A prayer like this, once spoken, belongs to humanity.

Beautiful prayers such as the one by Yellow Lark may be admired as literature. Yet there is no Native American prayer book. Only prayers offered spontaneously from the heart and soul are effective in transforming one's own spirit, touching the spiritual powers, and getting results.

MIRTHFUL MEDICINE

A merry heart doeth good like a medicine.
—*Proverbs* 17:22

Native Americans love to laugh. Even during healing ceremonies and counseling sessions, participants sometimes tell jokes. Among the Diné, a baby's first laugh is considered an important first stage in emotional and social development. It is a cause for celebration and gift-giving. In her excellent book *Navajo Lifeways: Contemporary Issues, Ancient Knowledge*, anthropologist Maureen Trudelle Schwarz describes laughter and tears as important expressions of empathy and kinship. "At all subsequent stages of life," writes Schwarz, "the developing Navajo person will continue to express empathy for others through laughter or tears because these are acknowledged as culturally appropriate forms of communication in the Navajo world."[9]

Perhaps you thought that the faces of Native elders are wrinkled because they have been out in the sun too long? It is just as likely that, to paraphrase Mark Twain's famous saying, wrinkles mark the places where smiles have been. It is a terrible mistake to take oneself too seriously. Look at yourself in the mirror or think of your behavior over the past day or two. If you are not laughing, someone should tickle you!

I am not talking about humor as a form of avoidance. Laughing at our troubles as if they weren't important, or masking painful emotions with a joke, is a form of denial. Rather, I recommend the laughter of deeper acceptance and understanding. Painful events need not sink us into depression. They become debilitating because of how we interpret and react to them. An emotionally upsetting event can be a catalyst for positive change if we reinterpret it as:

- A *lesson* that brings new understanding and that need not be repeated
- A *challenge* that spurs one to find new sources of emotional strength and ultimately new and hardier growth
- A *directive* to change or avoid a situation
- *A good reason to laugh*

We laugh when we suddenly see things in a new and unexpected way. *I was recently surprised and delighted to discover that my brain is far more valuable than Einstein's. After all, mine is hardly used!* The ability to see or create comedy requires sympathy for many kinds of people and life situations, and understanding of what makes people tick. A good joke makes people question their assumptions, including the assumed meanings of words and situations.

Two Lakota Indians were visiting New York City for the first time. "I'm hungry," one of them says. "Let's get something to eat." Just then, his friend notices steam rising from an outdoor food stand. "Look, the sign says HOT DOGS. Lila Wasté yelo. This is really good. Imagine being able to eat one of our ceremonial foods so far from home." They each buy a hot dog but are hesitant to take a bite. With a perplexed look, one friend says to the other, "What part of the dog did you get?"

Some of my favorite one-liners are in *The Rez Road Follies,* Anishinabe author Jim Northrup's wise and often humorous reflections on his life and on Indian life in general:

Are you really an Indian?
No, I'm a spirit. I just look real to you.

Do Indians have psychic powers?
I knew you were going to ask me that, I just knew it.

Are you a full-blooded Indian?
No, I'm a pint low, just came from the blood bank.[10]

I also enjoy the bilingual one-liners, a relatively new genre of humor among Native Americans:

In the summer of 2001, I was on my way to visit a medicine man north of Saskatoon, Saskatchewan. My Cree brother, Joseph, was driving. He asked me, "Do you know how we Cree treat our elders?" I replied, "No, tell me." He said, "We Mush-em and we Cook-em." (Mosom means "Grandfather" *in Cree; Kohkom means* "Grandmother.")

Do you know what Lakota people call an enemy?
Un-kola. (Kola means "friend.")

What do they say to a fat person?
Diet-kola.

Laughter teaches us how to make molehills out of mountains—a very important coping skill for people who are ill, in pain, distressed, or persecuted. Psychologist and former president of the American Association for Therapeutic Humor Steven M. Sultanoff, Ph.D., who describes himself as "a recovering serious person," says that humor encourages the mental resilience necessary for lessening the impact of stressors.[11] It is impossible to feel angry, resentful, or afraid and laugh at the same time. Here is a true-life example of how humor helped defuse tension in a potentially tragic situation:

A minister and his Indian friend were traveling on a 747 jet from Edmonton, Alberta, to Chicago. About halfway into the trip, one of the plane's engines went out, forcing the captain to fly at a lower altitude and look for a nearby airport at which to land. Soon, the other engine also began to make strange clinking noises. After a few minutes, the captain announced that they would be making an immediate emergency landing. As everyone assumed the folded-over crash position, the minister called out, "Pray to God. Everyone pray in your own way. He is the only one who can save us now." Immediately, the minister's Indian friend unbuckled his seat belt and stood up. He took off his cowboy hat and, holding it upside down, began to walk down the aisle, pointing it at the passengers. The minister called out, "Steve, what are you doing?" "You told everyone to pray," Steve answered. "I'm passing the collection box." (The passengers lived to tell the story: the plane landed safely at the next airport.)

Research conducted by the U.S. military shows that people with a good sense of humor are often the most likely to survive in dangerous circumstances. They can find hope in apparently hopeless situations, and because humor inspires creativity, they are more likely to find solutions. Military and civilian survival experts know that panic is the mind's worst enemy.

E. Paul Torrence, a consultant for the Air Force Personnel Training and Research Center at Stead Air Force Base, Colorado, found that when 165 subjects were asked to evade capture over a thirty-six-hour period, "those capable of generating humor were significantly less likely to be captured, compared to those who were unresponsive or used aggressive profanity."[12] In *Humor & Health Journal,* Jim Mitchell, Ph.D., chief of psychology for the Air Force Survival School, confirms that "[h]umor boosts our sense of self-efficacy by making threatening situations seem more manageable. . . . It shifts what we monitor and attend to away from potential threats and reasons to be fearful or miserable and focuses our attention on ironic or amusing aspects of the situation."[13]

Unfortunately, the times we need humor the most are often the times when it is most difficult to muster. Psychiatrist and stand-up comedian Clifford Kuhn suggests a "HA, HA, HA Prescription"—humor attitude, humor aptitude, and humor activity—for anyone who would like to develop the healthy humor habit.[14] These categories can also help us better understand Native American humor. I use some poetic license to interpret them below.

Humor attitude is the willingness to lighten up, be playful, and laugh. It is an important prescription for health care providers, who, without making light of a patient's pain, can help their patients wear their pain more lightly. Native counselors demonstrate their humor attitude often. Many years ago, I attended a course in Mexican *curanderismo* at the Boulder School of Massage Therapy in Boulder, Colorado, taught by Curandera Diana Velazquez. After she mentioned her fee for exorcisms, a young man in the class asked, genuinely worried, "What if I cannot afford it?" "Give what you can," she replied. "I don't repossess."

Many Native American tribes recognize the special power and importance of "sacred clowns, contraries, and tricksters," who learn their vocation from a vision, or calling, from spirit. As with clowns everywhere, the primary task of sacred clowns is to get people to laugh and lighten up. They act in unpredictable and unconventional ways in order to help free people from mental rigidity, even during sacred ceremonies or normally serious activities. A Lakota *heyoka,* or contrary, may say "Yes" when he means "No," clean himself with mud, walk backward, attempt to jump into a puddle for a swim, and worship Dog in ways that purge the overly pious of religious stink. The *heyoka* are considered medicine people and frequently also practice counseling. The famous Lakota medicine man Black Elk was a *heyoka.*

When Hopi sacred clowns, *tsukuwimkya,* accost dancers during a sacred ceremony with mockery, caricature, rude behavior, and ritual transgressions (such as asking a ritual leader for a Cadillac and girlfriends), they remind onlookers of their own faults. "The fact that no one, regardless of age or station, is immune from these vignettes of ridicule further strengthens this aspect," writes Barton Wright, former curator of the Museum of Northern Arizona, in his book *Clowns of the Hopi*. Because the clown shows us our flaws and how *not* to behave, "[t]he result is that the clown is the ultimate keeper of tradition."[15]

Humor aptitude is honing your capacity to learn, appreciate, and generate humor by constantly reminding yourself of the humorous perspective. Look for a cartoon of the day and attach it to your refrigerator. Keep a clown nose in your handbag so you can admire yourself in the mirror when life gets tough. Study comedians, watch funny movies, and practice telling jokes. Challenge yourself to tease a smile from the most serious person you know. One of the simplest ways to develop humor aptitude is by making a decision to reflect on funny memories when they are needed. Here is one of my personal favorites and most embarrassing:

Realizing that I couldn't speak accurately about hunter-gatherer cultures without first-hand experience, I asked my Assiniboine friend Marty to take me into the bush. We hired a float plane to take us to a lake in northern Saskatchewan. After landing, we hiked about five miles through the forest, until we came to the edge of a small meadow. The conditions were perfect: a clear sky glowed purple in the sunset, there were relatively few mosquitoes, and the wind was blowing toward us rather than from our backs, which would have carried our scent into the meadow. Marty said we would be certain to spot moose, and within minutes, as if responding to his prophecy, a large buck rustled through the undergrowth directly across from us and then stepped a short distance into the meadow. He was only about fifty feet away from where we stood.

I braced the rifle against my shoulder and steadied my hands. I was quite nervous. I had only shot a .22 before, never a high-caliber hunting rifle, and although I was sure of my aim, I was anxious about the recoil. Already, I was anticipating a sore shoulder. Now here's the embarrassing part. As I ever so gently stepped forward into what I thought would be a more stable stance, my foot touched uneven ground, and I tripped, falling flat on my back. I had the presence of mind to keep the rifle pointed directly up—safely away from my hunting partner—but as I hit the ground, I accidentally squeezed the trigger. At precisely that moment a flock of Canada geese passed overhead, honking. My wild shot had hit one! and it plummeted down, landing on a low pine bough nearby.

The combination of my fall and the gunshot must have startled and confused the moose, who immediately turned and bolted, his antler hitting a large dead spruce that was resting on an overhanging tree limb. The spruce landed on the moose's spine. He crumpled to the ground dead. By this time, I was on my feet, aware that I had initiated some sort of cosmic Indian domino game. I thought that the moose was "playing" dead or hiding—so little did I know about moose behavior. But the story doesn't end here. As the moose fell over, his final death spasm was a tremendous kick that dis-

lodged a rabbit, which was indeed hiding. The rabbit shot toward me like a bullet. I froze in disbelief. It hit me in the chest, and I tumbled head over heels down a small gully just a few paces to my right. When I picked myself up out of the river at its bottom, there was a large trout splashing about in my shirt.

A moose, a goose, a rabbit, and a trout . . . and all without aiming!

The third "HA" is *humor activity,* which means finding practical ways to apply your humorous attitude and aptitude. Create amusing and humorous situations as a way of spreading good medicine and to demonstrate greater acceptance of human foibles. I was once chauffeuring a group of famous artists to an exhibition when someone broke wind. Wishing to assuage the embarrassment of the guilty party, I said, "Thank you. My car was low on gas." Everyone cracked up. Jokes based on biology have universal appeal.

When Native medicine people speak about serious matters—such as personal or planetary illness—they sometimes use humor to provide comic relief. I have personally found that sacred teachings spiced with humor are also more easily remembered. For example, I once heard Johnny Moses tell a story of an Indian grandmother who kept a sacred stone in her medicine bag. She knocked out an attacker by swinging her medicine bag at his head, proving the power of "stone medicine." Every time I wonder why the spiritual path is often so steep and difficult, I remember an elder who said, "You have to reach high for your medicine. Don't gather it close to the ground where the drunks like to piss!"

Nurse Patty Wooten, author of the delightful *Compassionate Laughter: Jest for Your Health,* recommends five ways to find and generate humor:

1. Exaggerate and overstate the problem.
2. Look for irony . . . the difference between how things are and how they should be.
3. Recognize the incongruities and the nonsense of a difficult situation.
4. Learn to play with words.
5. Learn to appreciate SURPRISE![16]

Native American counselors may be interested to know that science has *proved* that humor makes people healthy and happy. (Of course, before science, humor only made people sick and miserable.)

Sustained laughter, the kind that shakes the entire body, helps vibrate away muscular tension and worry. A good belly laugh works the diaphragm muscle to stimulate deeper breathing, improved oxygen delivery to the cells, and a slower respiratory rate. As the body convulses with tension and relaxation, we get a cardiovascular workout, and blood circulation improves. According to humor researcher Dr. William Fry Jr., "twenty seconds of guffawing gives the heart the same workout as three minutes of hard rowing."[17]

Laughter also changes the body's chemistry. It helps to prevent and combat disease by stimulating immune cells, activating T lymphocyte cells and increasing the number and activity of NK (natural killer) cells, both essential in fighting viruses and some types of cancer.[18] Laughter increases the levels of salivary immunoglobulin A (IgA), an antibody that is the body's first line of defense against colds and upper respiratory infections.[19] In 1996, researchers Dr. Stanley Tan and Dr. Lee S. Berk found that people who watched a funny video had higher levels of interferon gamma (IFN), a chemical produced by the natural killer cells that fights parasites and viruses, controls cellular growth, and helps to regulate healthy functioning of the immune system. This effect was still significant twelve hours after watching the video.[20] Laughter has also been found to lower the blood levels of hormones and neurotransmitters associated with stress, hyperactivity, and fight-or-flight response, including cortisol, epinephrine, and dopamine.[21] It increases levels of beta-endorphins, the brain chemicals associated with euphoric or ecstatic moods.[22]

DIAGNOSTIC AND HEALING IMAGERY

Long before Freud or Rorschach, Native American counselors worked with a patient's dream imagery as well as any images he or she might report seeing on natural objects—for example, a human face carved by the elements into a cliff face—to find important diagnostic information. Counselors also teach patients how to work with their own intentionally created mental images to boost self-confidence and improve health. Some healers can use the power of their minds to project their own healing images directly into their patients.

— FIELDS OF THE MIND —

One of the most common Native American methods for gaining insight about oneself or a patient is to gaze at nature, looking for suggestive images. Passing clouds, stones, whirls of tobacco smoke, the dancing shapes in a campfire, any interplay of light and shadow, or the patterns in a waterfall or on the windswept surface of a lake become an amorphous field from which the mind crystallizes distinct and meaningful shapes.[23]

The "mind-field," as I call it, may draw out information from the unconscious, like a blank screen on which a patient projects his or her inner "movies," perhaps seeing a monstrous representation of personal fears or a beautiful dove to symbolize hope. Sometimes, the image is considered a message not from the patient's mind but from the Great Spirit and is thus a source of "objective" and transpersonal guidance. The image *wants* to be found or seen; it is seeking the patient as much as the patient is seeking it.

I once counseled a Native man who had just been released on parole after serving time for assault and battery. I had asked him to bring to his appointment a natural object that was spiritually meaningful to him. He presented me with a palm-sized oblong stone with numerous cracks on its surface. As I held and examined it, Spirit gave me the information I needed. When I suggested that these cracks might be places where his heart had been chipped and hurt during his childhood, he broke down and told me about his abusive parents. Each crack on that stone held a painful memory. At the end of the session, I gave him an "Apache tear," a smooth and round piece of black obsidian, to encourage him to continue seeking wholeness and as a reminder that it is always possible to find light within darkness.

This technique is similar to, but fundamentally quite different from, a tool widely used in Western psychotherapy, the Rorschach test. In the Rorschach test, a patient looks at a series of standardized black-and-white inkblot designs and tells the therapist what he sees. His responses, especially when they fall outside of the "normal" range, may give the therapist clues to the patient's mental functioning, or uncover repressed, painful emotions. It is not uncommon for the therapist to keep the "results" to himself, factoring them into the diagnosis but not sharing them with the patient. Unlike the Rorschach interpreter, the Native American counselor is not looking for any "correct" answer and is working with the patient's own images, not standardized ones. A Native healer would never presume to judge or totally understand a patient's symbols. He or she knows that images may reflect personal or cultural myths and derive from dimensions of reality that transcend the individual. The healer may interpret the mind-field herself, or a patient may interpret it with or without the healer's guidance. It is common for the healer and patient to examine the mind-field at the same time and to discuss its meaning. The images indicate not only the source of illness but the way back to health.

A Cherokee woman named Joyce, who was a sophomore psychology major, called me to arrange a traditional counseling session for help with a recent bout with depression. She had been sleeping poorly, she told me, but otherwise her basic physical health was fine, and she had a satisfying social life. "I just want to understand where this depression is coming from," she pleaded.

I asked Joyce to take a "medicine walk" in the forest the day before our appointment. "Smudge yourself and ask the Creator for guidance and help to find a good direction in life. Then take a walk and allow a rock along the path to find you. You will recognize your rock by your feeling. It will attract your attention or call to your mind in a special way. Before picking up the rock, offer some tobacco in gratitude. Bring the rock to our meeting."

The next day Joyce and I spent some time looking at and discussing her stone. Joyce saw its brown color as a symbol of the earth and a message that she should spend more time in nature. "I also see some kind of bird on the rock," she added. When I asked her, "What kind of bird?" she replied, "An eagle, I think. Yes, it's an eagle." I allowed the eagle to speak through me: "Joyce, I feel that you are in a rut and may be studying psychology out of prior curiosity but are now finding this subject too 'left-brained' and boring. The eagle reminds us that we are always free to choose. There is no track in the sky to follow; all directions are open. Perhaps you can use your spirit eyes in a way that is more fulfilling. Do you have an interest in art?" I knew that I was on target, because Joyce suddenly perked up and her eyes sparkled. She told me that she loved art but had always been warned by her parents that she could never make a living as an artist. "I then thought of studying art therapy, but by the time I'm done studying Freud and statistics, I doubt if I'll have any creativity left." I explained to Joyce that I couldn't tell her what to do, but to continue meditating on and with her stone and perhaps it would give her further clarification.

A few months later, Joyce called me to say that she had switched her major to fine arts. She told me that she felt as though the medicine walk had been the first "step" out of depression. The depression had lifted, and she was feeling optimistic about her future.

To interpret an image, the healer or patient enters a state of mind known as *hypnogogic,* meaning the condition of dreamlike awareness or reverie between waking and dreaming or between the ordinary consensual (and sensual) reality and the spiritual dimension. In this state, the brain slows down from the rapid *beta* brain waves (13–25 hertz, cycles per second), indicating that the mind is racing with thoughts or worries, to the slower *alpha* (8–13 hertz) and *theta* brain waves (4–8 hertz), a state of greater calm and intuitive awareness. During intuition, the unconscious—both hidden recesses of one's own mind and the transcendent powers beyond it—becomes conscious. The unconscious includes aspects of the self beyond conscious knowledge.

One of my favorite historical examples of insight derived from observing natural objects concerns the origin of a revered Absarokee medicine bundle. The following incident took place in approximately 1840, about twenty miles south of Columbus, Montana.

An Absarokee woman, One-Child-Woman, felt depressed and neglected by her husband, Sees-the-Living-Bull. She decided to leave him.

Taking her favorite horse, One-Child-Woman left the Absarokee camp and rode toward the mountains. After a distance, she let her horse free, determined to die on the prairie. One-Child-Woman continued on foot, following the path of a creek up a hill. At the top, she stopped to rest, and a glittering object caught her attention on the ground next to her. It was a stone that nature had carved into what looked to One-Child-Woman like four faces. One was a human face that resembled her husband. It pointed east, the direction of new light. She also saw the faces of a buffalo, an eagle, and a horse. One-Child-Woman sat near the stone and cried.

One-Child-Woman picked up the stone and examined it more closely. She saw the hoofprints of the horse and buffalo, as though these sacred animals had left their tracks across the stone's surface. She carried the stone down the hill, where she discovered a buffalo wallow and some buffalo wool, which she used to wrap the stone. Then, sliding the stone under her dress against her chest, she began a slow walk toward camp.

Along the trail, she met her father, Mad-Bull-Wolf, who, aware of his daughter's difficulties, had been out looking for her. Mad-Bull-Wolf put One-Child-Woman on his horse and took her back to his own tipi. Mad-Bull-Wolf examined the rock and saw that it was a powerful medicine. He told his daughter to pray to the rock, think about its meaning, and return home. He predicted that she would have no more trouble with her husband. He said he would hold the rock for safekeeping.

One-Child-Woman returned to her tipi. When Sees-the-Living-Bull heard about the rock, he took it from his father-in-law's tipi and used it as a good-luck charm during gambling. He had previously lost a great deal of property, but now his luck changed, and he won every time. This made him regret his petty use of the sacred medicine. Following his father-in-law's advice, he took the stone to the mountains to fast and pray. Ethnologist William Wildschut described Sees-the-Living-Bull's experience in his 1927 report *Crow Indian Medicine Bundles:*

> *For three days and nights he fasted in vain. But on the morning of the fourth day he saw a vision. He seemed to waken and saw around him a circle of light. Then he heard a voice telling him that he now possessed a great medicine. He was told to make the stone into a rock medicine bundle, to open that bundle only when the moon was full or when the birds migrated in spring or fall.*[24]

As a result of this vision, Sees-the-Living-Bull's family became happy and affluent. Sees-the-Living-Bull became a pipe carrier, a camp and war-party leader, and a powerful medicine man and prophet.

Any natural phenomenon can be a source of imagery and guidance. Medicine people among many southwestern Pueblo nations use quartz crystals to make both diagnosis and prognosis. A Diné medicine man told Donald Sandner, M.D., former president of the C. G. Jung Institute of San Francisco, "[c]rystal gazing is pretty sure. I just look at the crystal and see what is wrong with the patient."[25] According to Cherokee teachings, quartz crystals are the scales of the great Uktena, a dragon-like creature that once inhabited the sacred lakes in the Southeast, the Cherokee homelands. Crystals retain some of the Uktena's power and must be handled with great care. Some Cherokee healers look for or visualize an image of the patient in the crystal to determine the nature of a disease. For many ancient cultures, the stars are heavenly crystals. Diné stargazers diagnose by looking at stars or at the light of stars reflected in a quartz crystal held in the hand.

Reflective, transparent, or translucent objects are among the most powerful aids to spiritual vision. A healer may make a diagnosis based on images reflected on a lake or seen in a mirror. The powerful Lakota medicine man Brave Buffalo used a four-by-six-inch mirror in an unpainted wooden frame as a diagnostic tool. On the mirror was a drawing of a star and a new, crescent moon. Brave Buffalo told ethnographer Frances Densmore that to diagnose a patient, "I hold this mirror in front of the sick person and see his disease reflected in it; then I can cure the disease."[26] Some healers look at a patient *through* the quartz crystal or smoke. Many years ago, a Kiowa friend gave me a black silk cloth that works in a similar manner. When placed over a patient's body, it reveals disease-causing forces or spirits. I call it my Indian X ray, and like many traditional healing tools, it is inexpensive, lightweight, portable, and causes no harmful side effects.

I met Sam, a Maliseet Indian, whose people are from Maine and New Brunswick, during my book signing at an alternative medicine conference. A few weeks later, he called me to ask for a traditional healing. After offering me a pouch of tobacco, Sam told me his story. He is a forty-five-year-old high school teacher suffering from liposarcoma, a rare and highly malignant cancer of the fat cells and connective tissue. For the past twelve years, Sam has required surgery every one to two years to remove large tumors. His oncologist has recently told Sam that a new tumor, weighing nearly thirty pounds, was squeezing his kidneys and liver. Sam needed another operation, soon. He was terrified.

I smudged Sam with a mixture of sage, cedar, and sweetgrass, then covered him with my black cloth and prayed. Looking through the cloth with both my physical and spiritual eyes, I saw several images at once: I could see a wooden object shaped like a snake. The snake was inside Sam and eating his organs and life energy. My spirit powers informed me that Sam had enemies in the past who wanted to harm him, one of whom had given him the wooden snake. I also saw a group of women around Sam who were singing and praying to the sun. Although Sam had not told me about his life before cancer, as soon as I saw that image, I knew that the women were spiritual healers who had once attempted to heal him of a serious illness. The third image was of a house inside Sam's body. The letter G was inscribed on a wooden pillar of the house. I knew that this image related to a person who had hexed him.

I removed the X-ray cloth. I waved and then slowly coiled a feather fan over his abdomen as I visualized the snake uncoiling and winding around the fan. With a flick of the wrist, I discharged the snake into Divine Light. Then, I held my hands about six inches above Sam's abdomen and moved them slowly through the cancer's energy-field, or "aura," to disperse toxicity and stimulate his immune system. I sang healing songs and prayed for Sam's further release from negative forces.

After the ceremony, Sam and I discussed what we had each experienced. I told Sam about my vision and recommended that if he owned a wooden snake, he discard it. I also felt that he needed to sing and pray to the sun for the power to heal his cancer. I explained to Sam that I had removed the spiritual and energetic components of the illness, but there were still physical imbalances that were best handled by conventional surgery and Western medicine.

Sam said that both during and after the treatment, he felt power flowing through his body and a new confidence about the surgery. He confirmed what I had seen. While living among tribal people in Africa, he was given a carved snake walking stick by a man who vacillated between healing and sorcery and who acted jealous of Sam's education and relative wealth. Although the man had offered the stick as a token of conciliation or even friendship, Sam had never felt comfortable about its presence in his home. Shortly after receiving the gift, he contracted malaria. As he lay in a fever-delirium, a group of African sangoma *(female spiritual healers) whom he trusted sang invocations to the power of the sun. Sam recovered and returned to his reservation in the United States. Here, he had another encounter with a jealous sorcerer, a mixed-blood Native American whose surname was Boisvert. Boisvert means "Greenwood," a name that I knew was related to the G I had seen on the wooden pillar in my vision. Sam had his first bout with liposarcoma a few years later.*

Sam had the surgery and recovered without complication. He was in remarkably good health when I saw him three months later. His cancer went into a three-year remission, the longest since his diagnosis twelve years earlier. In spite of his cancer, Sam maintained an exuberant spirit and found the strength to return to work and to pursue his passionate love of hiking and canoeing. He lived for another eight years.

– DREAMS: AWAKENING THE INNER COUNSELOR –

In the seventeenth century, Father Jacques Frémin, a French Jesuit missionary to the Senecas, declared, "The Iroquois have, properly speaking, only a single Divinity,—the dream. To it they render their submission, and follow all its orders with the utmost exactness. . . . The people think only of that [the dream], they talk about nothing else, and all their cabins are filled with their dreams."[27] Although Father Frémin got it wrong—the Haudenosaunee worship the Great Creator and respect all of his messages, whether from the ordinary or dreaming reality—the statement does reveal how important dreams were and are in Native American culture.

Native American counselors were practicing dream interpretation many millennia before Freud. Like today's psychologists, they recognized that dreams commonly express, in narrative and symbolic form, people's conflicts, fears, hopes, and desires and help them work through the residue of thoughts and emotions that are seeking completion and resolution. Some Native American tribes practiced dream-enactment, in which dream stories were acted out and, if necessary, brought to a positive conclusion. For example, if a person dreamed that he was captured and killed by an enemy, his friends might stage his capture but then free him before he came to harm. Or if he dreamed that his home caught fire, he might build a fire out-doors and then extinguish it. In the West, *dream psychodrama,* role-playing based on dreams, is a feature of several modern and "innovative" schools of psychotherapy, including Virginia Satir's family therapy, Fritz Perls's Gestalt therapy, and Roberto Assigioli's psychosynthesis.

Dreams do not always come from within. They are sometimes visitations from the Spirit World: perhaps the voice or vision of a departed loved one, an ancestor, or a guardian spirit power. There is also a common belief that a person's dreaming soul may wander outside of the body and visit other places, people, or realities. The Zuni say *An Pinanne allu'a,* "His or her breath is wandering," to describe a dreamer. The word *pinanne* means "wind" or "air" and connotes psyche, soul, breath, and life force. Because *pinanne* is not bound by time, the dreamer may experience events in the past, present, or future.[28]

Helen, a white twenty-six-year-old business manager in a large electronics company, was climbing quickly up the corporate ladder, determined to be a millionaire by age thirty. Her stressful lifestyle seemed to collide with the spiritual interests that were buried in her subconscious, but it took an actual collision, a car crash, to slow her down. While driving home from work one day, she skidded onto a patch of ice and was sideswiped by a truck. She suffered multiple injuries—a broken shoulder and collar-bone, whiplash, and a mild concussion; she needed reconstructive surgery to repair her fractured and scarred face.

I saw Helen two years after the accident. A testament to the miracle of Western medicine, she was a beautiful young woman, fully recovered physically, but mentally confused. Helen consulted me in hopes of finding direction in her life. After the accident, Helen realized that she could not return to her previous way of living. Despite her achievements, she had been unhappy. Each accomplishment left her striving for a new goal. She realized that she couldn't remember a time when she felt relaxed and content in herself or with what she was doing. Like Joyce, the client mentioned earlier, Helen was looking for meaning and purpose in life.

I suggested a regular practice of "entering the silence," so her mind could be empty and clear enough to recognize guidance when it came. A few months after she began meditating, she had a powerful dream. Helen saw herself in a meadow, where she met a great brown bear. The bear asked her to stand with him inside a circle of stones that she knew was a place where people or spirits held council. The bear gazed steadily into

Helen's eyes for a few powerful moments and then moved to the center of the circle, where he traced four claw marks on the ground, moving from the center to the perimeter in each of the four directions. At the same time, Helen saw flashes of purple-colored lightning illuminating distant mountains, although she couldn't tell for certain whether it was the lightning that was purple or the mountains. Then the bear looked again at Helen and gave her a translucent green crystal. Helen woke up.

Helen realized that she wanted to learn more about healing, perhaps to help other car accident victims or recovering workaholics. The bear, the lightning, and the green stone became important healing symbols for her, representing her desire to learn about the role of nature and natural bodily or environmental electricity in healing. After the dream, Helen enrolled in a school of natural healing, where she earned a degree in naturopathy. She became a naturopath, using herbs to help balance her patients' life energy, and not long thereafter discovered the "purple mountains" of her vision: the beautiful Maroon Bells near Aspen, Colorado. She returns there each year to hike and camp and for spiritual renewal.

We can classify dreams in two major categories, *personal dreams* and *spiritual or visitation dreams*. Helen's dream fits into both. It resulted from her personal longing for a more spiritual way of life. It was also a visitation from the Bear Spirit, the symbol of healing and herbal medicine, and prophetic of her future vocation and an actual place that she would visit. It is not uncommon for a spiritual dream to contain prophetic elements, perhaps warning the dreamer of a danger to avoid or advising a path to follow. In the dream world, all of time and space is present. You can "remember" the future as well as the past.

A Native American counselor helps the patient interpret either kind of dream, using the same intuitive skills and psychological insight that are necessary to interpret images on a stone. According to anthropologist Anthony F. C. Wallace's *The Death and Rebirth of the Seneca,* dreams express the wishes of the soul. If these wishes were unclear to the dreamer, he would consult a medicine person, who "diagnosed the wish by free association in reverie, by drinking a bowlful of herb teas while chanting to his guardian spirit, by consulting his guardian spirit in a dream or trance. . . ."[29] Although Wallace was writing about seventeenth-century Seneca culture, these methods are still practiced today by medicine people throughout North America. Sometimes, the counselor seeks the diagnosis and proper therapy by dreaming *for* the patient. With the patient's permission, the healer prays and asks his or her own spirit powers for nighttime guidance.

Counselors may also instruct a patient in methods that create or attract more meaningful dreams or that improve the ability to remember them. For example, dreaming can be enhanced by smudging the bedroom and praying. Simply asking the Creator for help and guidance and saying to yourself "I will remember my dreams tonight" is often the most powerful way to open the dream-door. As we have seen, there is no rigid boundary between dreaming and visioning, and the difference between them may only be a matter of intensity. Thus, the process of seeking powerful dreams resembles the Vision Quest. Many tribes believe that important dreams are most likely to come to people who spend solitary time in nature or during a partial or complete fast. The Western Mono and Yokuts of California sometimes drink tobacco juice before retiring, to induce vomiting and empty the stomach in preparation for dreaming. People commonly observe that eating shortly before going to bed often causes disturbing dreams or nightmares and may account for dreams that hold little personal meaning.

Meaningful dreams often follow purification and spiritual rites, such as the Sweat Lodge or Pipe Ceremony. Native counselors frequently invite their clients to attend these ceremonies with them. Some California tribes practice night bathing in a sacred lagoon, pond, or other body of water as a specific dream-inducing technique. The seeker might bathe two or three times a night for a month or longer. Night bathing attracts the pity of helping spirits and exposes the seeker to the power of nature, the night, and nocturnal spirits. Very important for people today, it breaks the monotony and rigidity of a life ruled by the clock. Not that I would advise an insomniac to practice night bathing or suggest that anyone interrupt normal sleeping patterns on a regular basis. But as an occasional spiritual practice, I have found night bathing to be very powerful indeed. "Dream spirits," the elders say, "don't like regimentation."

Dream interpretation is not the exclusive domain of counselors. Native American people share dreams with friends and family and discuss together how to implement a good message or avoid a potential danger. Native people sometimes pray and meditate on their dreams in order to clarify their meaning. If you have had a powerful spiritual dream, acknowledge it by expressing your gratitude. I like to go outdoors and say out loud to the evening sky, "Thank you!" I live in the mountains, where this is easy to do. But you can find a way to say thank you no matter where you live. Some people like to burn a bit of cedar and send grateful thoughts up with the smoke.

It is important not to brag about your dreams or make a show of knowledge or power. Talking too readily about helping spirits is as dangerous as ignoring their advice. In both instances, the spirits may depart or withdraw their protection and guidance. Some dreams can only be shared with a spouse or close friend. Some dreams are only for the dreamer and must remain secret.

— DISTURBING VISIONS —

Like positive dreams, negative or disturbing dreams may be personal or transpersonal: expressions of the subconscious or visitations from evil spirits. A Native counselor can usually tell whether a "bad" dream is an indication of repressed fears or whether it was caused by a frightening spirit. Both kinds produce a negative psychic energy that must be released to restore happiness. If negative images preoccupy the mind, they may attract evil spirits who, like human bullies, are on the lookout for people who are weak, disempowered, and perceive themselves as victims.

Native American counselors know that recurring nightmares or disturbing dream images can sometimes be talked away. Discussing them unfolds partial or repressed memories and awakens acceptance and forgiveness. Smudging and prayer with the intent to release negativity are also effective in helping to lessen the hold of disturbing images and may make a person more relaxed and comfortable talking about them. Traumatic images may so occupy the mind that they cause fragmentation of the self, necessitating soul retrieval. Or they may have the power of what anthropologists call "harmful intrusions" that must be exorcised with prayer and releasing ceremonies.

When Phil was an army doctor in Vietnam, he was once ambushed by a Vietcong soldier. Seeing Phil walking through the jungle near the U.S. army base camp, the soldier suddenly emerged from behind a tree and held up his rifle to fire. During the second that the soldier hesitated, perhaps because he recognized Phil's medical attire, Phil pulled out his pistol and shot him. For more than thirty years, Phil had been haunted by the image of the man's eyes before he died. In dreams, Phil frequently saw the soldier holding a gun to his wife's head. He woke up terrified, just as the soldier was about to pull the trigger.

I felt that Phil was in desperate need of forgiveness for himself and from the soldier and his family. I told Phil that it was time for him not only to move on with his life but to let go of the soldier, so that he could enter the Spirit World in peace. As I held a shell of smoldering sage, I asked Phil to sprinkle some tobacco on top and pray to God for forgiveness. Then I prayed, "We ask for your pity and forgiveness, Great Creator. May this soldier's spirit be freed to join his ancestors. May the cords that bind Phil to the past be severed and released and be replaced by your light and love. May Phil continue learning his life lessons without this pain and have the strength to walk on with your guidance." After this healing session, the frightful dreams never returned.

I always pray when I discharge a negative image or power. Frequently, I also sing a specific releasing song or chant. I have learned releasing songs from elders in the Northeast and Northwest, and such songs are widespread among Native nations. Counselors who practice "hand doctoring," described in the next chapter, may use their hands to grasp and pull out the intrusive power. "Sucking doctors" use their mouths or a "sucking tube" to suck out and sometimes regurgitate the intrusion.

Both of these methods require special training to prevent the negative power that is released from harming oneself or others.

— THE IMAGE OF HEALTH —

Because the human body is an expression of mind and spirit, a person's dreams, images, and thoughts can have a direct effect on his or her biology. Brain chemicals called neuropeptides allow the mind to communicate directly with the body by bonding with cells and changing how they function. Thus, a positive image can create positive health, and negative images—the kind we see on the evening news—can contribute to illness.

The effectiveness of healing imagery is now well established in Western medical practice. For instance, imagining calm ocean waves can lower blood pressure. An image of warriors piercing and destroying cancer cells can stimulate the immune system. If an arthritis patient imagines that he is polishing and smoothing the femur, he may walk with less pain. The power of imagery is implicit throughout Native American healing. A Si.Si.Wiss healer sings a swan medicine song to invoke the image of a beautiful swan floating on a lake. This song has the power to calm a patient's mind and induce loving compassion. He sings a snowflake song and asks the patient to imagine her problems dissipating as snowflakes fall and melt on the trees or ground. Sometimes, the healer's appearance creates a dreamlike image in the patient's mind that positively affects his or her health. He may wear the hide or mask of an animal and dance, move, or gesture like one.

Native American healers also recognize the power of the mind's images to affect another person's physiology, which psychologists call "transpersonal imagery." If you look at someone in a positive way, he or she is more likely to act positively, not only because of the psychological influence of your expectations but because of the power of your mind to directly influence physical reality. Transpersonal imagery may be combined with self-healing imagery. Some healers imagine a healing power or project it to a patient and ask him or her to also think about or imagine it.

Jack had been in pain for months before his daughter convinced him to see a doctor. He was diagnosed with prostate cancer shortly after his sixtieth birthday. The doctor's words were devastating to him. His own father had died at age sixty-three from complications after cancer surgery. The doctor wanted to perform surgery immediately.

As we discussed his problem, I somehow knew that with a positive outlook and just a little spiritual help, Jack would be OK. As he spoke, I saw four spirit-buffalo surrounding him on all sides. When I told Jack what I saw, he said that one of his fondest childhood memories was traveling with his father to the Black Hills of South Dakota to admire the buffalo. That was all the confirmation I needed. I sang Jack four buffalo songs and sent this spiritual power into him. I told him to go ahead with the surgery. The surgery was successful, and five years later, Jack remained in excellent health.

Healing images have more than symbolic power. They *are* powers. For example, a healer might wave a vulture feather over a patient's cyst. The vulture, a scavenger that consumes dead tissue, symbolically eats the cyst. Yet once invoked by the healer, the Vulture Spirit has a life of its own, and its power does not depend on any-one's imagination. It actually enters the patient's body and consumes the cyst. It is possible that, as Carl G. Jung once suggested, images may act like transformers that change psychic energy into healing powers.[30] Or perhaps the mind tunes in to and calls forth a healing power that already exists in the Spirit World.

Rosa, a twenty-five-year-old Mexican-American, had been working for several years in a large computer firm and was increasingly frustrated and unhappy. She felt that her boss disliked her for no apparent reason, and he prevented her from getting a raise or a promotion. "Nothing instigated the problem," she told me. "It's just bad 'chemistry.' He writes negative evaluations, and when I complain, he makes demeaning comments or tells deliberate lies about me to my coworkers." Rosa had few friends at work. The other employees kept away from her because they wanted to stay on good terms with the manager. Rosa told me that during her childhood, a Mexican curandero *had once helped solve a dispute in her family. She heard that I was like a* curandero. *Could I help?*

I did a healing ceremony for Rosa to boost her self-confidence. During the ceremony, I saw a mountain lion. This image could have been influenced by my knowledge that the puma was a sacred symbol in ancient Mexico. When I asked Rosa if she felt close to or dreamed of a particular animal, she said that she loved cats. I sang a mountain lion song and asked Rosa to imagine herself as a mountain lion. "From now on, when you go to work, be a mountain lion. Be the hunter rather than the victim. It's espe-cially important that you maintain this image and feeling when you are around your boss or when you talk to him. Don't let anyone know about it; the mountain lion is a secretive animal and prefers to remain invisible."

A few weeks later, Rosa told me that everyone's attitude at work had changed. People were friendlier to her. Her boss rarely spoke to her, and when he did, he seemed a bit anxious or frightened. Within a month, Rosa was transferred to another depart-ment and promoted. She was very happy with her new job.

Although Native American imagery interventions tend to rely on the visual sense, the practice of healing "imagery" in both Western and indigenous medicine may in-clude any of the senses. The healer or patient may evoke sights, sounds, smells, feelings, tastes, or kinesthetic perception. Some people find that the most powerful images incorporate all of the senses. In her class notes to psychology students, Saybrook Graduate School professor and pioneering mind-body medicine researcher Jeanne Achterberg, Ph.D., recommends the following key points to develop a healing imagery script for a client:

1. Pacing—don't flood the client with images.
2. In the beginning, base imagery on the client's strongest sensory modality; gradually, over time, incorporate imagery based on other senses.
3. Use your client's images; insert your own only if he or she has none, or has weak or harmful images.
4. Although images are symbolic, the *process* [symbolized by the imagery] must be appropriate to the biology and nature of the problem.
5. To develop effective symbols, consider the client's skills and resources, including hobbies, interests, relationships, and spiritual guides.
6. Use language appropriate to the age, sex, and cultural and socioeconomic status of your client.
7. Stay in communication with the client during and after Guided Imagery. After the session, ask, "What worked? What didn't? What was clear? What was useful?"
8. Symptoms are the best biofeedback [clues about the nature of the problem and the effect of therapy].[31]

Dr. Achterberg's points also apply to anyone who wishes to develop a more effective self-healing imagery script. I would add the following clarification to points 4 and 6:

4. The action symbolized in imagery should be appropriate to the problem. For example, don't pump your immune cells with energy if your problem is an overactive immune system.
6. Use terminology that is personally meaningful.

— ARE HEALERS CRAZY? —

If you are beginning to suspect that Native American healers have active imaginations, you are right. This does not mean that they are losing touch with reality. When the imaginative faculty is an agent of healing, it is not aimless, as in a daydream, but rather is used to create mental images that both represent and evoke spiritual powers. These powers are real, but they are "seen" with the eye of spirit. From the Native American perspective, imagination is a powerful tool for healing and counseling only in the hands of people grounded in tradition and close to the earth. The simpler and quieter a person's mind, the more "real" and effective her images.

Unfortunately, today many people use their imagination to avoid their everyday reality rather than to perceive a deeper one. People who fantasize excessively or who cannot distinguish between the imaginative and material realms are psychotics, not healers. Healers control the imagination; disturbed people are controlled by it. Healers shift in and out of altered realities and expanded states of consciousness at will; people with mental illness are stuck in limited perspectives and fixed self-images.

Native American cultures' strong emphasis on autonomy is a key to understanding the difference between Native American healing and such phenomena as channeling, mediumship, or possession, which may or may not be pathological. The Native healer is in a state of voluntary communion and mystic awareness, not possession. Anthropologist Felicitas D. Goodman hypothesizes that the altered states of consciousness induced by channeling are related to but different from those induced by indigenous rituals. In her unpublished paper "Ritual Body Postures, Channeling, and the Ecstatic Body Trance," Dr. Goodman discusses scientific experiments that document the distinct neurophysiology of these states.

Indigenous mystical experience is characterized by low-frequency, high-amplitude theta brain waves—an indication of mental quiet and focus; decreased blood pressure; an initial increase in pulse followed by a radical decrease; a decrease in stress hormones; and a long-lasting rise in the levels of beta-endorphins (brain chemicals that create euphoria or positive mood). "[T]his finding is consistent with the euphoria reported throughout the literature and from the writings of the mystics." In comparison, during trance channeling, blood pressure dips only at the end of the experience, and the pulse tends to be steady. Blood levels of stress hormones and endorphins are constant but spike at the end of the channeling experience. Brain-wave data was not measurable because of chaotic electrical patterns created by a channeler's body movements. Although this is only preliminary data in need of replication, it does confirm the understanding of many Native Americans, who say that possession is different from invoking and speaking with a spirit. I once asked my medicine teacher, Keetoowah, why Cherokee healers do not practice mediumship or try to incorporate the souls of the deceased. His answer was simple and to the point: "Dead don't make you smart!"

The few Western researchers who have administered psychological tests to traditional Native American healers have confirmed that healers are frequently healthier than average "nonhealer" members of their communities. In the late 1950s, psychiatrist L. Bryce Boyer received a U.S. National Institutes of Mental Health grant to study the interaction of social structures and personality on the Mescalero Apache Reservation in south central New Mexico. When he and associates administered Rorschach tests to Apache medicine people and non–medicine people, results indicated that the medicine people had sharper awareness and greater capacity for humor and were more philosophical. The researchers concluded that medicine people were less neurotic and generally "healthier than their societal co-members."[32] When psychologist Richard Noll compared medicine people's accounts of their experiences with the criteria for mental illness outlined in the third edition of the American Psychiatric Association's *Diagnostic and Statistical Manual,* he found no indication of mental illness.[33] Noll did, however, find evidence that medicine people had "fantasy prone personalities."

How do we reconcile fantasy proneness with my view that healers perceive deeper spiritual truths and multiple levels of reality? It really hinges on how we define *fantasy.* Native healers *are* fantasy-prone if we define *fantasy* as intuitive perception. Native healers are *not* fantasy-prone if, by *fantasy,* we mean a faculty to produce images that delude the mind or that represent reality inaccurately, perhaps for the purpose of escape from unpleasant feelings. For example, there is a quantum difference between a Native healer's "fantasies" of a helping spirit and a person who "fantasizes" a negative outcome every time he encounters a situation similar to a past trauma. The former is an indication of deeper awareness; the latter is a symptom of phobia.

From another viewpoint, I hypothesize that Native healers and the patients who reap the strongest benefits from their interventions are probably high in hypnotizability. This means that they are adept at receiving and using images to change and influence emotions, behavior, and physiology. Hypnotizability does not mean, as is popularly believed, willingness to be controlled by others or gullibility. Because Native people recognize the power of thought and suggestion, they are extremely leery of any attempt at mind control or manipulation aimed at weakening willpower. A person should be open to the power of healing images only when he or she so chooses. This balance that Native Americans strike between healthy skepticism and deliberate openness to suggestion is sometimes a difficult point for non-Indians to grasp. Perhaps philosopher Bishop Berkeley said it best when he commented that excessive credulity and excessive skepticism are both children of "imbecility."

Dr. Ian Wickramaskera, professor of psychology at Saybrook Graduate School and visiting professor of psychiatry and behavioral science at Stanford Medical School, brilliantly analyzed the health benefits of high, but not excessively high, hypnotizability compared to "lows" in a 1998 article published in *Advances in Mind-Body Medicine.*[34] He notes that "low hypnotic ability is a personality feature that contributes to increased risk of organic disease," including higher resting heart rates and longer recovery time after cardiac surgery. "Lows" are characterized by rigid, skeptical, and critical cognitive style and a diminished ability to use feelings and imagination to reinterpret stressful events. They have less ability to feel, recognize, or cope with psychosocial threats than "people who approach their experience with a wider emotional range."

Scientists have discovered that hypnotizability is partially genetic. Is it possible that natural selection eliminated a disproportionate number of "highs" in European society while encouraging them among Native Americans? The intuition and sensitivity of highs were necessary for Native Americans to survive in nature. A hunter who has to *think* about the direction of the wind, the velocity of the arrow, and his distance from the prey misses his mark. On the other hand, European culture's emphasis on intellect, the written word, and both legal and religious codes favors Wickramaskera's lows. Of course, the proportion of highs to lows in any culture results from more than natural selection; society influences which traits will be transmitted to future generations. Imaginative people have always been accepted and honored in Native American society. By contrast, through much of post-Christian European history, spiritual healers or people who were considered too intuitive or imaginative—frequently, women—were shunned, persecuted, or burned at the stake.

10

— MASSAGE AND ENERGY THERAPIES —

THE NEED FOR TOUCH

You don't have to be a licensed massage therapist or a medicine person to practice healing touch. Just patting a person's shoulder or kneading someone's tight back muscles is a universal method of communicating caring and affection that can melt away stress.

Well-intentioned, loving touch begins at birth. It is the primary way that a parent bonds with an infant and expresses love. Infants and toddlers learn about their environment through touch. Numerous studies have shown that children who are touched often and appropriately are healthier, with greater self-confidence and capacity for intimacy, than children who are denied touch. In the old days, Native American parents carried their infants everywhere in a cradleboard, made with soft buckskin attached to a wooden frame. When parents were involved in camp activities, they generally propped the cradleboard upright against a tree or other sturdy object, where the baby could view the proceedings. The cradleboard gave infants a wonderful sense of security and comfort, as though arms were continuing to hold them even when their parents were busy. In addition, the infants' upright position increased curiosity and alertness to the environment. By contrast, in the European cradle, the infant is prone, helpless, and cut off from the activities and life of the community.

Adults do not lose their need for touch. Unfortunately, today many people have denied or repressed it and are unsure how to touch appropriately, with love and respect. In the United States, elementary school teachers are afraid to give their students a hug, lest it be "misinterpreted" as a sexual advance. Psychologists are forbidden by the ethical standards of their profession to hug or touch their clients.

215

(I believe that this rule is only justifiable if the patient has a history of physical abuse.) Surgeons do not hesitate to probe private body parts, yet many consider a healing hug to be unprofessional. Lack of touch reinforces the impersonal nature of Western society and leads to loneliness, alienation, and mistrust. Mariana Caplan summarizes the need for touch beautifully in her book *Untouched: The Need for Genuine Affection in an Impersonal World:* "Touching has to do with the acknowledgment of our shared humanness. It has to do with the recognition of the inherent vulnerability and intense wish for contact that is present in each of us."[1]

"You need at least three hugs a day to remain sane," an indigenous Mexican healer once said to me. This wonderful healer applies her philosophy to the treatment of long-term-care patients in an American psychiatric hospital, where her daily visits include a prescription of herbs, prayer, and healing touch. "Generally, the patients have received every kind of medicine except the most important: the warmth and caring of physical affection. I usually ask the patients, 'When was the last time you were touched?' " Tragically, for most of them, the answer is "a long time ago."

The healer worked with one anorexic and catatonic young man who had not spoken a word in three years. For a week, she spent an hour each day sitting with him by his bed, not talking, just gently cradling his head in her hands. At the end of that week, he began to speak. The healer's effectiveness in treating serious mental illness astonishes the physicians who refer patients to her in the hospital. Does this mean that psychiatric nurses or other health care providers should hold their patients' heads or hands? Not at all. I believe that touch should be neither encouraged nor forbidden. Rather, as in Native American medicine, its appropriateness may be determined on a case-by-case basis.

NATIVE AMERICAN MASSAGE

Native American healers use massage therapy to correct physical, energetic, and spiritual imbalances and to increase the patient's self-healing power. It is also used to prevent disease by creating an energetic/spiritual field of protection, a semipermeable boundary that allows good influences in and keeps harmful forces out. Massage techniques include kneading; rubbing; pressing (including applying pressure to specific therapeutic points); laying on of hands; physical, symbolic, or energetic removal of harmful forces ("psychic surgery"); and various noncontact healing methods in which the healer holds his or her hands near but not on the body. Native American massage treatment differs from Western massage therapy in that it is never used by itself but is rather supported and enhanced with prayer, song, or ceremony. Sometimes, both healer and patient prepare themselves by fasting, to demonstrate their dedication to the Great Spirit and to clear their bodies of physical and energetic obstructions to healing power.

While not all healers use every massage technique, most healers know and practice some form of massage. Like other practices, massage techniques may be learned from other healers or received directly from waking or sleeping encounters with spirits. In 1935, anthropologist Robert H. Lowie reported that the Absarokee practiced massage with a "stomach kneader," a wooden stick about eighteen inches long that widened into a semicircle on the bottom, which healers would push against a patient's abdomen to treat stomachache. According to Lowie, the stomach kneader was a gift of the Seven Stars of the Pleiades, who taught it to a woman.[2]

Some healers invoke the presence of a helping animal spirit before massaging the patient. It is perhaps the bear or wolf that doctors the patient *through* the healer. The Shoshone *puhagan,* "medicine man," John Trehero derived healing power from frequent dreams of the beaver. The beaver showed Trehero his front paws and taught him how to use their power. "If a person has pain I feel with my hands on him, and that pain comes in my hand. I use my own hands for beaver paws."[3] Bull Lodge (1802–1886), a powerful medicine man of the A'aninin (White Clay People, or Gros Ventre) of Montana, received and renewed his power during yearly visions of the red flicker. To "operate" on tumors, he placed the tip of a red flicker feather on the skin over the tumor, and then, as Bull Lodge imitated the bird's call, the feather entered the body like a knife. Bull Lodge then held the cut open with one hand while his other hand, spiritually transformed into a flicker, reached in to pull out the tumor. He sealed the cut by blowing smoke on it, after which only a small scratch could be seen.[4] Diné "hand-tremblers" locate and treat disease through the gifts of the Gila monster. Some Salish healers from the Pacific Northwest believe that the vibratory power of the bumblebee creates healing energy in the hands. Alaskan Yup'ik hand-healers (*unatelek,* "one with hands") acquire their power from magical worms gathered from a mouse cache. Or in the most subtle forms of healing, a Native healer may project his helper invisibly to a near or distant patient. No obvious physical gestures are required because the spirit does the healing.

Just as Western massage therapists often use oils or lotions, Native American healers massage the body with oils, mineral pigments, raw herbs, or herbal preparations. Bear *grease* (a common Native term for oil derived from bear fat) and buffalo fat are probably the most common indigenous massage oils. Traditionally, Cherokee mothers rubbed a newborn's body with bear grease to bestow strength and health, to toughen the skin, and as a protection against insect bites. (Similarly, the Yup'ik of western Alaska rub the newborn with seal oil to confer health and long life.) I sometimes treat chronic back pain by massaging bear grease directly on a patient's spine. Bear grease can also be combined with beeswax and various herbs to make healing salves. Virgil J. Vogel, author of *American Indian Medicine,* writes that the Pawnee treated digestive disorders by rubbing the abdomen with a mixture of buffalo fat and pulverized wild indigo seeds (*Baptisia bracteata*).[5] Earth pigments such as red ocher mixed with grease are sometimes used as sacred paints to anoint and bless the patient during massage. Earth from a sacred site—coarse and unmixed with fat or other substances—may be lightly rubbed on the body for general well-being or to treat specific disorders.

Many healers rub herbal teas or infusions, herbs steeped but not boiled in water, directly on the skin. Nineteenth-century anthropologist James Mooney documented that Cherokee healers treated rheumatism by reciting a prayer to the directions while blowing breath and rubbing a warm mixture of ferns and roots onto the affected area.[6] To treat jaundice, a Cherokee healer would rub his hands together in wild cherry bark tea. Then, while reciting the appropriate prayer, he massaged the patient's abdomen.[7] In Diné sandpainting rituals (called *'iikááh,* a term that suggests a place where the gods and spiritual forces enter and leave), the patient sits on sanctified images of sacred plants (corn, beans, squash, and tobacco), spirits, clouds, animals, or other objects, drawn with natural pigments on a one- to three-inch-thick bed of sand. The singer-healer summons powerful spirits, the "Holy People," with beautiful, poetic songs. Then, after moistening his hands in herbal medicine, the healer presses his palms on the patient's body. He also presses corresponding areas on his own body. In her book about the Diné *Earth Is My Mother, Sky Is My Father,* Professor Trudy Griffin-Pierce writes, "Thus, the physical contact the patient receives from the singer reinforces the process of identification with the supernaturals, so the patient becomes strong and immune from further harm."[8]

— ENERGY MEDICINE —

Native American massage can be considered a form of *energy medicine,* an important branch of complementary and alternative medicine (CAM). In both Western and indigenous science, energy can be defined as (1) the capacity to act or to cause change from one state to another and (2) usable power such as heat and electricity, or a feeling or perception of power in the body. Energy medicine is concerned with how energies interact with the mind and body to affect health.

One of the early pioneers of energy medicine was Harold Saxton Burr, Ph.D., professor of anatomy at Yale Medical School from 1933 to 1973. Using sensitive voltmeters, Dr. Burr discovered that humans and other living beings emit electric fields that vary according to their state of health and state of mind. He called them L-Fields, "Life Fields," and believed that they were the underlying blueprint of life.[9] During the last quarter of the twentieth century, scientists discovered that healers could intentionally increase the strength of the L-Fields around their bodies or hands. In experiments conducted from 1983 to 1995 by the Menninger Clinic in Topeka, Kansas, when nine spiritual healers—I was one of these—attempted to transmit energy using only the power of their minds (no physical movement), they generated huge voltage spikes on the surface of their skin (measured with an electrode on the ear), in their brains (measured by the electroencephalograph), and on copper panels several feet from their bodies (measured with sensitive electrometers). Unusual voltages were seen among all nine of the healers tested but in none of the six hundred control experiments with "ordinary" untrained subjects.[10]

It is possible that healers transmit powerful electrical signals to their patients, perhaps encoded with loving prayers. The energy can have an effect even if the patient doesn't believe in it. Thousands of experiments in China have proved that healers can use their energy fields to positively influence the health of animals and the number of bacteria or cancer cells in tissue cultures.[11] We can presume that neither the animals nor the microorganisms believe in the healers!

Native American healers speak frequently of "healing energy." They have always understood what today's physicists call particle physics and wave theory, that energy may travel as particles—discrete photonlike units that move beyond the laws of time and space—or in waves, having observed waveforms in currents of wind and water and in wavelike vibrations and resonances produced by the drum. Thomas Buckley, associate professor of anthropology at the University of Massachusetts, writes in his essay "Doing Your Thinking" that in the Yurok language of California, "The Universe, *ki wes'onah,* is energy. It moves against itself and creates waves and these waves go through everything."[12] Native healers can sense the energy of the human body as a field that originates in the soul but that passes through the body, carrying information from both realms, the physical and spiritual. According to Anishinabe philosophy, every person has a unique *cheejauk,* "soul" or "spirit," and *chibowmun,* "aura." In *Ojibway Heritage,* Anishinabe author Basil Johnston writes that a man's aura is "a substance emanating from his 'cheejauk,' through his body by which the state and quality of his inner being was sensed and felt."[13]

Some healers draw on the power of lightning, indisputably an electrical energy. Rolling Thunder described his hands as "two lightning rods" or "poles of a magnet." The Creek healer Bear Heart holds his hands near a patient's body and makes pushing and pulling movements to generate "electrodes within the [patient's] body—the patient can feel energy build up and there is a cleansing of the area that alleviates pain."[14] Even with their eyes closed, patients can often sense a healer's hands as they move over the body. It is very common for a healer's hands to become hot as soon as he or she starts healing, and patients feel the heat penetrating the diseased area.

Native American healers use their hands to transmit life energy, healing power, and spiritual blessing. In the mid–nineteenth century, a Coast Salish medicine woman from the lower Fraser River predicted that her son would someday become a medicine man. As an adult, he described how his mother trained him. One morning when he was three years old, after bathing him in an icy river, "[mother] clothed me with her power; she passed her hands over my body, from head to feet, draping her strength over me to shield and fortify me for the trials that she projected for me later."[15] In the Sunrise Dance, an Apache rite of passage for pubescent girls, the initiate lies on her stomach as an older woman "molds" and sculpts her body to make her healthy, strong, and beautiful. She massages the young woman's legs so that she will be able to walk far, her back so that she will not be bent with age, and her shoulders to give her the strength to carry things for the welfare of her family.

A spiritual healer believes that only God knows what kind of healing technique is required, and only God's power, invoked by or transmitted through the healer, can heal. Native American massage is effective because the body is a creation of Spirit, and it can be re-formed by Spirit at any time.

MASSAGE TREATMENT

Many Native American healers make use of conventional massage techniques—rubbing, squeezing, tapping, and kneading—and individual healers commonly add their own unique methods to this basic repertoire. The methods I present here reflect my own interpretation of tradition based on my training and clinical experience. Over the years, I have found them to be quite effective. Other healers may not describe massage methods in just the same way.

Clothing cannot block the power of Spirit. Unless liniments are applied or the healing is performed in a Sweat Lodge, the patient is almost always fully clothed during massage. The patient may be seated or supine. I know some Native massage therapists who treat their clients on a massage table, but the traditional way is to use Mother Earth as your "table"—perhaps a soft bed of sand or a blanket or an animal hide spread on the ground. In Si.Si.Wiss tradition, a person may sit in proxy for a patient who is not physically present. He or she maintains a meditative link with the patient throughout the healing. In various traditions, either one or any number of healers may treat a patient at the same time. Everyone present is expected to pray and to think good thoughts.

Most of the following techniques are performed with the hands either on the body or near it, at a distance that allows the healer to "tune in" to the patient's energy, generally about six inches away.

— LAYING ON OF HANDS AND "PRESENCE" —

In laying on of hands, the healer places one or both hands lightly on the patient's body, generally on the diseased or painful area. "Presence" is a noncontact method in which the hands don't touch the body and are instead held steady above or on either side of a distressed area. These are the gentlest forms of massage therapy and the ones that can most quickly build a trusting and caring patient-healer relationship. The healer uses her hands to entrain the patient either to the healer's own psychospiritual state or to a divine power that sustains them both. A practitioner of energy medicine might say that the healer's energetic field resonates within the patient, and they begin to vibrate together, as when one tuning fork causes another to vibrate at the same frequency.

To increase their "charge," some Native healers imagine energy moving back and forth, from one hand to the other. The effect seems grounded in a scientific principle: an oscillating current of electricity generates a magnetic field. This treatment is especially appropriate for nervous system disorders and paraplegia. Cherokee healer Keetoowah and I once worked together on a patient who was paralyzed from the waist down. Keetoowah placed his hands on the patient's head while I held his feet. We sang a healing song and, holding our hands perfectly still, sent waves of energy back and forth. He and I could feel the energy moving, and so could the patient! In addition, the patient's legs sweated slightly, a rare occurrence in a paralyzed person. Unfortunately, the treatment did not restore movement.

The Iñupiat medicine people of northern Alaska also use the principle of polarized energy moving between the hands in their healing work. In *The Hands Feel It: Healing and Spirit Presence among a Northern Alaskan People,* anthropologist Edith Turner writes that according to Iñupiat healers, a person who is physically and spiritually balanced has good blood circulation and healthy internal organs. "Normally, when the blood flows well, and when the stomach and organs are in tune, well disposed, well aligned, well positioned, they are able to contain the spirit and maintain it happily."[16] Iñupiat healers can feel the difference between healthy tissue and sick tissue. In order to sense the differences more clearly, they touch healthy and sick areas of the body at the same time. The left hand is placed over a healthy organ while the right hand manipulates the sick, displaced organ into alignment. Turner explains that the hands form a bridge of communication between the two parts of the body—the spirit of one organ "speaks" to the other.

Here, indigenous and Western science are very close indeed. Western medicine agrees that a person becomes ill when internal organs fail to communicate with one another (through appropriate biochemical messengers). Practitioners of the Feldenkrais method, a modern Western system of massage and physical/neurological therapy, also hold sick and healthy parts of the body at the same time so that both practitioner and patient can feel the differences. Healthy body parts can "teach" sick, tense, or misaligned parts how to heal. For example, if a patient's shoulders are stiff and chronically raised, a Feldenkrais practitioner may massage only one shoulder and then let the patient rest for a few minutes to fully experience the difference between the two. Amazingly, the other shoulder often relaxes and drops by itself.

– CIRCLING –

The late-nineteenth-century Cherokee medicine man A'yuⁿini, "Swimmer," advised the following treatment for snakebites: The medicine man recites a Cherokee chant in which the poisonous snake is called "a common frog" in order to lessen its power. At the same time, "Rub tobacco (juice) on the bite for some time, or if there be no tobacco, just rub on saliva once. In rubbing it on, one must go around four times. Go around toward the left and blow four times in a circle."[17] Swimmer explains that snakes coil to the right when resting; by circling in the opposite direction, the healer uncoils the snake and energetically releases its poison.

Circling gestures are common in Native American massage, as the circle is the shape of wholeness, harmony, and balance. Circling a hand on or above the body creates a feeling of harmony and comfort. It can also "unwind" toxic forces and break up stagnant energy that may be at the root of tension, cysts, blood clots, and inflammation. Keetoowah taught me to warm my hands over a ceremonial fire and then, while praying, to circle my palms either on or at a distance from a diseased area. Clockwise circling adds energy and strengthens weak or depleted areas. Counterclockwise circles reduce or remove congestion, fever, infection, and inflammation.[18]

— SWEEPING —

In sweeping, a healer sweeps the patient with the fingertips or, sometimes, the whole hands, in large, rapid strokes, as though brushing away dust and dirt from a garment. The fingers are held a few inches from the patient's body or may be lightly touching the body. Sweeping is used to cleanse the patient of impurities and is also an effective treatment for headaches, lethargy, and pain. When the movements are slow and heavy, as though an energetic projection of the fingers were moving *inside* the body or through an invisible viscous substance surrounding it, then the healer's intent is to strongly discharge an intrusive energy or spirit. Sweeping may be performed over a specific area of the body or in broad gestures, from head to foot.

Sweeping can also be used to brush healing power *into* the body. According to anthropologist Jay Miller's excellent account of the ancient Lushootseed Spirit Canoe Ceremony, after the healers retrieved a patient's lost soul, it was "put back into the proper body, the shaman lightly brushing it into place using both hands with the palms out. As a result, these patients were immediately restored to health, singing and dancing their power songs."[19]

— PULLING, GRASPING, CUPPING, AND TOSSING —

Like slow sweeping, pulling, grasping, cupping, and tossing gestures of the hands are also used to remove disease-causing intrusions. The healer imagines subtle, energetic extensions of her hands reaching into the patient's body or the patient's energy field ("aura"). She grasps, pulls out, or cups harmful forces in her hands and then tosses them away. These gestures are also used in other spiritual healing traditions, such as Philippine psychic surgery and African tribal healing. A Filipino healer, Nonoy, told me that intrusions may "materialize" as feathers, hair, bones, thorns, insects, or flint. In Richard Katz's *Boiling Energy: Community Healing among the Kalahari Kung*, an African tribal healer explains, "I pull little pieces of metal out of my wife's legs and hips, like little pieces of wire. These bits of metal are tying her leg ligaments up."[20] Even if these objects are produced by sleight of hand, they are nevertheless powerful healing symbols that facilitate a cathartic release of disease.

Many of the healing gestures discussed in this chapter are also practiced in the Indian Shaker Church (no relation to the Shakers of the eastern United States), a Christian sect founded in 1882 by the Squaxin spiritual leader John Slocum, in the upper Puget Sound region of Washington State. The Indian Shaker Church combines Christian with Northwest Native American beliefs and practices. At weekly evening prayer meetings, people who are ill or in need of spiritual help are healed by members of the congregation. The "healers" use their hands to sweep, pull, grasp, cup, and toss spiritual power, sometimes with shaking or trembling movements. The services are accompanied by bell ringing, singing, and prayer. Robert H. Ruby, M.D., a physician and history teacher from Moses Lake, Washington, and John A. Brown, professor emeritus of history at Washington's Wenatchee Valley College, describe the Indian Shaker Church rituals in their richly documented book *John Slocum and the Indian Shaker Church*: "[S]everal people gathered around the sick man and slowly brushed him with their hands from head to foot and from foot to head. They passed their hands close to his body without touching. . . . A sharp exclamation announced that one of them had caught the 'disease' in his cupped hands above the patient's head."[21] The disease might then be put in a crock of water and buried. During or after this process, some Shakers clap their hands softly three times, to acknowledge the Holy Trinity's power to release disease. Shakers and northwest tribal healers may also capture disease in their fists and then suddenly open their hands and toss the disease out.

— TREMBLING AND SHAKING —

In Native American massage therapy, shaking and trembling are involuntary vibrations in any part of the body or in the body as a whole that occur when spiritual energy surges. Not all healers shake, but those who do generally shake only when they feel full of healing power, as though "buzzing" with electricity. In response to massage, the patient may also shake or, more rarely, tremble even if the healer is still. I once received a treatment from a Native American healer whose hands vibrated quickly one to two inches back and forth while he slowly swept my arms, legs, and torso with light touch. From my own experience, I can say that shaking "shakes up" a patient's reality and causes a healer's energy to enter more deeply into his body, mind, and spirit. It loosens the patient's hold on the mundane, so that he may join the healer in an alternate spiritual reality.

In his book *Shaking Out the Spirits,* psychologist and shaman Bradford Keeney, Ph.D., notes that shaking gestures are found among indigenous healers throughout the world.[22] The ancient Siberian word *shaman* originally meant a state of spiritual ecstasy and its physical expression through dancing, jumping, twirling, or shaking. African Kung-San (Bushmen) healers shake as they shoot arrows of *num,* "healing power," into their patients. Diné healers known as "hand-tremblers" experience involuntary trembling of their hands or entire arms when they locate and treat disease. Author Thomas Waterman described in his 1922 report to the Smithsonian Institution that Lushootseed healers in the Pacific Northwest "would shake and tremble in every limb."[23] The Indian Shaker Church is named for "the shake" that seizes healers who are "under the Spirit." The shake is a sign that the healer is ready to transmit power and spirit to the patient. According to Ruby and Brown, "Shakers claim to have cured many medical problems, ranging from arthritis to infections and trauma and including respiratory ailments, fevers, cramps, and weakness."[24]

Shaking may announce the arrival of spiritual forces in a place. In the Shaking Tent Ceremony, spirits grab hold of a tipi or other lodge and shake it vigorously when they are ready to give a medicine man a prophecy or information about how to cure a disease. The ceremony is found among the Absarokee, Anishinabe, Assiniboine, Blackfoot, Cree, Innu, Kiowa, Kutenai, Dakota, Tsistsistas, and many other tribes.

Shaking can also occur during other ceremonies, such as the Sweat Lodge or the Sacred Pipe. In 1879, Sir Cecil Denny, one of the original members of the Canadian Mounted Police, and Billy Gladstone, a white Blackfoot-language interpreter, visited a Blackfoot camp on the Red Deer River in Alberta. One evening, they decided to visit a medicine man in his tipi. They entered the tipi and sat down on the ground. The medicine man was smoking a sacred pipe and seemed completely uninterested in them. The visitors sat there for a while until the silence was suddenly broken by the sound of a bell ringing overhead, even though there was no bell anywhere to be seen. Then the tipi began to rock, and one part of it, behind Denny, even lifted off the ground. Ethnographer Claude E. Schaeffer describes the incident in his paper "Blackfoot Shaking Tent": "Commenting upon the number of poles in the lodge structure and the weight of the buffalo hide cover, Denny noted that it seemed nearly impossible to lift one side, for no wind could blow a lodge over. The rocking motion ceased after a time and Sir Cecil went outside to see if anyone had been playing tricks on them, but no one was in sight."[25] When Denny sat back down, the tipi began to rock again, this time even more violently, one side of it lifting several feet in the air. Meanwhile, the medicine man remained unperturbed, perhaps because he had expected this demonstration of power. The two men had seen enough. They left the tipi and the camp, frightened and mystified.

— NATIVE AMERICAN ACUPRESSURE AND ACUPUNCTURE —

Acupressure (pressure applied with the fingers to specific points on the skin in order to relieve pain or to stimulate healing) and acupuncture (puncturing these same points with a needle or some other sharp, pointed object, such as a thorn) have been practiced in China since the seventh century B.C. and in Japan since the sixth century A.D. But Asians may not have been the first acupuncturists. The indigenous peoples of Europe and North America may have practiced acupuncture and acupressure at the same time or first.

On September 21, 1991, two hikers in Austria's Ötztal Alps discovered the frozen body of a 5,300-year-old male hunter. Scientists identified fourteen sets of tattoos on the body of the "Iceman," the majority arranged in vertical lines, from the man's lower back to his feet, which had been made by injecting ash under the skin with a wooden or bone needle. Several of the tattoos were in the shape of crosses on the anklebones and knees. Did the vertical lines mark paths of energy flow, like the Chinese acupuncture meridians? Were the crosses used to mark or locate specific healing points? Was the puncturing process intended as therapy, and were the tattoos a mere side effect? Scientists conjecture that the answer to all three questions may be yes, but no one can be certain.[26]

Scientists agree that the tattoos were not decorative. The Iceman lived during a period of severe cold, and no one would be likely to see the designs under heavy furs. The tattoos appeared over the back, knees, and ankles, areas of the body that, for an arctic hunter, would be especially prone to aching, pain, and inflammation. Radiological and forensic exams showed that the Iceman suffered from arthritis of the neck and hip, and his intestines were infested with whipworms, a parasite that causes abdominal pain and diarrhea. It is remarkable that several of the tattoos cover acupuncture points traditionally used in Chinese medicine for treating arthritis, pain, and stomachache. Max Moser, a physiologist at the University of Graz, Austria, supports the evidence for ancient, indigenous acupuncture. Reporter Josie Glausiusz quotes him in *Discover* magazine: "At the time when Otzi [the Iceman] was around, I'm sure that many shamanistic cultures worldwide might have practiced it."[27]

The Iceman is not the only evidence of primitive acupuncture. A frozen body found in southern Siberia and dated to approximately 400 B.C. also has tattoos along its spine that may mark energy channels and acupoints. I believe that ancient hunter-gatherers, whose senses were sharpened by the challenge of survival, had a sensitivity that is hard for modern people to imagine: they could see and feel subtle energy in the body, and they discovered how acupuncture or other therapies could influence it. Native American healers have practiced acupressure and acupuncture for millennia. Unlike Europeans, however, they never permanently tattooed points on the body, nor did they illustrate them in books like the Chinese. Yet concurrently with the Chinese, they preserved the location of acupuncture points and methods of treating them in oral teachings passed down through the generations.

Archie Sam, a prominent Cherokee healer, told author Thomas Mails that some Cherokee practice acupressure. In his 1988 book *Secret Native American Pathways,* Mails writes, "[I]t appears that the Cherokee used fewer pressure points [than the Chinese] but worked in the same ways."[28] Mails describes how Archie's father, White Tobacco Sam, advised healers to apply pressure in a slow and relaxed manner and never to apply pressure to a spot for more than two minutes at a time. White Tobacco Sam said that "this should be done with utmost gentleness and love." The areas to be massaged would depend on the presenting symptoms. To induce general bodily relaxation, Cherokee healers commonly pressed points on the cheeks, arms, legs, back, and neck.

Native healers also apply heat to points on the skin or to diseased areas. Melvin R. Gilmore reported that Omaha healers would moisten the stem of the shoestring plant (*Amorpha canescens*), place the stem on the patient, and burn it down to the skin.[29] For arthritis, the Cree sometimes roll the birch tree fungus (*Inonotus obliquus,* Latin; *Posakan* or *Wisakecak Omikih,* Cree) into a matchstick shape, place it on the skin over the painful area, and burn it. James Willard Schultz, who lived with the Blackfoot tribe of Montana during the late nineteenth century, wrote that to treat acute pain, "sometimes dried prickly pear thorns are inserted in the flesh, and burned, the thorn being consumed to the very point."[30] According to adopted Blackfoot Adolf Hungry Wolf, the renowned Blackfoot holy man Eagle Plume healed his son's knee injury by pushing a dried rose thorn into his son's leg. "He just put the thorns in my leg and he burned them—they burned right down to the bottom." After a second treatment, "the swelling went right down and I was able to walk."[31] Similar techniques were practiced by the Choctaw, Pima, and Maricopa tribes. Hungry Wolf correctly observes that the procedure seems to be a kind of acupuncture. Indeed, it is advanced acupuncture, similar to the Chinese practice of inserting an acupuncture needle into the skin and then attaching a ball of *moxa* (mugwort) to the other end and burning it. Heat travels down the needle to stimulate healing. Chinese healers sometimes roll the *moxa* into a needle shape and burn it directly on the acupuncture point.

The first time I explained to Rolling Thunder the function of acupuncture and *moxa,* he looked at me incredulously and said, "You mean the Chinese know about that? That's Cherokee medicine."

~ DON'T STEP ON MY FOOT! ~

Observing such techniques, some anthropologists have dismissed Native American acupuncture and acupressure as "counterirritants": step on someone's foot, and his broken finger stops hurting—at least for the moment. Such characterization is notable mainly for the ignorance it reveals of both the positive clinical results of such treatments and the growing body of scientific evidence that supports their efficacy. Both the Chinese and Native American methods illustrate a principle of natural healing found in many cultures throughout the world—including India and Africa: disease causes life energy to become congested or blocked at specific areas of the body, and pressure or heat can open and disperse the blockage.

It may be more reasonable to ask whether these methods work because of the *placebo effect,* the power of positive expectation. I am certain that placebo usually plays some role in healing, and master healers of any persuasion are adept at its induction. Since pressure, heat, and other Native American massage techniques work on nonbelievers and animals, placebo cannot be the only explanation, however. To keep the matter in perspective, we should remember that experiments conducted in the United States during the 1950s demonstrated that mock chest surgeries—the chest cut open but no procedure performed—often healed angina as effectively as the actual surgery.[32] A placebo or counterirritant, perhaps?

BOOSTING THE POWER OF MASSAGE

Just as Western therapists use a wide variety of gadgets to enhance the effects of massage, Native American healers also have various tools. Unlike the tools used in conventional massage therapy—heating pads, muscle vibrators, and infrared or electric stimulators—a Native healer's tools are fueled by the Spirit. They only work when plugged in to the ultimate power source.

~ BREATH ~

Because the breath, like the hands, transmits life energy, Native healers use special breathing techniques before, during, or after massage or in combination with other healing methods to blow away disease or to blow spirit and healing power into the patient. In *Black Elk Lives: Conversations with the Black Elk Family,* Olivia Pourier, granddaughter of the famed Lakota holy man, says that when her grandfather healed people, he "would blow on whatever he was doing." Sometimes, his breath would sound like the hard blowing snort of a horse. "We didn't know if it came from him or if the spirits did it,"[33] Ms. Pourier comments.

The most powerful Tsimshian healers are called "blower shamans" (*swansk halait*), a reference to their ability to concentrate the breath. To blow on or near a patient is to invite the power of the wind to cause motion and dissipate stasis, thus allowing growth and transformation. In the midst of a healing ritual, healers may blow spiritual force to a patient or blow an aura of protection from disease around the patient. In *Midwinter Rites of the Cayuga Long House,* ethnographer F. G. Speck describes the Dark Dance, a ritual practiced by the Cayuga of Ontario, Canada, one of the six nations of the Haudenosaunee Confederacy. It is performed in a private home to cure people of illness and weakness, and as the name suggests, much of it is performed in the dark, with lamps extinguished and house lights off. At the end of the ritual, "The patient may be brought out into the middle of the floor, where the performers dance around him or her while singing six verses of the [Dark Dance] song. They all blow their breath on the patient at intervals as they circle around in the short shuffling step of the dance."[34]

"Sucking doctors" make use of the power of the breath by sucking out intrusive forces and physical toxins—pus from a wound or poison from a snakebite—either by putting the mouth directly on the patient's body or by using a "sucking tube," such as a hollow horn, bone, or plant stem. Some sucking doctors vomit the intrusion into a basin that contains a secret substance that absorbs and neutralizes the harmful power. The contents of the basin are then burned, buried, or otherwise carefully disposed of to prevent toxic energy from being released and harming others. In author Peter M. Knudtson's book *The Wintun Indians of California and Their Neighbors,* noted Wintu healer Flora Jones explains that of the various kinds of Native California healers, sucking doctors are the most powerful. "They cured by extracting minute pathogenic spirit-missiles, or 'pains.' They removed the pains by sucking while in a trance—a procedure that presumably affected local blood flow as well."[35] In Ann Fienup-Riordan's account of Alaskan Yup'ik healing:

> *Along with sucking or lifting illness out of the human body, the* angalkuq *[shaman] might breathe on the affected area. People referred to a person with such power as someone with "strong breath." Angalkuq might combine various healing techniques, drawing the sickness out of a patient's body with their hands and then breathing on their hands to dispel the illness from their own bodies.*[36]

Breath is related to speech and prayer. To speak is to combine thoughts or feelings with sacred breath. In the Pawnee language, *tsiksu,* "throat" or "windpipe," is the stem of the word for thinking and feeling, *-atsiks-.* When we think good thoughts and speak good words, we spread blessings into the wind. When the mind is clouded or confused, we exhale pollution. Healing songs sometimes blend specific breathing methods with words and vocables. Wind-honoring songs from diverse tribes include "whooshing" sounds that imitate a howling wind and evoke the wind's power to dispel impurity. A purification song from the Pacific Northwest is punctuated with exhalations that chase away obstructions to healing. In Philippine psychic healing, a tradition with many parallels to Native American medicine, healers believe that *oraciones*, "prayers," that are not puffed away with a strong exhalation will cause power to stagnate in the mouth and rot the teeth.

— GRANDFATHER FIRE —

The light and warmth of fire—whether from a campfire, a candle, or sunlight—are universal symbols of life energy. Smoke, the visible breath of fire, also represents this power. Methods of using fire include:

Warming the Hands

Some healers prepare for massage therapy by warming their hands over a fire, either an ordinary campfire or a *sacred fire* built with certain kinds of wood and a specific number of kindling pieces and "fed" with ritual offerings, commonly tobacco. Here, we see another interesting parallel with ancient Chinese medicine. Taoist priests from the Longmen sect prepare for noncontact healing by warming their hands over a ceremonial fire in which have been burned talismans, or *fu,* pieces of paper covered with geometric patterns and Chinese ideograms that invoke the gods.[37]

The benefit for the patient is obvious and immediate. Warm hands are comforting, and they enhance relaxation. When they touch the skin, blood vessels dilate, improving circulation and oxygen delivery to the cells. More important, however, warming infuses the hands with the spiritual and life-giving power of fire, enabling the healer to be more effective. Based on the Native principle of "like treats like"—things of a similar nature can influence each other—the healer uses his hands to balance the patient's fire, his energy of life. James Mooney gives a historical example. Cherokee healers believe that toothaches are caused by an "intruder" identified as a worm that has wrapped itself around the tooth. The healer calls upon the Red Spider of the Sunland, the Blue Spider of the North, the Black Spider of the West, and the White Spider above to let down threads to trap and take up the intruder. The healer then recites a prayer to "Ancient White," the ritual name for fire. The healer warms his hands over a fire and presses his thumb against the jaw over the aching tooth, transmitting healing power. The healer may also blow a disinfectant herbal tea on the spot.[38] Equally sophisticated and beautiful hand-warming rituals are found throughout Indian Country.

Lighting Up

Native healers use their hands to wave sunlight or campfire light into the patient, or they may scoop red light from heated Sweat Lodge stones into their hands and then send it to a nearby or distant patient. In the Pacific Northwest, hand-healers draw on the power of fire by waving candlelight into a patient's body, "lighting him up," or by sweeping disease into the candle flame. Patients may also use these methods to heal themselves.

Holding Coals in the Mouth

The medicine of holding coals in the mouth combines the powers of wood, fire, and breath and was given to me by a Kiowa healer. Like surgeons who share new techniques, Native healers share methods with their colleagues. I taught the Kiowa man Cherokee hand doctoring, and he taught me how to place red-hot coals from a sacred fire in my mouth. I blow the heated breath onto sore or diseased spots. The method does not involve any tricks or protective salves in the mouth.

Tsistsistas (Cheyenne) oral history records the existence of ancient shamans who were unharmed by fire. Karl H. Schlesier, Ph.D, an anthroplogy professor who has been a close associate of the Tsistsistas since 1969, writes in his superb book *The Wolves of Heaven,* "During special performances, they [the shamans] ate burning coals, drank boiling soup, and walked through fires with naked feet."[39] Creek healer Bear Heart says, "Our medicine people use live coals—we put them in our mouths and blow on the patient."[40]

"Smoking" the Patient

Smoke is associated with cleansing in cultures throughout the world. The English words *fume* and *fumigate* are related to the Latin *fumus,* "smoke," and *februa,* "cleansing," from which we derive the word *February,* the Roman month of purification. Smoke from a campfire is the most ancient cleansing smudge. I talked about the importance of smudging the healing space in Chapter 5. The Comanche medicine woman Sanapia treated infants for any condition related to the head by placing a white otter fur on live coals and then waving the infant through the smoke. According to author David E. Jones, "This medicine smoke is believed to enter the infant's head, where its curative qualities work their effects."[41] Sanapia learned the technique from a Shoshone woman near Fort Washakie, Wyoming.

The practice of blowing tobacco smoke on a patient is also extremely common and widespread. Anthropologist A. L. Kroeber described how the Maidu Indians of California used smoke in his classic *Handbook of the Indians of California:* "Smoke [from a pipe] is blown on the patient while orders are given to what resides in him to depart. This treatment seems to be particularly favored for headache."[42] Tobacco amplifies the power of the mind and the efficacy of many massage techniques. Some healers use their hands to work on the physical side of disease and tobacco smoke to disperse spiritual and energetic toxins. Because of its power, traditional Native Americans try to avoid negative words or thoughts when they are around tobacco, including cigarettes. I was once sitting in a restaurant with an eccentric Manchurian

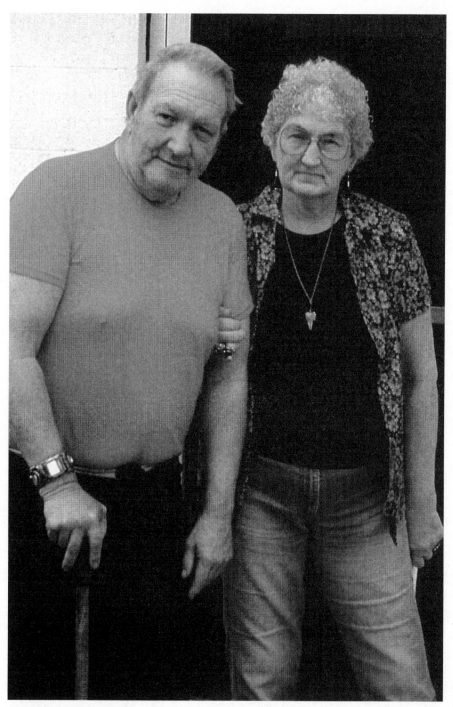

War Eagle and his wife, Helen, 1989.

shaman who picked up his empty plate and fanned it in the direction of some smokers sitting across from us. They probably thought we objected to the smell. He confided, "I can't stand what they're thinking." You will find more information about this versatile healing plant in Chapter 13.

In contrast to other patients described in this book, with War Eagle's permission, I have used his actual name in the following anecdote.

War Eagle, a Cherokee healer and close friend, had been diabetic for many years, and now, at age sixty, he was beginning to experience complications from the disease. He had been diagnosed with congestive heart failure. He had lost a foot due to infection, and recently, his prosthesis caused him so much pain that he was bedridden most of the time. He could only walk with the aid of a walker. Faced with so many serious, debilitating problems, it had become difficult for War Eagle to maintain a positive outlook on life. He requested that I do a healing, not as an attempt to cure his ills but as a way of asking the Great Spirit for a blessing. He knew that the outcome of a healing was always unpredictable.

First, I smudged War Eagle with a mixture of Colorado sage and North Carolina cedar, sacred plants from my home and his. As a helper beat a drum, I sang healing songs and used a noncontact healing technique. I waved my hands to sweep away disease and pulsed my palm rhythmically over his heart to strengthen his heart muscle— a kind of spiritual pacemaker. As I worked, I could see that his physical and emotional heart were both ill.

I lit a sacred pipe and blew tobacco smoke over his body. I told War Eagle that spirits were present and advising him not to dwell in negative thinking, that he needed to pray more frequently and every day to spend at least some part of the morning outside in the sunshine. When the ceremony ended, War Eagle was inspired to stand up. Holding on to the bedpost, he raised a hand to the sky. He prayed in Cherokee to express gratitude to the Creator.

The next day, War Eagle decided to try to meet me at a restaurant for breakfast. He was in good spirits and grateful: his old craving for southern biscuits and gravy had returned! Although this high-fat food was not the best for his heart condition, I knew that it would do his spirit a world of good. I was first to arrive at the restaurant, a spacious dining room in a hotel near War Eagle's home, and was sitting at the table when—with slow, measured steps—War Eagle walked in and sat down. Then it hit him. He had left his car without the walker and was pain-free! The twinkle in his eye that had been missing for years was back. War Eagle asked me if I had ever eaten a Cherokee breakfast in a restaurant. When I said no, he turned to the waitress, who was waiting to take our order, and said, "Give me ham, ram, bear, and beef. Also two bluebirds on toast and persimmon juice." Before the astonished waitress could reply, he said, "OK, I was just kidding. How about biscuits and gravy?"

The pain never returned to its previous levels, and War Eagle was able to walk unassisted for the rest of his life. He succumbed to heart failure two years later.

~ GIFTS FROM THE EARTH ~

Objects from nature, placed on the body or held near it, are sometimes used as massage instruments. To transmit healing energy, the healer may cover the patient with an animal hide, wave a feather at the patient or fan him with an entire wing, paint the patient's face with a natural earth pigment such as red ocher, throw or spray water on the patient, sweep the body with a cedar branch, or rub or place stones or plants on diseased areas. Seminole healers will scratch a patient's arm, deep enough to draw blood, with an eagle claw, a rattlesnake's fang, a thorn, or some other pointed object to improve muscle tone and enhance vitality. To bring relief from lower back pain, they make four light scratches at the base of a patient's spine with a sharp fragment of a turtle shell, similar to methods practiced by indigenous healers from other continents.[43] Among Pacific Northwest tribes, common basalt rocks are lightly rubbed on an infant's skin to confer strength and health. I sometimes warm stones for a few minutes in a fire and then place them on sore muscles to aid relaxation. Many Native healers see stones or other healing tools in their dreams, where they also receive instructions about proper use.

Leslie is a white American accountant and aerobics instructor in her early thirties, and a multiple trauma victim. Three years earlier, she had been thrown twenty feet in the air in a motorcycle accident. Landing on her head, she suffered a severe concussion, a broken leg, and multiple fractures. Then, six months later, while recuperating in a mountain resort, she was struck by lightning. Within that same year, she was a passenger in a car that was rear-ended by a drunk driver. Although the last accident only resulted in a mild whiplash injury, it exacerbated her previous injuries. By the time I met Leslie, she was in severe chronic pain, with daily migraines, frequent bouts of nausea, and insomnia.

Knowing very little about alternative medicine and, predictably, skeptical of its benefits, Leslie was surprised, to say the least, when her neurologist referred her to me. (I had met him while lecturing at a medical conference.) Despite her multiple traumas, when I saw her, she could walk normally, but she seemed to be in a hyperalert state. Leslie claimed to sometimes go twenty-four hours without sleep. In fact, she had not slept for more than three hours straight since the first accident. Once every three or four days, she would experience a frightening narrowing of her field of vision, followed by a period of total blindness and paralysis of the entire right side of her body, usually lasting about an hour. During the rest of the time, she experienced multiple vision, seeing everything in triplicate. Leslie was hopeful and still possessed a sense of humor. "Since there are three of you," she said, "I expect you to be three times more effective with me than with other clients."

With Leslie's permission, I spoke to her physician and various specialists. Her diagnosis was consistent with severe head injury: fibromyalgia, migraine, torn ligaments and tendons on both sides of the neck, the first to fifth cervical vertebrae tilted forward out of alignment, and sporadic left vertebral artery spasms. The latter caused a reduction in cerebral blood flow that may have accounted for the spells of blindness.

Leslie said that since her second accident, painkillers had been ineffective. Her surgeon wanted to fuse four of her cervical vertebrae to immobilize her neck, preventing further degeneration of the vertebrae and probably reducing the pain. She had so far been unwilling to take this extreme step. While she was in treatment with me, she was also seeing a biofeedback therapist, who was trying, unsuccessfully, to teach her to use meditation and visualization to warm her hands. (Biofeedback therapists teach techniques that help patients become aware of and control aspects of their metabolism, such as blood pressure, muscle tension, and skin temperature. Voluntary control over hand temperature can help a patient relax chronically constricted or spasming blood vessels and is often an effective treatment for migraine.)

I decided on four treatment modalities with Leslie, to take place once a week for an undetermined period of time: therapeutic exercises to correct her posture, relieve pain, and strengthen her legs and lower back muscles; noncontact hand healing and healing imagery to further reduce pain, mend damaged tendons, nerves, and bones, and to enhance relaxation and overall health; and traditional healing ceremonies to seek a blessing from the Great Spirit. We began to notice significant improvements after the first session. I held my palms on either side of her cervical and lumbar regions. To Leslie's surprise, she felt warmth rising to her head. She also said that her torso felt relaxed and that she felt that she was breathing abdominally. Leslie returned home and slept for ten hours continuously. *During the second session, I held my hands in front of her face, sending energy directly to her head. Leslie remarked that my hands felt "like a heat lamp, as if I'm lying on a beach in the hot sun, only the warmth goes through my skin into my brain." She also noted, "The pounding in my head is gone." Thereafter, her migraines became less frequent and their pain less intense.*

The real breakthrough came two weeks later, during Leslie's third session. Leslie told me that the evening of the previous session, she had had a frightening experience. After another unusually long and deep sleep, she woke feeling a heavy presence lying over her and squeezing her hands. She felt that it was a bear. The bear was not malevolent, she said. She was frightened only because the experience was so strange. "I just don't believe in visions," she told me. "Or at least, I didn't." Before the image of the bear faded, Leslie saw two letters appear in her mind, A and S. She didn't know what they meant. I suggested that they stood for Arkos, the Greek word for Bear. The Bear is a symbol of healing, and this powerful helper was making herself known, as if to say, "I am here. Do not fear. I will help you." This explanation was very satisfying to Leslie,

*who told me that she loved bears and hoped she would see a real one someday. I re-
minded her that she had already seen one!*

*Taking a cue from her vision, during the following fourth session, I drove Leslie to
a special place in the mountains where bears have been spotted. Spreading a bear hide
on the ground, I asked Leslie to lie down on it. I smudged her with sage and placed
stones on or under her body: thin, flat, and smooth river stones (basalt) under her neck
and each thigh for strength and balance; a North Carolina emerald, for improving vision, on each eyelid; and a large, clear quartz crystal on the ground, with the tip touching the crown of her head. The crystal would transmit healing energy to every cell in
her body. I sang several healing songs and prayed.*

*After the ceremony, Leslie exclaimed, "You are a lot better than Tylenol. My pain is
almost gone, and I am only seeing double rather than triple." I told her that I trusted
she would soon be "seeing single" but not less than that! Leslie had an appointment
with her biofeedback therapist the next day and was able to warm her hands by ten
degrees.*

*Leslie continued to improve during the following six weeks that we met. I am sure
that the other therapists' interventions worked synergistically with mine to create a
greater overall effect. I followed Leslie's case for the next four years. At the end of that
period, she was entirely without pain, headaches, or discomfort and was functioning
normally. Her healing had brought a shift in priorities. Leslie decided not to resume
her previous employment and was training to be a massage therapist.*

Stones are nature's elders; the lines on rough stones are like the wrinkles on the
face of a very old person, each taking perhaps a million years to form. Smooth stones
also show the effects of time; their surfaces were polished by millennia of erosion by
wind or water. When a healer places stones on a patient's body, the patient feels a
deep sense of peace and connection with ancient forces.

Native American, indigenous, and Western mystical traditions[44] recognize that
clear quartz and geologically related crystals such as rose quartz, amethyst, and obsidian have powerful healing effects on both physical and psychological disorders.
Since 1988, neurosurgeon and founder of the American Holistic Medical
Association C. Norman Shealy, M.D., Ph.D., and colleagues have been researching
quartz crystals as an adjunctive therapy for depression. One of their most interesting experiments, entitled "Non-pharmaceutical Treatment of Depression Using a
Multimodal Approach," was reported in the peer-reviewed energy medicine journal
Subtle Energies.[45] Although Dr. Shealy does not mention indigenous therapies that
use quartz crystals, his experiment is highly relevant to understanding how science
validates their efficacy.

Shealy treated 141 chronically depressed patients who had been unresponsive to antidepressant medication in a forty-four-hour program over a two-week period. Therapy included twelve hours of lectures on topics such as stress, exercise, nutrition, and other methods of improving health; two hours each day of listening to relaxing music; daily stimulation of the crown of the head using a minute electrical current (one milliamp or less, shown to raise the levels of the neurotransmitters serotonin and endorphin, important mood regulators);[46] and daily light stimulation to produce harmonious brain waves.[47]

In addition, every day each patient wore either a quartz or lead (glass) crystal in a pouch suspended from the neck. Patients were randomly given either quartz or glass by drawing coded slips from a box. Neither the project director nor the patients knew which kind of stone they received. The patients were instructed to "program" their stones by breathing onto them while thinking of a personal affirmation such as "I am happy and joyous" and to reprogram their stones periodically. Dr. Shealy hypothesized that the holistic "multimodal" approach would reduce depression and that quartz crystal would have a positive effect on mood and be more effective than glass.

After therapy ended, for the following three months, the patients continued listening to music, practicing self-healing meditations, and wearing their crystals. The patients' mental states were measured with standard psychological tests. Blood levels of neurochemicals were measured before and after the two weeks of intensive therapy and again after the three-month follow-up. Results confirmed both of Dr. Shealy's hypotheses. After the initial two weeks, 84 percent of all patients improved, whether they were wearing quartz or glass. After three months, 70 percent of those who wore quartz remained improved, compared to only 31.5 percent of those who wore glass. When subjected to statistical analysis, the probability that the improvement was *not* due to the quartz was less than one chance in one thousand. In the *Subtle Energies* journal article, Dr. Shealy writes, "Actually, no drug has been reported to give 84% of patients improvement in depression within two weeks. Furthermore, the three-month follow-up results in the quartz crystal group are almost twice as good as can be expected with most antidepressants, and without the side effects." In his popular book *Miracles Do Happen,* Dr. Shealy reports that he continues to find significant improvements among depressed patients who use quartz crystals as "reinforcers" of other therapies.

In Native American medicine, quartz has a wide range of healing properties. Being clear and capable of refracting all colors of the rainbow, it can, according to the healer's intent, act like any colored stone. Quartz can stimulate like the ruby or calm like the aquamarine. It also amplifies the power of affirmations and, perhaps for this reason, was effective in Dr. Shealy's experiments.[48]

MORE MIRACLE CURES: A WORD ABOUT THE EFFICACY OF NATIVE MASSAGE TECHNIQUES

Leslie's story is fascinating because of the extent of her injuries and the rapidity of the cure, but I have had many other clients who experienced similarly dramatic improvements. For example, a fifty-year-old airline pilot, Jay, once attended a Si.Si.Wiss healing ceremony in which several people prayed and did laying on of hands simultaneously. I was both the "orchestra leader" in this ceremony, meaning I supervised and coordinated the actions of participants, and one of the healers. None of the healers was aware that Jay had a medical condition, nor of the ceremony's effect, until I met Jay in a grocery store two years later. Jay told me that five years before the ceremony, he had been in a car accident that had herniated two lumbar spinal discs and left him with continuous radiating pain. Since the ceremony, he had been pain-free. He remained asymptomatic during the eight years that I followed his case.

When we analyze the efficacy of a treatment, we must consider the natural course of the disease. Would time have healed it? Was the disease already in remission or likely to go into remission? If so, did the intervention accelerate the expected rate of healing? Musculoskeletal conditions, such as Jay's and Leslie's, are especially impressive examples of the efficacy of Native American medicine because they are frequently degenerative. Western doctors know that anti-inflammatory drugs, vitamin and mineral supplements (such as niacin and glucosamine sulfate), and range-of-motion exercises can reduce pain and slow down the degeneration of an arthritic joint, but physicians do not recognize any therapy other than joint replacement surgery that can almost immediately restore healthy functioning, as sometimes—albeit rarely—happens in Native American medicine.

Some diseases infiltrate the body's genetic code and become alternately symptomatic and aysmptomatic throughout the patient's lifetime. Examples include herpes, lupus, rheumatism, and multiple sclerosis (MS). There are instances in which Native American healing causes such rapid improvement in these diseases that it borders on the miraculous. Over the past twenty years, I have witnessed several such events in my own practice. In one, Jon, a European man in his forties, came to a healing ceremony that I was conducting. The only thing I knew about his health history was that he was disabled from multiple sclerosis. He used a walker, inching forward with excruciating difficulty. He relied on the strength of his arms to keep his buckling legs steady.

I helped Jon to a chair. A group of helpers began to sing healing songs as I doctored him with my hands. I reached energetically and spiritually into his body, gently stroking the damaged myelin sheath that surrounds the nerve cells. I brushed away toxic information from his nervous system and asked the Great Spirit to help me wave in a healing gift. The ceremony lasted approximately forty minutes. When it was over, and after Jon rested for a few minutes, I extended my hand to help him to a standing position. Jon clung to my arm, but as I was about to move his walker closer, he asked me to wait. Jon took a small step without losing his balance. He took another step. His legs were steady. He continued stepping with the same ease, while crying, "My God, I can walk!"

Frankly, if I had been watching this scene, I would have thought it was a setup. I did not trust the healing that I had personally witnessed until the next week, when Jon's previous level of disability was confirmed by my personal interview of various people who knew him. The owner of a local business said, "It's a miracle. Everyone in town has seen Jon walking for the first time in ten years." Jon remained completely free of pain or disability for six weeks. After that, some of the symptoms returned. He became depressed and convinced that he could not maintain the improvement on his own. Yet for the following five years, the MS never returned to its original level, and Jon no longer needed a walker.

The reader might wonder whether these cases are the exception rather than the rule. How many failures occur before one significant healing? This is an excellent question because healers have a tendency toward *observation bias* and *selective recall*. They may observe and remember their successes but ignore and forget their failures. If we define "success" as healing, curing, and/or satisfying our patients, then Native healers can accurately report a very high ratio of success. Although not every patient is permanently cured, nearly everyone is helped along his or her path to spiritual wholeness.

WILL I EXHAUST MY RESOURCES BY GIVING TO OTHERS?

Of course it was not I who cured. It was the power from the outer world,
and the visions and ceremonies had only made me like a hole through which
the power could come to the two-leggeds. If I thought that I was doing it myself,
the hole would close up and no power could come through.
Then everything I could do would be foolish.
—Black Elk[49]

I have heard many alternative healers complain that when they attempt to transmit healing energy, they use up their supply and become sick. This has not been my experience. From the Native American viewpoint, the human body and mind are not closed systems. They are part of the great web of life, and healers who are aware of this web do not exhaust their own energy or spiritual resources.

The healer is a hollow tube for the Great Spirit's power. It is the Great Spirit who touches the patient and sends healing energy. The healer must be in a state of prayer so that he or she stays linked to this power. Seneca healer Moses Shongo held one hand raised above his head while healing with the other hand. The raised hand linked his mind and body to "the Creator's light of love" and reminded Grandfather Shongo that he was not the source of healing. I was taught a nearly identical technique by spiritual healers from China and the Philippines, who keep one hand pointed to the ground while healing with the other hand. The "grounding hand" reaches meditatively through the earth's surface to an ever-present current of healing force. Healers who are connected to this life current are never in danger of losing personal energy when they interact with a patient. Nor are they in danger of "picking up" toxins or evil spirits, since during the healing, they no longer exist as separate individuals. They are in a state of spiritual unity with life.

A little-explored dimension of indigenous healing is the effect of grounded posture on grounded being—that is, how the posture of ancient peoples created the physical, mental, and spiritual state necessary for healing. A healer who can stand and move with balance and grace is a clearer channel and better communicator of the Great Spirit's healing power.

II

— THE PALEOLITHIC POSTURE —

The phrase "Live in balance" summarizes Native American spiritual ideals, but it is used so often by people who write or speak about Native spirituality that it has become, regrettably, a cliché, which hides a deep and perhaps unexpected meaning. To live in balance means harmony with the web of life and, as Rolling Thunder used to say, "moderation in all things." But there is also another side to the expression. To live in balance is as much a physical state as a state of mind. A physically balanced person has good posture, relaxed breathing, mental alertness, clarity, and vitality. Physically balanced healers can generate more energy to heal themselves and others. Good posture creates good circulation and warm "healing" hands. If a healer's massage gestures say "heal" but his posture says, "I am sick," the treatment won't be effective.

I call the ancient, natural way of standing "the Paleolithic Posture." In the Paleolithic Posture, the knees are slightly bent, the spine is straight and long, the breath is deep and quiet, and the eyes are open and alert. The body feels like a tree with deep roots for balance and tall branches for grace. Although we usually think of a "posture" as a static pose, it includes our carriage in movement as well. Since a straight and tall stance confers the greatest balance, sensitivity, awareness, and alertness, we see it in a scout standing still on a mountain lookout or walking through camp to a council meeting. We see it in a mother who keeps a watchful eye on her children; if she slouches, she might not see an enemy or a predator. (Naturally, some postural elements vary according to circumstance. For instance, while stalking, silently and invisibly following the prey, a hunter keeps a low profile and sways in harmony with nearby trees when the wind blows.)

The Paleolithic Posture is an attitude of mind and body that was a matter of instinct and survival among ancient hunters, warriors, mothers, and healers. A person who lives in the wilderness must adapt to his or her surroundings in order to survive. A subsistence hunter would never walk with a rigid gait in the stiff, unyielding shoes of a modern city dweller. His survival does not depend on standing out in a crowd or "getting ahead." On the contrary, he wishes to be invisible. He needs to listen to the ground through his moccasins, lest he snap a branch and scare away the prey. He does not want to make an impression on the earth. He allows the earth to make its impression on him. This requires a stance of utmost relaxation, balance, and alertness. Because his schedule is determined by nature's cycles—the rising and sinking of the sun, the seasonal migrations of animal herds—the hunter's mind is focused on present experiences rather than on distant goals.

The hunter moves, breathes, and lives slowly in order to conserve energy for when it is needed. His heart does not race from imaginary threats to his physical safety and well-being but only from real, actually perceived ones. His body's "fight or flight" stress response is never prolonged because of persistent pessimism or negative expectations. He does not shrink from life for fear of an unknown future or death. He accepts death as an inevitable and natural part of the life cycle.

The Paleolithic Posture was and is practiced among hunter-gatherers on all continents. Our ancestors could not afford to miss the sound of a rustling leaf, the sight of a moon ring, or the sensation of frost in the nighttime air. Living in nature requires listening with one's whole being, even to the subtle signs and omens presented in dreams. Today, people often feel that their psychological well-being depends on their ability to shield themselves from a world filled with excess and disturbing stimuli such as the rattle of subway trains or machine noises. Omens and dreams are shut out because we have little time for them, and they make us question our values, belief systems, and identity.

POSTURAL PIONEERS

In her book *Where the Spirits Ride the Wind*, trailblazing anthropologist and sage Felicitas Goodman, Ph.D., shows that ancient religious art throughout the world portrays humans in similar postures. She describes persistent postural motifs in Stone Age European cave paintings, ancient Egyptian hieroglyphs, and modern Puget Sound totem poles that she believes are part of an ancient, universal language of posture and gesture related to *specific* psychospiritual states. Dr. Goodman has found specific poses associated with divination, healing, and transformation, each of which maintains a fairly consistent symbolism across geographical and cultural boundaries. Most important, Dr. Goodman discovered that if modern non-Native people imitate the postures, they automatically experience their meaning.[1] She calls these "trance postures" because they induce a highly intuitive state of consciousness in which the practitioner feels as though he or she is contacting sacred forces. For example, the Bear Posture—found in two-thousand- to six-thousand-year-old artworks from Spain, Crete, Mexico, Israel, the United States, and many other places—depicts a man or woman standing upright with bent knees and hands resting on the lower abdomen. It always seems to symbolize healing power and wisdom and helps to awaken these feelings when a modern person holds it as a meditative stance.

The link between posture and consciousness is actually not so far-fetched. Try to imagine a happy feeling while you are stooped over with hunched shoulders and sunken chest. On the other hand, how easy is it to remain depressed if you are standing tall and poised? When someone says, "I can't stand it," notice the locked knees. A person who is "uptight" is tense in the upper body; over time, his posture and gait become rigid and distorted. If you stand in an uptight posture, you become uptight! Posture structures and may even alter perception.

The Paleolithic Posture came naturally to peoples living in nature, as a matter of necessity. Today, however, we must practice it quite deliberately to reap its benefits. One particularly inspiring story of the rediscovery of the ancient wisdom of posture concerns a German woman named Elsa Gindler. In 1910, Gindler, then in her twenties and teaching physical education in Berlin, developed tuberculosis. The doctors pronounced her "terminal" and advised her to spend her remaining days at a sanatorium in the Alps, something Gindler, a poor working-class woman, could not afford. Instead, Gindler decided to devote her full attention to the only source of healing that she truly understood—her own body. She taught herself to sense her diseased lung and to maintain it in a state of complete rest while breathing with only her healthy lung. According to *Sensory Awareness: The Rediscovery of Experiencing,* Charles Brooks's classic exploration of Gindler's work, "Since breathing involves more of the large musculature than any other basic life activity, this meant an awakening to her own inner flexibilities and processes on a very general scale. Indeed, it meant an alerting of the entire sensory nervous system, for, like a pebble dropped in water, an excitation at any point in the organism tends to set up reactions everywhere."[2] As Gindler became more sensitive to her body's functioning, she learned how to "cease interfering with the organism's innate tendencies to regeneration." To the bafflement of her physicians, after a year of such self-treatment, her tuberculosis was cured.

From the time of her healing until her death in 1961, Gindler taught her new, yet very ancient, approach to physical education—how to sense, appreciate, and awaken each part of the body and, through that awareness, restore healthier functioning and greater aliveness. She called it simply *Arbeit am Menschen,* "Work on the Human Being." A woman of great integrity, compassion, and courage, Gindler gave special classes in her method for German Jews during the Second World War, some of whom she concealed in her basement.

The influence of Gindler's work can be seen in the West's human potential and humanistic psychology movements. During the 1940s, her best-known student, Charlotte Selver, taught what she termed "sensory awareness" to the famed psychologists Erich Fromm and Fritz Perls (founder of Gestalt therapy). Selver also had a profound influence on Wilhelm Reich's understanding of the breath, thus laying the foundation for both Reichian and bioenergetic therapy. In 1963, when Selver began to teach at the newly founded Esalen Institute, she influenced a generation of innovative therapists who coined terms like *sensitivity training* and *encounter groups*.

I studied with Charlotte Selver during the early 1970s, and she remains a major influence on my life, my work, and my understanding of indigenous spirituality. She taught me that one cannot feel in touch with the earth without standing sensitively on the ground: "Many of us have been taught to stand on our own two feet. But sadly, we have not learned how to stand on the ground. We do not trust its support," she said. "To trust the ground is to live with confidence." I consider sensory awareness to be a return to natural and primal wisdom. Selver once summarized her approach to me: "An animal knows how to take care of himself when ill—what plants to eat, where and how to rest. People can also awaken this natural healing potential."

My exploration of the Paleolithic Posture is based on a number of sources, including the work of Felicitas Goodman and Charlotte Selver; a study of human postures in Native American petroglyphs and pictographs; my observation of common postural traits among healers, hunters, and warriors; my experiences as a practitioner of indigenous healing; and thirty years' training in qigong, a Chinese system of posture, exercises, and breathing techniques to improve health. Warriors in both Native American and Asian traditions use the Paleolithic Posture to better launch an attack or to sense and defend against one. It is seen in ritual dances such as the Northern Plains Shield Dance, in which two warriors fight a pantomime battle, as well as in Chinese martial arts. As a martial arts judge in international competitions, I have observed that a competitor's posture is directly related to combat skill.

I witnessed an inspiring example of the connection between Chinese and indigenous wisdom during a seminar I taught at a mountain retreat center. The seminar focused on deer qigong, a series of deerlike postures, each held for about ten minutes at a time, designed to increase strength, improve health, and cultivate nature awareness. One afternoon, while my students and I were holding a deer stance in a mountain meadow, we noticed a deer at the edge of the woods standing perfectly still, her head turned, gazing alertly in our direction. She stood with us during the ten minutes that we held the posture. Then, when we relaxed to discuss our experiences, the deer, losing interest in these deer-now-turned-people, walked slowly back into the bush.

Inspired by this experience, I invited a Lakota elder and his wife to be guest lecturers on the final evening of the seminar. After my students and I demonstrated the deer postures, the elders shared with us a beautiful message: "*Wasté!* 'It is good!' These exercises are part of our tradition. They are part of the original way of the Earth People (*Maka Oyate*). Our Chinese relatives remind us of a beautiful way of healing."

HOW TO PRACTICE THE POSTURE

The best way to learn about the Paleolithic Posture is by practicing it as a static meditative pose. Before practicing it, I would like to invite you to first try a simple experiment. Place one palm on your lower back with your fingertips lightly touching your tailbone. Begin to walk about, feeling how your lower back and spine naturally accommodate the act of walking. Notice how your spine seems to open and close, gently resonating with each step and each shift of weight. Continue walking, but now, lock both knees as you walk. This is, of course, an artificial and unnatural way of walking. Nevertheless, it makes clear, through exaggeration, a common, unconscious habit. Many people lock one knee after the other as they walk. As you do this intentionally, how does it feel? What do you feel under the palm on your back? Do your back muscles have as much play? Does the spine still respond to your steps and shifts? How has locking the knees affected your breathing? If you are unclear about the answers to these questions, try walking naturally again, this time being careful never to lock either knee. (Each foot steps down before the leg reaches maximum extension.) Notice your back and your breath. Then stand higher and walk while keeping both knees locked. Be clear about how these different ways of moving affect your levels of comfort or dis-ease.

You don't need a degree in physical therapy to realize the damage that could result from a chronic habit of locking the knees. The knees and the cushionlike cartilage within them act like shock absorbers. When we walk with the knees locked, there is no spring in our step. Our movements become slow and cumbersome. In Karl W. Luckert's book *The Navajo Hunter Tradition*, Diné hunter Billie Blackhorse says, "The hunters feel very lightfooted; they become fast runners."[3] Here is one of their secrets: "You walk, sit, and sleep with knees bent at all times. In that posture the hunter never tires."[4]

When we lock the knees, every step shocks the lower back, resulting in pain and gradual degeneration of the spine. Locking the knees locks the back, increases lower back pain, weakens the joints and supporting muscles, speeds up the breath, and feels generally miserable. Why, then, do most Americans stand and walk with locked knees? The culprit is sidewalks! Straight, flat, unyielding surfaces do not require the knees to bend or extend, as would a natural varied terrain. Because we are confident that there will be no boulder in front of us or tree trunk across the path, we do not need to sense the ground or even to watch our steps. As a result, we suffer from an atrophying of the back, thigh, and calf muscles and a tendency to balance ourselves over locked bony structures.

Thus, the first step in the Paleolithic Posture is to stand with the knees slightly bent. If you are unable to stand because of arthritis or disability, sit in a chair but still imagine openness and "spring" in the knee joints. As a meditative exercise, I suggest keeping your arms in one of three positions:

1. *Natural Stance:* Let your arms rest naturally at your sides, with your fingers gently extended as though "listening" to the life energy of the earth.
2. *Bear Posture:* Your palms or gently closed fists rest lightly on the lower abdomen. This hand position stimulates abdominal respiration and mental quiet.
3. *Shaman's Pose:* This posture is commonly seen in Native American rock art. One hand is raised, fingers skyward at the height of your head. There is a ninety-degree angle in your elbow, which should position your hand about a foot away from your head. The other hand is pointed to the ground at your other side. It is raised to the height of your hipbone and also about one foot to the side of your body. The fingers of both hands are slightly spread and extended. The Shaman's Pose expresses reverence for the Great Spirit and Creation. It induces a state of communion with the forces of Earth and Sky. The upraised arm is a common gesture of prayer in many Native American cultures.[5] Be sure to practice it on both sides.

In all of these postures, the feet are relaxed and sensitively in touch with the ground. If the weather is pleasant, practice barefoot and outdoors (see the sidebar "The Importance of Feet"). Can you feel the earth's aliveness? Can you allow this aliveness to rise through you, so that your *whole body* is aware of standing on the ground? Many people unconsciously grip the ground with their toes, as though either grasping the earth for balance or pushing the earth away. Let go of these unnecessary tensions and simply trust the ground to support you. Indian runners imagine the ground pushing up against the feet and providing the energy they need. In Peter Nabokov's book *Indian Running*, anthropologist Thomas Buckley explains that runners "receive the trail as a being, letting it dictate the run. . . . Gradually you put more and more trust in the earth, and move into a light trance state when you're no longer interfering in the running."[6] The runners practice "effortless gliding," skimming the tops of the bushes as they cover huge distances in incredibly short periods of time. These principles apply equally to standing still. Standing is effortless if you allow the ground to hold you up and give you energy.

In balanced standing, you can feel the ground rising to support you. Paradoxically, you should also be aware of the weight of the body sinking down. Imagine that you can stand *through* your feet, *into* the ground, like a tree with deep roots. Both sensations—the upward and downward flow of energy and awareness—are maintained simultaneously.

Your body is as relaxed as possible while holding the erect posture. Relaxed does not mean slouched. It means using the minimum effort necessary to stand with grace and dignity. Your spine is straight but not stiff. It is gently extended, as though pushing your head up, like the branches of a tree, toward the sky. Your eyes are open, gazing wide and long into the distance without being fixed on any particular object. Your attention is focused completely on the present. Your eyes neither look ahead to what is not yet in view nor hold on to a previous image. They simply allow the environment in without grasping at particulars.

You allow your body to breathe at a quiet, relaxed pace. Do not *take* a breath; rather, allow a breath. You do not need to suck the air in or push it out: breathing happens all by itself. The healthiest and most natural way to breathe is to allow the abdomen to gently expand with the inhalation and retract with the exhalation. The chest hardly moves at all. Do not hold the belly in or try to flatten it, as this will interfere with breathing and diminish your healing reserves. Deep belly breathing brings the maximum amount of oxygen to your cells. In the presence of a full supply of oxygen, your respiratory rate can slow down. You need fewer breaths per minute to supply your body's energy needs. The average American draws approximately seventeen inhalations per minute while at rest. When a person is angry or anxious, the breathing rate jumps to more than twenty cycles per minute. Within a few months of practicing the Paleolithic Posture, most people find themselves slowing to an average of five breaths per minute! Your mind becomes calmer.

While holding the posture, be aware of your environment. Your senses are open. You notice sounds in your environment, smells, textures, colors. You sense your own body: your posture and breathing and the feeling of simple aliveness.

To review, the basic elements of the Paleolithic Posture are:
- Feet under the shoulders
- Slightly bent knees
- Receiving and feeling the ground
- Long, straight spine
- Relaxed as possible
- Eyes open with a wide, level gaze
- Slow, quiet belly breathing
- Awareness
- Whole body alive

The Paleolithic Posture, the common stance of our ancestors, awakens a quality of awareness that is both ancient and timeless. I recommend practicing the Paleolithic

Posture by holding any of the three stances as a meditative pose for ten minutes every day. You can also experiment with other arm and hand positions, while maintaining all of the postural principles. The Paleolithic Posture calms the mind, stimulates self-healing, and greatly increases vitality.

I recommend the Paleolithic Posture to people who practice any form of energy healing or massage. Use it to center and energize yourself before and during healing work. A healer familiar with the Paleolithic Posture automatically assumes it during periods of rest and at appropriate times during a treatment. It enhances her healing presence, which instills confidence and hope in patients. It also optimizes the healer's diagnostic sensitivity and helps her tap into the healing power of Nature and Spirit.

There is an easy way to tell if you are practicing the posture correctly and are "plugged in" to a source of healing power. You feel a comfortable warmth throughout your body, which is especially pronounced in the hands. The hands change color, becoming either mottled or slightly red. The fingers also tingle. From the physiological perspective, these changes occur when the body relaxes and small blood vessels open up to accommodate increased circulation. From the spiritual viewpoint, the hands fill with life energy and radiate an energetic field, like a wire with a strong electric current running through it. When the hands are warm and tingling, you are a more effective healer—better able to sense energetic disturbances in a patient and to project healing energy.

Energized hands are like dowsing rods that respond to invisible currents of power. A healer can use this sensitivity to locate invaders in the body or environment. In order to locate an enemy, the Apache medicine woman Lozen would move slowly in a clockwise direction. According to H. Henrietta Stockel's account, "Lozen halted when a tingling feeling or change in the color of her palms became noticeable. The direction she faced when she stopped was usually the place where the enemy was located."[7] We can see from this example the close tie between the skills of the healer and those of the warrior.

ANIMAL POWERS

You may model the Paleolithic Posture on various animals with whom you feel an affinity, such as the Deer, Bear, Badger, Sparrow, Eagle, Ant, Salmon, or any other creature teacher. Do not imitate the animal; be the animal! The postures are most effective if practiced in the environment where you would naturally find the animal. Don't practice a Buffalo Stance in Hawai'i or a Dolphin Posture in the Arizona desert. Animal gestures are common in Native American improvisational, choreographed, social, and ceremonial dances and are also used while doctoring patients.

Animal postures also serve a very practical use among hunting peoples. A hunter

— THE IMPORTANCE OF FEET —

Native people define life as the capacity for movement, perception, and/or communication. In Maureen Trudell Schwarz's *Molded in the Image of Changing Woman,* Diné elder Harry Walters of Tsaile, Arizona, brings an earthy concreteness to the definition of "being alive." It is "to have your foot, to have your feet, planted into the earth and your head in the sky. In your Mother Earth and Father Sky. Everything that is alive has its feet planted in the earth and its head in the sky."[8]

Earth and Sky also mean the earthly and heavenly, the physical and spiritual realities. In this special sense, even fish have "feet." Indeed, all of creation has feet: insects, birds, plants, even mountains. With a wisdom similar to that of Native Americans, Zen Buddhist texts speak of the "mountains constantly walking." They move at a slow pace, but they move! For a human being, to be fully alive is to move with awareness and dignity between Earth and Sky. This awareness begins at the feet.

My wife and I were married in an outdoor ceremony according to the traditions of the ancient Cherokee Keetoowah Society. When we were planning the ceremony with the medicine man, she said, "I will be barefoot. I want to feel the earth." Taking the hint, I added, "And I will wear my moccasins." This got me thinking. To what extent are people ungrounded because they cannot sense the ground?

Unfortunately, because of shoes, most people today cannot feel the earth even when they are walking on a trail rather than pavement. Numerous studies have shown that people who walk or run barefoot or in moccasins have extremely low incidence of foot disease, like fungi and bursitis, or other foot problems, such as flatfoot, bunions, and uncomfortable toe angulation, and also suffer few movement-related injuries compared to "shod" populations.[9] They develop strong and well-rounded arches that can successfully absorb the impact of the ground. By contrast, when the foot is immobilized in shoes, the arch, which is designed to be a flexible lever, weakens. Equally important, shoes' padding and cushioning prevent walkers and runners from perceiving incorrect weight distribution on the feet. As researchers Steven E. Robbins and Gerard J. Gouw write in the journal

> *Medicine and Science in Sports and Exercise,* "[A] perceptual illusion is cre-
> ated whereby perceived impact is lower than actual impact, which results in
> inadequate impact-moderating behavior and consequent injury."[10] The au-
> thors also point out that barefoot humans automatically bend their knees
> more than shod ones, which also lessens impact. "Better" running shoes do
> not help. In fact, research shows that more expensive running shoes cause
> significantly more injuries than inexpensive ones.[11]
>
> This does not mean that we should immediately throw away our shoes.
> They are necessary during cold weather, on dangerous surfaces (where
> there may be broken glass or other sharp objects), to enter most businesses,
> and sadly, for many social occasions. However, we should make an effort to
> walk barefoot whenever and wherever possible. It generally takes about six
> weeks of daily frequent barefoot walking for the feet to adapt.

may wear an animal robe and learn to imitate an animal so closely that observers cannot distinguish him from the four-legged. Bison-robed hunters would lead or lure the herd to other hunters or to steep ledges, where the animals would fall to their deaths. (An outstanding place to learn about these "buffalo jumps" is the Head-Smashed-In Buffalo Jump in Alberta, Canada, now a World Heritage Site and interpretive center that pays tribute to the lifestyle of Canada's First Peoples.) Or the hunter may imitate an animal's predator in order to scare it into an ambush—for example, a wolf-person stalking a caribou.

Native American warriors, like Chinese martial artists, have also used animal postures and meditations to develop combative skills. A Native American warrior who has the Hawk as his spirit helper may wear the hawk feather and has the swiftness necessary to avoid attacks and perhaps to dodge arrows. A warrior who attacks like a grizzly bear terrifies his enemies. A scout who moves like the mountain goat is surefooted in the steepest terrain. The warrior moves like the animal, is protected by the animal, may engage the animal helper to do combat for him, and in the deeper reality of dream and vision, *is* the animal.[12]

If the Paleolithic Posture is a traditional indigenous warrior's stance, then why do modern soldiers stand at "attention" with locked knees, stomach in, and chest out? The Paleolithic Posture seems the opposite of military posture. I had the same question until several years ago when I discussed posture with a retired U.S. Army general. He told me that he didn't trust a soldier who stood with bent knees. "He is likely to do his own thing." Interesting! Military posture produces an altered state of consciousness that makes the soldier most likely to follow orders. The forced, un-natural posture cuts off the feeling of the earth and the "ground" of one's own being. If you feel disempowered, you are more easily subject to outside authority. By contrast, the warriors of long ago were expected to practice a balance of self-determination, autonomy, and cooperation. In traditional Native American society, each person was a potential leader.

12

— UNFOLDING THE MYSTERY —
Sweat Lodge and Sacred Pipe

The word *ceremony* in the Native American tradition has a broad range of meanings. It is used to describe a sequence of prescribed actions, generally accompanied by prayer, songs, and music, often drumming, undertaken to influence, honor, or communicate with people, land, life, and/or Creator. It also has a timeless quality; while participating in a ceremony, one has the impression that it was preordained, received in whole from the Spirit World, rather than created by a person. To participate in a ceremony is to participate in a mystery.

Like meditation, a ceremony deepens the direct experience of sacred or hidden realms of being, but unlike meditation, which is private, a ceremony may be individual, such as the Vision Quest, or communal, such as the Sun Dance. Ceremonies generally include some activities that are relatively fixed—for example, offering cedar smoke to the directions—as well as leeway for personal variation, such as the specific prayers that a person makes while smudging. A ceremony may be as short as ten minutes of prayer, or it may last many years, such as the Nuu-chah-nulth preparation for whaling—praying and bathing at a sacred pool for at least five years, every day from January to April and several times each month thereafter.

Because they demonstrate reverence to the spiritual, life-sustaining powers, Native American ceremonies help to maintain the balance of life on earth. In *Masked Gods: Navaho and Pueblo Ceremonialism,* Frank Waters, the great writer on the American Southwest, describes the purpose of the Hopi Snake and Antelope Dances in terms that could apply to *all* Native ceremonies: "The specific function of the Snake-Antelope ceremonial is to bring rain. But it is rooted in the primary purpose of all Hopi ceremonials—to maintain the harmony of the universe. Not only physically in the outer world, but psychically in the inner world."[1] A basic principle of Native American philosophy is that inside and outside reflect each other; what happens on earth, including in people's minds, influences the Spirit World, and what happens in the Spirit World influences life on earth. In her excellent book *Medicine for the Earth,* shaman Sandra Ingerman writes, "When we remember our divine nature, nature will reflect that back to us."[2] Ingerman applied this principle to create rituals that can actually transform natural elements. She discovered that when a group of people imagine themselves transfigured into spiritual powers and then focus loving attention on a cup of polluted water, asking the Great Spirit to purify it, the pollution level drops dramatically.[3]

Yet living a spiritual life is even more important than ceremonies. Rolling Thunder put it best when he told me, "Some people are doing things in reverse. They believe that by participating in ceremonies, they will become spiritual. Instead, they should make their lives spiritual by respecting the Mother Earth, each other, and the Great Spirit. Then, when the time comes to attend a ceremony, it will be an expression of who they are." I certainly experienced the truth of this statement when I lived at Meta Tantay, the traditional Native community that Rolling Thunder directed. It was only after I'd spent many months of cutting winter wood, fixing outhouses, and milking goats that Rolling Thunder invited me to attend an herb-gathering ceremony. By then, it seemed so natural, it grew out of the way I lived.

That said, it is also true that modern society conspires against a spiritual lifestyle and mistrusts anyone who disconnects from its institutions. Ideally, one would not join any ceremony until one's way of life were in accord with its values, but today both Native and non-Native people must sometimes "do things in reverse." Native ceremonies remind us of the values that we need to apply to our everyday lives and reveal previously unrecognized layers of reality.

THE ELEMENTS OF CEREMONY

Healing and spiritual ceremonies of indigenous peoples throughout the world share common elements. According to West African Dagara healer Malidoma Somé, Ph.D., these are invocational, dialogical, repetitive, and opening and closure.[4] Here is what these terms mean in a Native American context:

1. Invocation: The ceremonial leader and helpers—which may include all participants—invoke the presence of sacred powers, commonly with music and prayer. The ceremonial leader may also welcome spirits by creating a ceremonial altar consisting of objects such as stones, candles, or animal skulls placed on a cloth or blanket spread on the ground. In the Northern Plains, it is common to place *tobacco ties* on the altar. These are tiny bundles of cloth filled with prayer-charged tobacco and tied one after the next on a single string. Specific colors of cloth or a set number of ties may be required for a ceremony. In some ceremonies, individual participants place their own altars in front of them. During group healing ceremonies, I generally create a community altar and invite participants to place personally meaningful sacred objects on a central altar blanket. As the ceremony progresses, the objects receive blessings. Participants take their "recharged" objects back at the end of the ceremony.

2. Dialogue: Each ceremony has a purpose; the leader and sometimes the participants commune and dialogue with spiritual powers to express gratitude, request help (better luck in hunting, an end to drought), or retrieve information—for example, how to heal, solve a personal or community problem, or find a lost object. No matter what the goal of a Native ceremony, however, there is always an aspect that is in a sense purposeless and beyond the personal. In his book *Myths to Live By,* Joseph Campbell, the great scholar of world mythology, wrote, "A ritual is an organization of mythological symbols; and by participating in the drama of the rite one is brought directly in touch with these, not as verbal reports of historic events, either past, present, or to be, but as revelations, here and now, of what is always and forever."[5]

3. Repetition: Though many ceremonies leave room for improvisation, they also include ritual actions that remain consistent in every performance. Entire ceremonies may also be repeated in detail if they are considered complete revelations or gifts of the Great Spirit that do not require revision or adaptation, such as Cherokee *i:gawé:sdi,* exactly worded chants to bring luck, protection, or healing, generally accompanied by physical procedures, such as turning tobacco in the palm. Repeated ceremonial actions may have either of two opposite effects. On the one hand, they may become stale, performed mechanically and without real feeling—in which case, they are ineffective and may shield the practitioner from the spiritual realm rather than open a door to it. Or because the physical gestures have been memorized—for example, the way Cree people circle a vertically held Sacred Pipe through the smoke of burning sweetgrass— the ceremonial leader and participants can concentrate on the spirit behind the actions. As a ceremony is repeated time after time, ceremonial actions become more and more refined, graceful, powerful, and transparent to the Spirit.

4. Opening and closure: A ceremony has a distinct opening and closing—such as smudging, a drumbeat, a song, or a specific way to enter or leave a ceremonial space, perhaps by circling clockwise around an altar—to set it apart from everyday concerns and to draw participants into *sacred space* and *sacred time*. During many Native ceremonies, there is a feeling that one is at the center of the universe; all of space seems to be encompassed within the ceremony. There simply is nowhere else. Time no longer exists, and the present is infinite.

To these four elements, Native Americans add a fifth: *sacrifice*. Sacrifice, which literally means "making sacred," is a form of devotion and worship in which people surrender a part of themselves, give up a comfort for a higher good, or make an offering to a divine power. Sacrifice is an underlying theme in most ceremonies. It is necessary before a healing can occur. The healer, patient, and helpers may prepare for ceremony by fasting, giving up food and water. People heal by sacrificing unhealthy habits and belief systems. Prayers are made with an offering of the breath. The Sacred Pipe is smoked by sacrificing tobacco to the fire of life. As the tobacco "dies," it releases its spirit in the form of scent and smoke. Probably the best-known Native American ceremony involving sacrifice is the Sun Dance, a ritual of supplication for the healing, cultural renewal, and well-being of the tribe, practiced by the Absarokee, Blackfoot, Cree, Arapaho, Lakota, and other Northern Plains nations. Dancers express their devotion to the Great Spirit by dancing under the hot sun and sacrificing pieces of flesh cut from their arms or chest.

To sacrifice is to participate in the mystery of death creating the compost for new life. "Except a corn of wheat fall into the ground and die, it abideth alone; but if it die, it bringeth forth much fruit" (John 12:24). According to the Cherokee, when Selu, the First Woman, died, corn shoots sprang wherever her blood touched the ground. Her body, sacrificed to the Earth Mother, rose as a tall Plant Person with beautiful corn-silk hair. Sacrifice is an everyday occurrence. Animals and plants sacrifice life to give humans food. Every earthquake, volcano, and tidal wave shaves off or burns away part of the earth's skin: Mother Earth sacrifices the old to make room for the new.

The elders say that good people should be willing to sacrifice money, time, effort, and comfort so that their children's children, "the seventh generation," will not only survive but have better lives. In Native American spirituality, a sacrifice is never injurious to or destructive of family or community. A human life is *never* sacrificed. A child's happiness is *never* sacrificed. What if a spirit commanded a Native American Abraham to sacrifice his son on a mountaintop altar? He would say, "No!" because such advice could never come from God.[6]

A PAN-INDIAN RELIGION

Ceremonies pervade Native American healing and spirituality. In earlier chapters in this book, I introduced many ceremonies, including smudging, Vision Quest, the Moontime Ceremony, the Giveaway (Potlatch), Winter Spirit Dances, healing rituals, puberty rites, and Shaker Church meetings. I have also referred several times to the Sweat Lodge and Sacred Pipe, the best-known and most widely practiced ceremonies.

The Sweat Lodge is the name of both a ceremony and of the man-made structure in which it takes place. (To avoid confusion, I will use lowercase—sweat lodge—when referring specifically to the structure.) In the Sweat Lodge, people sweat away their illness, unhappiness, and negativity and invite helping spirits with prayer and song. In the Sacred Pipe Ceremony, a person, individually or in a group, smokes a mixture of tobacco and natural herbs in a special pipe as a way of unifying the mind with nature and seeking power and wisdom from the Great Spirit. The Sweat Lodge and the Sacred Pipe have always been practiced by a majority of Native American peoples.

Although there are still many unique tribal and personal variations of these ceremonies, in recent years, as people of various tribes have met and shared traditions or tried to recover lost ones, these ceremonies have become truly intertribal or "Pan-Indian." I have been in Sweat Lodges with California elders in which the procedures were virtually identical to those performed by my Cree relatives. I know Cherokee pipe makers in North Carolina who make their pipes with the red pipestone common to the Great Lakes and Northern Plains rather than the local green steatite. More and more Native Americans are sharing the Sweat Lodge and the Pipe with people of diverse nations, including white people. In fact, among Native ceremonies, the Sweat Lodge and Sacred Pipe are the ones most likely to be open to respectful non-Indians. According to Arval Looking Horse, caretaker of the most sacred pipe of the Dakota/Lakota people, "The Pipe is for all people, all races, as long as a person believes in it. Anyone can have a pipe and keep it within their family."[7]

— SWEAT LODGE —

The Sweat Lodge, also called the Purification Lodge or Stone People Lodge, is possibly the oldest of Native American ceremonies. In the Lakota language, the Sweat Lodge is called *Initipi* (or *inipi*), beautiful words that mean "tipi or lodge of the life-breath," or *Oinikagapi,* "place where they renew life." The sweat lodge is generally a temporary structure, a bough-framed dome in the middle of which is a pit filled with red-hot stones. As many as a dozen participants at a time sit around the pit and purge themselves in heat and steam. Some California tribes build fires in permanent wooden structures that are partially underground, where they sweat and purify in dry heat.

The Sweat Lodge is a physical and spiritual purification and an occasion to commune with the forces of nature—earth, water, fire, and air—and the Great Spirit who created them. The Odawa Indians of the Great Lakes say that in the Sweat Lodge, one bathes in the breath of the Great Spirit and is reborn. The five main posts of the Diné Sweat Lodge are called "fingers." "When people are in the sweat lodge, it is said that they are in the hands of the gods,"[8] writes Robert S. McPherson, teacher of social sciences and humanities at the College of Eastern Utah.

Cold water is also cleansing and highly invigorating. Among many tribes, a cold water plunge follows immediately after the hot Sweat Lodge. Some tribes use the cold water by itself. The Cherokee ritual purification called "going to water" consists of plunging four or seven times in a river. The water is considered most potent when the red light of dawn is reflected on its surface and during the autumn, when fallen leaves turn the river into a medicinal infusion.[9]

Fire, water, or their combination are used for purification throughout North America. Natural hot springs and vapor caves, filled with the breath of Mother Earth, are universally considered gateways to the spirit. They are nature's sweat lodges, and when Native people bathe in them, they often consider it a kind of Sweat Lodge Ceremony. Unfortunately, many original "primitive" hot springs have been turned into commercial spas and resorts. However, even bathing in one of these can be a sacred experience if you remember to say "Thank you" to Mother Earth before bathing. I like to hold a pinch of tobacco in my palm as I approach a hot spring. I secretly drop it on the ground before entering the water.

A Northern Plains Sweat Lodge Ceremony

Although there are many tribal and individual variations of the sweat lodge and its ceremony, the style of the Northern Plains is the best known and most widely practiced, even outside of its area of origin. The lodge is a low, dome-shaped structure, about seven feet in diameter and four or five feet high at its apex. It is framed by twelve to twenty one-inch-diameter willow saplings tied together and covered with various materials that completely shut out light. Willow is used because it is supple yet strong, is associated with water (it grows in proximity of rivers and lakes), and as the first plant to turn green in the spring, is a natural symbol of renewal. Depending on availability, some tribes make the sweat lodge poles from cherry, piñon, cedar, or other wood saplings. In the past, sweat lodges were covered with animal hides, bark, and packed earth; today, blankets, canvas, and tarps are common. The lodge's entrance is an arch covered with a flap to block light and hold the heat. The entrance faces a specific cardinal direction, depending on tribal tradition. The earthen floor of the lodge is covered with a blanket of sweet-smelling sage.

The best sweat lodge stones are round igneous rocks, about the size of a man's head, gathered on a hillside. Igneous rocks can be heated to extreme temperatures without splitting or exploding (unlike sandstone, granite, or quartz). They are heated in a sacred outdoor fire that is carefully tended by a firekeeper, who does not enter the lodge, though he is a respected and equal participant in the ceremony. His sacred task is to take care of the ancient Grandparents—the Stone People—and the Sun (fire) in a symbolic tipi made of branches and logs of the fire. The red-hot stones will be placed in a round pit, called the "fireplace" or "firepit," dug in the center of the lodge. The fireplace symbolizes the center of the universe, the dwelling place of the Great Spirit and his Power. As the firekeeper carries the stones to the lodge, he walks an "umbilical cord," tracing the path of life from Creator to Creation.

Traditional sweats are not cogendered or "mixed," as Native people say; men and women sweat separately to honor their unique medicines. Participants humbly crawl into the lodge and find a place to sit cross-legged around the fireplace. They are naked, except for a towel or bathing suit covering their private parts, ready to face life without the coverings, masks, and roles that are the source of identity in the outer world.

The firekeeper uses a pitchfork—or if he is following the old tradition, deer antlers—to carry the red-hot stones to the entrance and pass them into the lodge. The medicine person, already seated inside, supervises their placement and may use a small antler to help load them in the pit. The first four stones invite, honor, and symbolize the four directions; the next three represent the sky or up, earth or down, and center. More stones are placed on top of these, as many as thirty in all, and the firekeeper closes the door flap. The lodge becomes pitch-black but for the faint glow of the stones. Sacred herbs such as sage, sweetgrass, cedar, or osha are placed on the stones to make an intense smudge that quickly fills the small space. Participants take turns pouring ladles of water over the rocks, creating searing heat inside the lodge. All of the senses expand and open to the natural elements.

Sitting in a darkness illuminated only by the mysterious red glow of the rocks, with the air hot and humid, participants feel that they have returned to the beginning of life on earth, the womb of creation.[10] The Sweat Lodge is the place of spiritual rebirth. (Not surprisingly, the Sweat Lodge plays a prominent role in Native American creation stories. According to the Diné, the Holy People planned the creation of the world in a Sweat Lodge.) Participants sweat away disease, pollution, negativity, and all forms of physical, emotional, mental, or spiritual obstructions to Truth and Power. The group sings healing and sacred songs, including some that are specific to the Sweat Lodge Ceremony. The ceremonial leader asks each person to pray out loud, one after the next. If it is an intertribal Sweat, participants pray in their own language. The ceremony is generally divided into four sections or "rounds," after each of which the door flap is briefly opened to let unneeded forces out and to allow refreshing energy in. Participants smoke the Sacred Pipe within the lodge, and sanctified water is passed around and drunk by each participant.

Nowhere is the Sweat more beautifully described than in the poem "A Circle Begins" by Santo Domingo Pueblo poet Harold Littlebird:

in the surround of snow-touched mountains
a circle begins
in a meadow by a snow melt creek

where hands weave a house of thin green saplings
it is a way of song
    a way of breathing
    a pure womb to center oneself through sweat
a way of blessing and being blessed
a circle of humility, prayer and asking
and there are no clocks to measure time
but the beating of our singing hearts[11]

The Blessings of the Sweat Lodge

To enter the Sweat Lodge is to be blessed by the ancient spirits of nature. Some people practice the ceremony as a regular weekly purification. It is commonly held before and sometimes after an important activity or event, such as a Vision Quest, hunting, healing, or naming ceremony. Because the Sweat Lodge is such a powerful place in which to pray, a person may host the ceremony in order to pray for a specific purpose—for example, the well-being of children, protection from misfortune, peace in the country or the world, or victory during times of war. The Sweat is usually a communal event that, through the sharing of wisdom and prayers, strengthens ties of mutual support. There is nothing wrong with a private Sweat Lodge, held whenever the need arises, however.

The Sweat Lodge is also a powerful purification after a painful, disturbing, or negative experience. The Sweat can help bring us solace after the death of a loved one, and it can renew our faith in Spirit during periods of hardship. Several of my Native American friends lament that so many Indian veterans—particularly Vietnam vets—could have been spared the psychologically and spiritually devastating effects of warfare if they had prepared for and closed their military service with the Sweat Lodge, other traditional warrior ceremonies, and the advice of elders. Thanks largely to the misrepresentation of Indian life by Hollywood, few non-Indians realize the wealth of rituals of peace and exculpation that were once commonly practiced among Native American peoples. When Maricopa warriors from the Gila River in Arizona returned from battle after killing a human being, they were isolated in a hut for sixteen days to heal and cleanse after the trauma. During this period, they bathed daily before dawn and ate only a small portion of mesquite bean gruel each morning. Elders visited the warriors every evening to remind them of the importance of societal obligations and traditional values such as kindness to others.[12] Without these rituals, post-traumatic stress disorder would have been as common in the past as it is today.

The Sweat is a common way for both healer and patient to prepare, individually or together, for subsequent counseling and doctoring. When the body is purged of impurities, the healer's energy can flow more strongly, and the patient becomes more sensitive and receptive. The Sweat Lodge is also considered a healing intervention by itself. Negative energies (including hexes), fears, insecurities, alienation, and apathy are sweated out and dissipate in the steam; poisons pour out the pores. The intensity of the Sweat helps participants express their prayers directly and powerfully; those spoken by others enter more deeply into the soul. Many healers bring their patients into the Sweat with them. Patients receive blessings, guidance, power, and information about the cause or cure of disease through the mediation of the healer or healing spirits. A healer may also bring sacred objects or medicines into the Lodge to bless and empower them for use either during the Sweat or at a later time. Spirit animals sometimes enter the Sweat: a buffalo may physically shake the lodge from the outside; an eagle may fly through the darkness and fan a patient with its wings.

The Sweat Lodge is itself a very powerful spirit, and it is this spirit that heals the patient. A medicine person who has this spirit as a helper—acquired like all helpers through Vision Quest but also through frequent participation in the Sweat Lodge—may be able to call on it to heal a patient, even outside of the actual ceremony. Mourning Dove (1888–1936), a member of the Colville Federated Tribes of eastern Washington State, wrote in her autobiography that no individual guiding spirit or animal power can overcome the Sweat Lodge Spirit, because it combines "five special strengths: wood for ribs, fire for heat, stones for stamina, earth for support, and water for cleansing."[13]

Many Like It Hot: Ancient Saunas throughout the World

Fire and water purification methods are found throughout the world. Not surprisingly, Central American Indians have practices closest to those found in North America. When the Spanish invaded Mexico in 1519, most Native homes had, nearby them, beehivelike sweat lodges, called *Temazcal* (Nahuatl, Aztec, for Bathhouse), made of mud or stone. *Temazcal* were also common in Guatemala and Belize and are still used today. The Aztecs believe that to enter one is to return to the warmth, humidity, and darkness of the mother's womb. The *Temazcal* is presided over by Tonantzin, the mother of all gods and humans and the goddess of herbs and healers. In it, a healer, usually a woman, fans a patient with a switch of therapeutic herbs and then massages him. The *Temazcal* is used to treat many conditions, including skin conditions, arthritis, pain, congestion, infertility, cysts, gout, and menstrual problems such as PMS and irregularity.[14]

Natural hot springs are common in Japan and China, where they have always been used to relax, to prevent disease, and, as part of religious discipline, to purify and strengthen the body. Because hot springs are usually in areas of great scenic beauty, Chinese people like to go to them to enjoy nature and write poetry.[15] Author and storyteller Joseph Bruchac reports that tribal healers in Liberia, Ghana, Nigeria, and other African countries use heat and steam for healing and purification.[16] The Vedas of India, religious hymns composed during the second millennium B.C., speak of *tapas,* a word that is usually translated "asceticism" but that literally means "extreme heat." In the eighth century B.C., Indians sometimes practiced a form of *tapas* called "the Five Fires" in which a person would sit in the center of four fires set in the four directions while a fifth fire, representing the sun, heated him from above. According to the Jain religion, interior concentration is also a form of *tapas;* it burns away seeds of past actions—*karma*—that stain the clarity of the soul. Some scholars believe that the word *shaman* is derived from an Indian word for an ascetic, *sramana,* from the Vedic root *sram,* "to heat oneself."[17]

In 425 B.C., Herodotus described wooden sweat bath houses of the Scythians, in present-day Russia. The Russians still practice therapeutic steaming; their word "to bathe," *paritsia,* literally means "to steam oneself." The ancient Greeks and Romans enjoyed baths of water and steam. The Finnish sauna and Scandinavian steam baths probably predate Christianity and, like the Native American sweat lodge, were enjoyed for physical and spiritual purification. In Iceland, there are many places where the ground visibly steams from underground geothermal activity. Icelanders build wooden, floorless shacks on these sites, to allow people to bathe in the concentrated natural steam that rises directly from and through Mother Earth. In one such site that I visited near Reykjavík, it is possible to conclude the sweat by jumping in a pure, cold lake just outside the "sweat lodge." As if this weren't enough of Paradise, there is a gourmet seafood restaurant a hundred paces away. (The idea of sacrifice and fasting is not incompatible with experiencing life's pleasures; it's all a matter of balance. I have attended a few nightlong Native American ceremonies that concluded when participants sang a song with the refrain "We've prayed long enough. When do we eat?")

In an article in *American Anthropologist,* Ivan Alexis Lopatin writes that the steam bath may have originated in northern Europe and spread, perhaps from Iceland, across the Atlantic to North America. We know that Leif Eriksson explored the New England coast, which he called Vinland, "the Land of Grape Vines," in A.D. 1001. He was probably not the first Norse seaman to visit these shores. It is also likely, however, that during this same period, Native Americans from Maine, Labrador, and Baffin Island journeyed to Iceland and Greenland. Perhaps the Finnish sauna was inspired by the North American sweat rather than the reverse. As anthropologist Robert L. Hall points out in *An Archaeology of the Soul,* "This Maritime Archaic culture dates from around 3000 to 1000 B.C. and was at least as well oriented toward exploiting sea resources as the contemporary cultures of northwestern Europe."[18]

The Benefits of Heat

The healing benefits of heat have been documented by Western medical science and clearly described in Dr. Jeanne Achterberg's landmark work *Imagery in Healing: Shamanism and Modern Medicine:* "[T]he sweat or sauna may act as a sterilization procedure, killing bacteria, viruses, and other organisms that thrive at body temperature, but are susceptible to heat."[19] The HIV virus, which causes AIDS, and the rhinovirus, responsible for the common cold and half of all respiratory infections, are especially sensitive to heat. External heat mimics fever, the body's natural reaction to toxins. It is reasonable to assume that as heat opens pores, dilates blood vessels, and stimulates circulation, impurities may be more quickly flushed out of the body. In addition, hyperthermia increases heart rate and improves blood flow to the skeletal muscles, effects associated with exercise and cardiovascular conditioning. (Certain viruses, however, such as herpes, may proliferate when heated. *Hyperthermia,* heat therapy, is not without risks to heat-sensitive people or those suffering from certain conditions, such as heart disease and seizure disorders.)[20]

At least fifty medical centers in the United States have experimented with using hyperthermia to kill cancer cells and to make remaining cancer cells more vulnerable to conventional therapy. Cancer researcher Ralph W. Moss, Ph.D., writes in *Cancer Therapy,* "For many types of cancer, heat therapy increases the chances of controlling the disease by 25 to 35 percent."[21] When the whole body is heated to 107 degrees Fahrenheit (42 degrees centigrade) or higher—as happens in the Sweat Lodge—cancerous cells, which are much more sensitive to the heat than surrounding tissue, are destroyed, and those that remain stop multiplying as quickly. Heat has the strongest effects on cancers of the head, brain, neck, breast, and skin.

More than half of United States Indian Health Service facilities promote the Sweat Lodge Ceremony as a complementary therapy. The Sweat has become an essential element of Indian-directed alcoholism treatment programs such as the White Sage Institute for Sustainable Health, a branch of the Four Worlds Development Project at the University of Lethbridge, Alberta. When the Sweat is combined with other therapies for alcoholism, such as counseling and health education, treatment outcomes are improved. There is evidence that hyperthermia can also benefit adult-onset diabetes, epidemic among Native Americans. In 1999, Philip L. Hooper, M.D., reported in the *New England Journal of Medicine* that diabetic patients who sat in hot tubs for thirty minutes a day, six days a week, for three weeks lost weight and had lower blood glucose levels. One patient reduced his insulin dose by 18 percent. The patients reported improved sleep and a general sense of well-being. Dr. Hooper concluded that hyperthermia should be further evaluated and "may be especially helpful for patients who are unable to exercise."[22]

— SACRED PIPE —

The Native American "Sacred Pipe" is part of a spiritual path that I call "the Way of the Pipe," in which a specially made pipe is used to communicate with spiritual powers and the Great Spirit. The pipe mixes the power and breath of one's body with the breath of nature (air) and the "breath" (smoke) of a plant such as tobacco. It may be smoked by an individual or shared with a group. A Pipe Ceremony can be considered a kind of meditation; the Sacred Pipe has the power to induce an expanded state of consciousness among participants. As soon as the ceremony begins, they feel as though they are one with all of life and are aware of realities that both underline and interpenetrate the ordinary.

Many tribes believe that the pipe and instructions for its use are a gift of the Great Spirit or a messenger from the Great Spirit. The Creator gave the Cree tribe sacred things that they could use to communicate with him: tobacco, fire, the pipe-bowl and stone of which it is made, the pipe-stem and the tree from which it is made, and sweetgrass. According to Blackfoot tradition, the Pipe was a gift of Thunder, brought to the people by his mortal wife. The Lakota say that the sacred White Buffalo Calf Woman gave the original Pipe to the Itazipco[23] branch of the Teton Lakota near Mato Tipila, "Bear Lodge" (incorrectly called "Devil's Tower" on U.S. maps). "With this sacred pipe, you will walk upon the Earth," she said, "for the Earth is your Grandmother and Mother, and She is sacred. Every step that is taken upon Her should be as a prayer."[24] White Buffalo Calf Woman advised the people to use the Pipe to "pray for and with everything."

You cannot purchase a sacred pipe in a store. You may find a pipe that looks like a sacred pipe, but it won't carry the spirit. *A pipe is only considered sacred if it is given to you by an elder who has blessed and "awakened" it in recognition of your worthiness to have it.* Criteria of "worthiness" vary from pipe carrier to pipe carrier. I personally feel that to receive a pipe, a person must first have performed many brave and good deeds for others. He or she may have raised ten orphans, volunteered at a hospice, brought peace between people or countries, saved fellow soldiers during an ambush, risked personal reputation to defend the truth, or performed other acts of courage and sacrifice. The most important "brave and good deed" is to live a good life, with integrity and responsibility, no matter what the pressure to live otherwise.

A person who has thus earned a pipe is called a "pipe carrier," though "pipe caretaker" probably more accurately describes the role. The pipe carrier is a male or female ceremonial leader who "carries" the pipe for the People. Some pipe carriers have more than one pipe, any of which may be dedicated to specific usages. For example, I have been given seven pipes. One of these is a personal pipe, which I do not share with others; another, which I call the "community pipe," I use with large groups; I also carry a pipe dedicated to world peace, a "disc" pipe, with a circular pipe-bowl, given to me shortly before the September 11, 2001 tragedy. Not everyone can be a pipe carrier, but anyone may be invited to smoke a sacred pipe in the Pipe Ceremony. The sacred pipe was called the "peace pipe" in many American Westerns from the 1950s. Some pipes, however, are "war pipes," smoked for success in battle. The pipe may be used as a counseling pipe, a council pipe, a healing pipe, a meditation pipe, and always, a prayer pipe. *Sacred pipe* is the best and most inclusive term.[25]

A Pipe Ceremony for All My Relations

The Way of the Pipe is my religion. I practice it in the church of Nature either by myself or with a circle of other worshipers. As I join the long wooden stem to the red pipestone bowl, I join the living, growing, green of the Plant People with the quiet strength of the mountain. As the bowl receives the stem, masculine and feminine are harmonized. I fill the pipe with a mixture of Indian tobacco and natural herbs that I have gathered with prayer: red willow bark, sage, bearberry, mullein, and other healing herbs that I have learned from elders and dreams. (Marijuana and recreational drugs are *never* smoked in the sacred pipe.) Holding each pinch of the mixture briefly in my fingers, then placing it in the bowl, I invite a spirit to enter the pipe and join the ceremony: the Four Winds, Grandmother Earth, the Sun, Moon, Stars, the Great Spirit. All of Creation is invited into the pipe-bowl.

I hold the filled pipe-bowl and point the stem to each of the helping powers, inviting them to smoke first. The pipe-bowl is carved into the shape of my animal ally, the face looking away from the stem, according to an ancient custom. As I offer the stem, I see this power facing me. When I smoke, the power will face away and help carry my prayers to Creator.

Then I place the pipe on an altar, cradling the T-shaped bowl in a small deer antler. I begin drumming and sing four songs. Then I pray. If I am sharing the pipe with my family or with a group, each participant gets a turn to offer a prayer. The prayers may be recited in any language or fashion the speaker chooses. Prayers may be long or short, but they are never a sermon. The purpose of prayer is to express deep feelings and to allow Spirit to speak through you. The shortest prayer is to simply say "All My Relations," meaning that the prayer is not for oneself but for the good of all. In a Christian church, worshipers end their prayers with "Amen." In a Pipe circle, each person's prayer ends with the expression "All My Relations," or this can be the prayer itself.

I lift the pipe carefully from the altar, always holding it in both hands, the bowl in one, stem in the other, and light it with a glowing braid of sweetgrass. I empty my mind to make my spirit hollow like the pipe, ready to be filled with the Great Spirit's breath. As I smoke, the separate "I" disappears. There is a sensation of merging with the breath of life; I don't know if I am smoking the pipe or if the pipe is a vehicle through which the Great Spirit smokes me. I puff seven times, rubbing some of the smoke on my chest to receive its blessing. If this is a healing ceremony, I may blow smoke on the patient while concentrating on healing power entering his or her body and chasing away disease. Then I pass the pipe to the person to my left. He or she takes seven puffs, and the pipe continues clockwise around the circle until all have smoked. If there is tobacco mixture left in the bowl, the pipe continues again around the circle until all of it has been smoked. The smoke makes our prayers visible and light and carries them up, out, and in to the Great Spirit.

When the ceremony is completed, I remove the stem from the bowl. The elements—wood and stone, male and female, sky and earth—have separated. We have returned from the always-present Sacred Realm, a state of being in which our minds can be one with one another and with Creation, to the divided dimensions of the everyday. The pipe is now just a bowl and a stem. I clean the pipe with a sharpened piece of wood and a long pipe cleaner and place it back in my moose-hide pipebag.

This has been a description of the basic elements of a Pipe Ceremony. It is not the whole ceremony, nor does it include the special instructions that are reserved for pipe carriers.

Sacred and Dangerous Power

Like the Sweat Lodge, a Pipe Ceremony provides protection from misfortune and more power to accomplish any goal. During a Pipe Ceremony, the power of good thoughts increases sevenfold, to more easily affect reality. The power of negative thoughts—not momentary, stray thoughts, but those deliberately maintained, with the intent to inflict harm—also increases sevenfold. Through the power of the pipe, the negative energy does not escape with the breath; it implodes, harming the thinker. I have heard elders describe the pipe, loaded with tobacco and ready for smoking, as a "loaded gun." It must be used with great care and respect.

The Sacred Pipe Ceremony is the most powerful way to make a vow or seal a promise because the Great Spirit is your witness and is always in the contract. Native Americans often recount a story about General George Armstrong Custer as an example of the pipe's power. Custer smoked the pipe with a Tsistsistas (Cheyenne) holy man, Stone Forehead, in the tribe's most sacred ceremonial lodge. When Custer asked the meaning of the ceremony, one of the Tsistsistas attending told him that he was swearing to keep his promises. As he smoked, Custer said, "I will never harm the Cheyennes again. I will never point my gun at a Cheyenne again."[26] When the tobacco was finished, Stone Forehead used his wooden pipe tamper to scoop some ashes from the pipe-bowl, deliberately causing them to fall on the general's boots, warning him, "If you break your promise, you and your soldiers will go to dust like this." Custer repeated his promise. The Battle of the Little Big Horn tells the story of the price Custer paid for his deceit.

Stems and Bowls: Types of Traditional Pipes

Individuals and tribes have their own ways of making and working with the pipe. The most common pipe-bowl is made of the beautiful red pipestone (*Inyan Sha,* "Red Sacred Stone," in Lakota), also called catlinite, after author and painter George Catlin, who visited the Pipestone Quarry in Minnesota in the 1830s. Pipestone is considered the blood of Mother Earth or the congealed blood of ancient people who were crushed in a great flood that once covered the prairies. It is quarried without power tools by hardworking and dedicated Native Americans. Some tribes make their bowls of black or green steatite (also called soapstone), gray shale, black slate, or clay. Clay pipes probably represent the oldest pipes made of nonperishable materials in the Americas. Olmec clay pipes have been dated to 1200–900 B.C. In the 1820s, the Haida and other northwestern tribes began to make entire pipes, stem and bowl, out of argillite, a beautiful soft black stone found only in Canada's Queen Charlotte Islands. Although, today, some Native people use them ceremonially, these pipes were originally made only for trade with the whites.

The pipe-bowl is generally shaped like either an *L* or an upside-down *T* and, like the stem, may be carved or decorated according to the pipe carrier's dream. From the thirteenth through the sixteenth centuries, a round, disc-shaped pipestone bowl with a shallow tobacco hole in its center was common throughout north-central North America and continued in use among the Osage and Iowa. It is still made by pipe makers at Pipestone National Monument.

The ceremonial pipe-stem is generally from nine to eighteen inches long. It may also be made of pipestone or other stones, though by far the most common material is wood. Sumac is a favorite because the soft pith can be easily burned out with a heated rod to make the smoke channel. Other woods such as the red osier, willow, and ash are also common. Pipe makers may use any wood that is local and that "speaks to them." Keetoowah was fond of using Osage orange wood and once made me a pipe-stem of aspen. While performing sacred dances, dancers sometimes hold wooden pipe-stems decorated with eagle feathers, ribbons, and other ornaments.

Although pipes with a separate stem and bowl are now the most common, in ancient times, simple tubular pipes were created from the leg bones of deer, antelope, or other animals. Tobacco was packed in the wider end of the pipe, and the entire pipe could be wrapped with sinew or rawhide to prevent the hot pipe from cracking and to make it easier to hold. A small stone placed in the tube prevented the smoker from ingesting pieces of burning tobacco. In California, tubular pipes were often made of polished manzanita or other hardwoods. The tubular pipe had the disadvantage of requiring the smoker to tilt his or her head back to prevent the tobacco from falling out. This problem was solved by creating a bent-shaped bowl in which one end held the tobacco and the other end was fitted with a stem. Small single-piece bent pipes of clay have long been common among the Haudenosaunee and Huron. They are generally not passed but rather are smoked by an individual as a contemplative practice that inspires good thoughts. This is not, however, an inflexible rule. Community pipes are sometimes smoked by a single person, and personal pipes are sometimes shared. I was once honored to smoke a personal clay pipe with a Huron elder in memory of one of his ancestors.

Two rare types of pipe ceremony allow several people to smoke a single pipe at the same time. In the first, smokers insert their own stems into a round bowl with multiple stem-holes. In the other, Earth-Pipe Ceremony, smokers lie on their bellies and place their stems into a common pit filled with hot coals and tobacco. The earth is the pipe-bowl. The Earth-Pipe is an ancient and widespread method of smoking natural herbs. It is a natural extension of the common practice of putting sacred herbs in a fire while praying. The Earth-Pipe Ceremony has been reported in South Africa and in West and Central Asia. It is still practiced by Native Americans.

Some readers may wonder why I have failed to mention the most common pipe in North America, the corncob pipe. According to Anishinabe elder and herbalist Keewaydinoquay (1918–1999), the corncob pipe was invented by Native Americans for smoking medicinal herbs; in other words, it was part of herbal therapeutics rather than ceremonial tradition. For instance, for headache relief, one might smoke a mixture of willow bark, sweetgrass leaves, and bearberry leaves; for bronchial problems, one could smoke mullein leaves. A smoking mixture, says Grandma Kee, "is placed in a clean pipe (one that has never been used for any other purpose) and smoked slowly by the patient. This is how corncob pipes came to be invented—to meet the need, in medicinal smoking, of a quickly prepared one-time receptacle easily disposed of after use."[27] Because mission school education had convinced Kee's mother that "no God-fearing lady would ever smoke anything for any reason," Kee often placed her headache herbs on the kitchen stove's hot iron, where she could inhale the fumes. She was determined to be a healer and a lady at the same time, a feat that Christians might have considered impossible!

Euro-Americans who commonly smoke a corncob, meerschaum, or briar wood pipe may also be aware of a pipe's potential for preventing disharmony. It is impossible to hold a pipe in one's mouth and argue at the same time! What William Thackeray said of the briar pipe a Native American could have said of the ceremonial pipe: "The pipe draws wisdom from the lips of the philosopher, and shuts up the mouth of the foolish: it generates a style of conversation, contemplative, thoughtful, benevolent, and unaffected. . . ."[28] Some of this effect is undoubtedly the result of the tobacco itself, which is nature's most powerful healing herb.

13

— TOBACCO —
Wicked Weed or Gift of the Gods?

SMOKING SPIRITS

According to creation stories and teachings from tribes throughout the Americas, spirits, like humans, love tobacco, and they placed it on the earth to help people communicate with them, with nature, and with the Creator. Tobacco is the sacred herb of prayer. Its smoke is offered to the spirits, to express gratitude to those who help us, and to protect us from those who can cause harm.

In the Diné creation story, Sky Father and Earth Mother planned the creation of the world while smoking tobacco. In the beginning of the world, say the Yokut of central California, Hawk Spirit chewed tobacco to become wise, after which he made the mountains. The Absarokee believe that tobacco is a star that descended to earth. The Kickapoo, originally from Wisconsin and Illinois, and the Cahuilla of southern California both say that the Creator took tobacco from his own heart. In the Cahuilla story, the Creator made the sun to light the first pipe, also taken from his heart. The Haudenosaunee tell a beautiful tale that symbolizes the relationship between tobacco and the spirit of the earth. Earth Mother, the first woman born on earth, gave birth to the twins Tarachiawagon, the good spirit, who made all the good things on earth, including people, animals, rain, and plants (except for the sacred plants corn, beans, squash, and tobacco), and Tawiskaron, the evil twin, who made monsters, diseases, and other evil things. When Earth Mother died, corn, beans, and squash—the three staples of life—grew from her body; tobacco, which calms and soothes the mind, grew from her head. Many Native tribes believe that tobacco is protected by the Little People, foot-high spirits who, like tobacco, act as intermediaries among the human, natural, and spiritual worlds.[1]

Some Central and South American tribes say that the Great Spirit smokes tobacco. Lacondon Maya of the Mexican rain forest say that the Lords of Rain and Thunder are passionate smokers. In physician and anthropologist Francis Robicsek's authoritative text *The Smoking Gods,* we read that "the comets (or meteorites) passing through the dark-blue tropical skies are still-glowing cigars they [the Mayan Gods] have thrown away."[2] Yucatec legends describe how the Balams, the Gods of the Winds and the Four Directions, strike huge rocks together to create sparks to light their cigars. We mortals hear the crashing rocks as thunder and see the sparks as lightning.

Because tobacco is such a sacred gift, it must always be smoked with awareness and respect. This principle applies as much to cigarettes, cigars, and Western pipes as to Native ceremonial use of tobacco. Rolling Thunder taught that after you light tobacco, with your first puff, you should think a good thought or make a prayer. With your second, quiet your mind; rest in stillness. With your third puff, you can receive insight related to your prayer—perhaps an image, words spoken by spirit, or an intuitive feeling. I often share this technique with people who are addicted to tobacco. By making them conscious of a previously unconscious habit and awakening, through prayer, the spirit of tobacco, they are freed from the addiction. Many cease smoking altogether or begin to smoke only on special occasions, when they are in a prayerful mood.

TYPES OF TOBACCO

Tobacco belongs to the genus *Nicotiana* (from which derives the word *nicotine*), named for Jean Nicot, the sixteenth-century French ambassador to Portugal who once sent a gift of tobacco to the queen of France. It is a member of the nightshade family, along with potatoes, tomatoes, and eggplant; hallucinogens like mandrake and belladonna; and some common garden flowers such as the petunia (from *petún,* a Brazilian tribal word for tobacco). The plant itself is quite beautiful. It grows from two to nine feet high with thick, moist stems; large, fleshy, oval-shaped green leaves; and funnel-shaped pink, yellow, or white flowers. There are nine species of tobacco in North America (including Mexico). The most common are the wild *Nicotiana rustica* or *Nicotiana attenuata* and the cultivated *Nicotiana tabacum* varieties. Wild tobacco, commonly called "Indian tobacco" or "real tobacco" by Native Americans, is considered the most spiritually potent and is used exclusively for ceremony.[3] All kinds of tobacco are sacred.

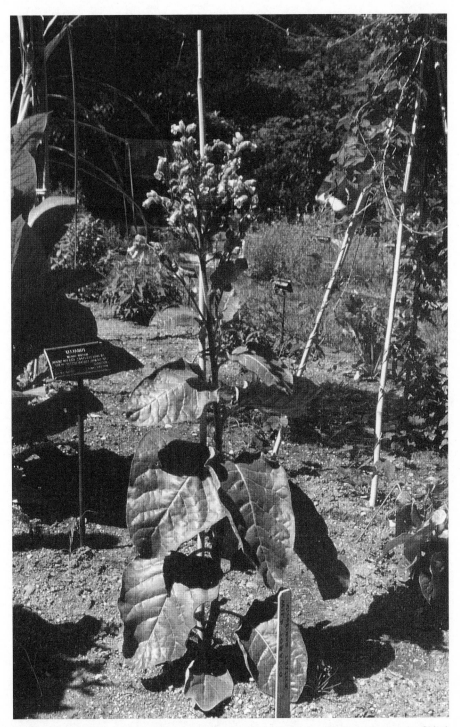

"Indian tobacco" (Nicotiana rustica) *in the Brooklyn Botanic Garden. Photo by Alessandro Chiari.*

USES OF TOBACCO

There is no way to catalog all of tobacco's uses, since these often vary from person to person. The most common include smudging a person or place by burning the dried leaves; smoking the leaf to induce a state of mental calm, expanded awareness, and prayerfulness; blowing tobacco smoke on a patient to enhance healing; sprinkling dried, crushed leaves on the ground, on an altar, or in a fire, as a gesture of gratitude and respect; and using the fresh leaves or a tea made from them in ointments, poultices, decoctions, and other healing remedies.

We cannot determine with certainty how much tobacco is smoked by Native people who identify themselves as "traditional" or how much was smoked in the past. I have a Cherokee friend who prides himself on "not smoking," by which he means he doesn't smoke cigarettes. He smokes tobacco only in his sacred pipe, perhaps once every month. On the other hand, I know a Cherokee healer who smokes a pack of cigarettes a day. He always prays with his first puff of each cigarette, but in spite of this brief homage to traditional culture, he uses tobacco primarily as a drug. Yet he is a pipe carrier, and when he loads tobacco in his sacred pipe, he clearly enters a sacred realm. Like many Native people, he lives in two worlds, the Indian and the white, and uses tobacco in both.

Although scientists studying ancient peoples have learned that they suffered from many modern illnesses, there is no evidence that ancient smokers experienced an unusual incidence of cancer or heart disease. On the contrary, the combination of *organic* tobacco leaves, moderation, and positive thoughts made tobacco a powerful agent of healing. In fact, the reasons why cigarettes cause cancer are not as simple as one might suppose. They have less to do with tobacco than with the chemicals used to grow and process it.

— HEALING THE SPIRIT —

The Indians of Haiti and Hispaniola gave tobacco its name. They purified themselves in a *tabaco,* a sweat lodge, with the smoke of an herb of the same name. Indigenous peoples throughout the world, including those who first received tobacco from European traders, consider tobacco an important ingredient in ceremony. Because it comes from the Spirit World, tobacco nourishes the human spirit with power and wisdom. It also "feeds" the spirit powers, some of whom live only on tobacco. Burning tobacco leaves in an outdoor fire or in the fire of a pipe is, of itself, an act of worship, similar to lighting a votive candle on a church altar. Smoking tobacco with a respectful attitude increases the smoker's sensitivity to healing forces. As Karuk author, artist, and tribal scholar Julian Lang writes in his beautiful article "The Divine Origin of Tobacco," "Tobacco and pipes go hand in hand with doctoring. At every healing ceremony in the northwest, the doctor danced and smoked her pipe. The pipe was the means for the doctor to 'get into her power.' . . . All doctors smoked, and the more they smoked the better the patient and his or her family felt."[4]

To prepare tobacco for healing or conjuring—which means to influence people, events, or natural phenomena with spiritual power[5]—Cherokee medicine people knead and turn tobacco in the palm while praying silently or out loud. The ritual, called "remaking tobacco," is most effective when performed at dawn by the edge of a river or other body of water, where water meets land and night meets day. The healer thus stands at the border between the spirit and mundane worlds and, like tobacco, is a bridge between the two.

Tobacco's power is naturally linked to breath. The healer blows tobacco smoke on a patient to encourage friendly spirits and dispel harmful ones, who detest its scent, and to seal healing energy in the body. The Pima or *Akimel O'Odham* ("River People") of Arizona say that *wústana,* the act of blowing breath or smoke on a patient, "illuminates" the disease—that is, it helps the healer to spiritually see its cause. Anthropologist Donald M. Bahr and his colleagues report in the classic *Piman Shamanism and Staying Sickness*, "Smoke is said to be the shaman's 'helper.' "[6]

Tobacco smoke is a powerful insecticide, and it may be blown on crops to help rid them of infestations. It also acts as a repellent to mosquitoes, gnats, and other stinging insects. On a spiritual level, tobacco smoke chases away pathogenic forces, including the insect spirits sometimes directed by sorcerers to their victims.

Tobacco opens the door to other realities. Both the smoke and the plant itself are a kind of passport, identifying the bearer as an Earth Person. As a gift, tobacco expresses gratitude, respect, and a sense of sacred connection. Before picking an herb, Native Americans talk to the plant and place a pinch of dried tobacco leaves near it as an expression of gratitude. Requests for a healing are often accompanied by a pouch of tobacco, and in the Northern Plains, one should always offer a pouch of tobacco or, if one is a pipe carrier, a tobacco-filled sacred pipe to an elder when asking for his or her guidance. I knew an elder who tested his students' commitment and sincerity by smoking the most awful-smelling tobacco in his corncob pipe. If you could sit through a conversation without choking, you had earned some good teachings by the end of your visit.

Tobacco ties may be placed on a ceremonial altar and are sometimes hung from the rafters of the sweat lodge. They are also left as offerings to special places in nature. When I first moved to the Rocky Mountains, I made a string of forty-nine tobacco ties—seven directions times seven—and carried them to a beautiful waterfall, where I wrapped them around the limb of a nearby pine. You are likely to find tobacco ties hanging from tree branches or resting on boulders at Native American sacred sites, including some that have, unfortunately, become public parks. Never touch or disturb them. Although tobacco ties are sometimes burned, many are left, like Tibetan prayer flags, exposed to the elements, to carry good thoughts, prayers, and blessings on the wind.

The spiritual meaning of tobacco was ignored by the early colonists. The English courtier Sir Walter Raleigh (1554–1618) helped to popularize tobacco as a recreational drug and commercial crop and developed a method of curing the leaf that is still used today. Many people have heard the famous story of how a servant saw plumes of smoke pouring from a clay tube sticking out of Sir Walter's mouth. Thinking that his master was on fire, the servant threw a barrel of beer over his head to "put him out." Such mishaps did nothing to dampen enthusiasm, however. Sailors and traders brought tobacco back to Europe, and by 1600, smoking was considered a mark of fashion, similar to playing cards and dancing. Smoking dens filled with "reeking gallants," as the smokers were called, sprang up all over England, where gentlemen would light one another's pipes with a coal on the point of a sword and practice blowing elegant smoke rings.

Yet when traders brought tobacco to the indigenous people of Siberia during the late sixteenth century, *the spirit of the plant told them that it was to be used in a sacred and ceremonial way.* Siberian shamans smoked tobacco in foot-long pipes with silver bowls and detachable wooden stems. They considered tobacco smoke an excellent offering to the spirits of place and to personal spirit helpers. Vladimir N. Basilov's essay "Chosen by the Spirits" contains a classic description of how Siberian Yakut shamans enter trance states. The shaman stares intently into a fire, and as it "... wanes little by little, darkness and quiet settle over the yurt [the standard Siberian tribal dwelling]. The shaman ... then takes up a lighted pipe and smokes a long time, gulping the smoke."[7] The shaman then half closes his eyes and reaches dreamily for his drum, which he begins to beat rhythmically. In her book *Chosen by the Spirits,* Siberian Buryat shaman Sarangerel says that when she brought a Native American sacred pipe to Siberian shamans, they knew how to use it ceremonially, and a Buryat shaman who had smoked with Native American elders felt that their practices were almost identical.[8]

Many anthropologists believe that Native American culture originated in Siberia and spread across the Bering Strait into Alaska and southward. I believe that the similarities in spiritual beliefs and practices point to the universal truths discovered by people who live close to nature. In his book *Soma: Divine Mushroom of Immortality,* renowned scholar of the world's religions R. Gordon Wasson supports this view: "Let it be noted that tobacco became adapted to Siberian Shamanism without the influence of the American Indian cultures. Here lies a wholesome object lesson for those who would lightly draw inferences of trans-Pacific contacts merely on the strength of parallel usages."[9]

— HEALING THE BODY —

The tobacco leaf is used in a wide variety of healing drinks, poultices, and smoking mixtures throughout the Americas. I do not recommend that readers try any of the following remedies themselves because I am only outlining basic ingredients or procedures, and as with other indigenous prescriptions, many are meant to be taken as part of healing rituals supervised by elders.

The Mayans drink a mix of chocolate, peppers, honey, and tobacco juice for fever, skin rashes, and seizures. For prostate problems and difficult urination, they make a drink consisting of fried tobacco leaves that are ground into a powder and combined with cane liquor. To cure bloating, Mayan herbalists prescribe eating the fresh leaves with garlic cloves. To prevent miscarriage, they massage a woman's abdomen with a mixture of tobacco and lime. The Aztecs apply tobacco as a poultice for abscesses and snakebites. The Cherokee and Haudenosaunee put the leaves directly against cavities to reduce pain.[10] In the southeastern United States, moistened tobacco leaves remain a common folk remedy, among Natives and non-Natives alike, for bee stings and snakebites.

Tribes west of the Mississippi steep tobacco leaves in bear grease as an ointment for swellings and skin conditions. Many tribes such as the Paiute, Shoshone, and the Haisla and Hanaksiala of central British Columbia use a poultice of chewed tobacco leaves for rheumatoid arthritis or apply juice squeezed from the fresh leaves directly over inflamed or painful areas. Mohegan healers blow tobacco smoke in the ear for earaches. The Nanticoke of Delaware and Maryland blow the smoke into a cup of water to make a medicine for stomachaches. The Shoshone make a decoction of the leaves to expel intestinal worms, a usage adopted by Western medicine in the eighteenth century. The Thompson of southwest British Columbia use the decoction as a hairwash for dandruff and to prevent falling hair. For spring and summer fevers, Cherokee healers make a warm decoction by placing four dry tobacco leaves in water with seven hot coals. While the patient stands facing the sunrise, the healer recites a chant, then takes some of the medicine in his mouth and blows a spray of it on top of the patient's head, followed by his right shoulder, left shoulder, and chest or back. A Cherokee healer may hold blossoms or a decoction of the blossoms of tobacco, lobelia, and wild parsnip (*Pastinaca sativa,* the root of which is poisonous) in his mouth while sucking out an evil or destructive spirit. Tobacco helps to neutralize the intrusion's harmful power. Tobacco is even used in indigenous veterinary medicine. The Catawbas feed a tobacco infusion to sick horses. Europeans were not blind to this powerful medicine. In 1573, Jean Nicot published a French-Latin dictionary that gave the following definition of tobacco: "This is an herb of marvelous virtue against wounds, ulcers, lupus of the face, herpes, and all other things."[11]

More recently, tobacco is valued in medical research. In "Tobacco Can Be Good for You," published in the *New York Times Magazine,* August 23, 1998, science journalist Thomas Maeder describes tobacco as one of the most useful plants in genetic engineering: "It's the lab mouse of the plant world, the plant on which a lot of original genetics work was done," says Arnold Foudin, a scientist with the United States Department of Agriculture, quoted in the article. Scientists insert human and animal genes into tobacco plants through a gene-splicing technique called recombinant technology. Tobacco thus becomes the raw material to create new:

- *Antibiotics:* An antibiotic, which literally means "to destroy life," kills or slows the growth of harmful, disease-producing cells, such as bacteria. It is commonly produced from living "host" cells, but the problem is that powerful antibiotics often kill their hosts, making the production process slow, difficult, and expensive. Antibiotics cannot easily destroy genetically modified tobacco cells. Tobacco is thus a potent source of the desired antibiotic molecules.
- *Blood products:* Tobacco is a source of genetic material to create human hemoglobin and anticlotting agents for treating stroke and heart disease.
- *Cancer vaccines:* Here's an irony: the plant that many believe causes cancer is being used to grow vaccines that may one day help cure it.
- *Dental rinses:* Guy's Hospital Dental School in London has successfully administered oral solutions of tobacco-grown microorganisms that prevent the *Streptococcus mutans* bacteria from causing tooth decay. The solution may someday be used as a mouthwash.
- *Eco-friendly plastics:* Henry Daniell, a molecular geneticist at Auburn University in Alabama, has used tobacco to synthesize a protein found in human connective tissue. Tobacco may someday be a source of materials for reconstructive tissue surgery and inexpensive, biodegradable plastics.

— HEALING THE MIND —

Moderate tobacco smoking induces a calm yet alert state of mind: qualities equally prized by Native Americans and by Asian meditators. According to Dr. Robert E. Svoboda, a practitioner of *Ayurveda,* the traditional medicine of India, "Tobacco can make task performance easier by enhancing alertness and concentration, improving memory (especially long-term memory), reducing anxiety, increasing pain tolerance and reducing hunger . . . ,"[12] depending on how much tobacco is consumed. A few puffs stimulate the nervous system; a five- or ten-minute period of smoking calms it and may produce feelings of euphoria. Excessive smoking is toxic.[13]

From the scientific viewpoint, these various effects are caused by tobacco's principal active component, nicotine. Nicotine is fat-soluble and easily absorbed by cells and tissues throughout the body, causing widespread and rapid physiological changes. It reaches a smoker's brain in seven seconds.

Nicotine closely resembles one of the body's natural chemicals, the neurotransmitter acetylcholine (ACH), which carries messages across the gaps (synapses) between nerve cells and, by attaching to *receptor cells* in the motor nerves, tells our muscles to either contract or relax. ACH receptors are also found in the medulla, hypothalamus, thalamus, cerebellum, and cerebral cortex regions of the brain. Like a skeleton key, nicotine fits all the ACH "locks." Inside the body, nicotine mimics ACH's actions. At first, nicotine acts as a stimulant. It accelerates the burning of glucose, the raw material for cellular energy, setting off quick, low-voltage brain waves to produce a hyperalert mental state. Nicotine also releases potent neurochemicals such as epinephrine, norepinephrine, serotonin, and dopamine. In excess, these chemicals cause restlessness, tension, high blood pressure, headaches, anxiety, and fear—all reasons to avoid recreational tobacco use.

A clue about potential calming effects of tobacco can be found in the smoking habits of schizophrenics. Many clinicians have observed that schizophrenics are often heavy smokers. A tobacco-stained index finger has even been used as a clinical sign of the disease. In "Schizophrenia and Nicotinic Receptors," published in 1994 in the *Harvard Review of Psychiatry,* Robert Freedman, M.D., and colleagues explored the biological effects of nicotine on schizophrenics and possible reasons why schizophrenics feel compelled to smoke.

The brains of schizophrenics lack the ability to effectively block or "gate" stimuli. For example, the sound of an electric fan or the hum of a refrigerator would not interfere with your ability to engage in a conversation. Your brain automatically filters out irrelevant or distracting stimuli in order to pay attention. For a schizophrenic, without such filtering action, a noisy or visually complex environment is a painful mosaic of stimuli, any or all of which may add to the confusion produced by delusional thoughts or hallucinations. Nicotine-sensitive ACH receptors in the hippocampus are responsible for healthy gating. Dr. Freedman and associates found that "[s]moking is probably the most effective way to provide the brain with brief bursts of high-dose nicotine that are most likely to activate the receptors, but even this treatment, in which the peak levels last less than 15 minutes, leads to desensitization and only transient improvement."[14] To put it simply, smoking cigarettes provides a brief filter that allows more appropriate awareness and focus.

Scientists have yet to explore what effect nicotine has when ingested during a ritual atmosphere of sage smoke, prayer, and drumming. Nicotine produces quick, low-voltage brain waves, indicating a state of extreme alertness, bordering on anxiety. Native American drumming stimulates slow, highly charged brain waves, indicating mental focus, intuition, and tranquillity. Do the effects of drumming override or modify the effects of nicotine? Does tobacco cause anxiety in some people but calm or even euphoria in others? Interestingly, as James H. Austin, M.D., points out in his monumental book *Zen and the Brain,* human subjects who receive nicotine intravenously "cannot distinguish between the euphoriant effect of nicotine and that of morphine or amphetamine."[15] Do the ACH receptors, filled by nicotine, cause a release of brain opiates? Perhaps the mind-altering effects of nicotine are a result of the resemblance between the chemicals it releases and certain hallucinogens, specifically norepinephrine to mescaline and serotonin to psilocybin. How does ceremony effect the behavior of these naturally occurring internal chemicals? All of these questions have yet to be answered.[16]

My hypothesis is that among healthy participants in Native American ceremony, tobacco filters a potentially confusing array of realities and perceptions. It allows a person to focus deliberately on any reality or aspect of reality, whether conventional or alternate. Tobacco invokes spiritual forces and strengthens the faculty to perceive them.

DOES TOBACCO CAUSE CANCER?
YES AND NO

How is it that such a powerful spiritual healing substance has become public enemy number one in the ongoing war against cancer? Certainly, there is a massive body of scientific research that shows the carcinogenic potential of tobacco. People who smoke cigarettes, cigars, and pipes have, respectively, 68 percent, 22 percent, and 12 percent higher mortality rates than nonsmokers. The conventional wisdom blames nicotine, but the culprit may be the way tobacco is processed for commercial production and the attitude with which it is used rather than the tobacco itself. From the Native American viewpoint, there are three reasons why smoking tobacco *may* be hazardous to health:

1. *Overuse and addiction:* People who smoke tobacco moderately, with prayer and attentiveness, do not become addicts.
2. *Absence of sacred intent:* When you use tobacco or any plant according to the Creator's plan, you receive a blessing; when you ignore the Creator's plan, you receive a curse. Not praying when using this most sacred herb is a sacrilege equivalent to stomping on a Bible. The payback may be cancer. And as I said earlier, praying with tobacco is a good way to become conscious of unconscious, habitual smoking, making it easier to stop.
3. *Adulterated crops:* Traditional Native Americans smoked only organic tobacco, and some evidence suggests that where tobacco is still grown naturally,

lung cancer rates are lower. According to the United States Surgeon General's 1992 report *Smoking and Health in the Americas,* the smoke-attributable lung cancer mortality rates throughout Latin America are consistently lower than those of North America. Mexico has about one-fifth the rate of the United States. Central and South American Indians, traditionally heavy smokers, have a low incidence of cancer.

Commercial tobacco, grown with pesticides and chemical fertilizers, is carcinogenic. Cigarette tobacco contains approximately one hundred carcinogenic compounds, including phenol, a poisonous, caustic acid that gradually destroys the bronchial tissue, and benzopyrene, an irritant found in both coal and tobacco tars. Though clearly harmful, scientists consider these substances to be relatively weak carcinogens and not the major cause of smoking-related lung cancer. Tars, for example, probably account for only 1 percent of smoke-attributable cancers. The chemical carcinogens in tobacco do not *cause* cancer; they *encourage* it, making it more likely to occur by weakening the lungs, damaging tissue, and making the cells more vulnerable to infection. Instead, it is the unusually high levels of radioactivity found in North American commercial tobaccos that are the direct link between smoking and cancer.

The amount of background radiation exposure from ordinary air, food, and water is small, about two hundred millirads per year, or five rads (five thousand millirads) in twenty-five years. By modest estimates, an average cigarette smoker is exposed to a minimum of twenty rads per twenty-five years, four times the normal background radiation. (See the sidebar "Radioactive Cigarettes.")[17] The lung tissues of chain smokers are continuously bombarded with highly carcinogenic alpha radiation particles. *These particles are the most likely direct cause of cancer in smokers, working in synergy with chemical carcinogens, viruses, genetic susceptibility, and emotional/spiritual factors.*

Given the extreme toxicity of radiation, if the radioisotopes found in tobacco were delivering highly concentrated radiation doses to lung cells, they would kill the cells rather than cause cancer. Instead, levels of radiation are just enough to corrupt the cells' DNA without destroying their ability to reproduce, creating ideal conditions for cancer cell growth. This level of radiation distributed throughout the lungs over an extended period of time is far more harmful than short-term, concentrated doses. In other words, contrary to what we might assume, radioactivity that is merely "warm" is sometimes more dangerous than that which is "hot."

Scientists who have conducted research confirming the radioactive components of tobacco smoke include Dr. Edward P. Radford Jr., former chairman of the prestigious Biological Effects of Ionizing Radiation Committee (BEIR) of the National Academy of Sciences; Dr. Vilma R. Hunt of the Environmental Protection Agency; Dr. Edward Martell, a senior radiochemist with the National Center for Atmospheric Research; and Dr. John B. Little, chair of cancer cell biology at

— RADIOACTIVE CIGARETTES —

For a comprehensive understanding of the biological dangers of tobacco radioactivity, we need to take into account the combined effect of various radioactive isotopes found in tobacco, the inefficient gaseous exchange in smokers' lungs (causing smoke particles to linger in the tissues), and radioactive "hot spots," such as the bifurcation of the bronchial tree, where the concentration of radioactive elements may be one thousand times greater than in the lungs. Considering all of these factors, a person who smokes one and a half packs of cigarettes daily may receive as much as 60 millirads of radiation each day, 21.9 rads per year, and 547.5 rads in twenty-five years: the equivalent of 547,500 chest X rays.[18]

Scientists have documented several reasons why tobacco produces dangerous levels of radioactivity:

- The chemical fertilizers used to grow tobacco contain calcium. Naturally occurring radium 226 is structurally similar to calcium and may fill its chemical bond, making these fertilizers radioactive.

- Because of wind direction in the United States, the East Coast, where most tobacco is grown, has high levels of airborne contaminants, including radioisotopes. For instance, radon gas produced across the continent blows east and is concentrated in the East Coast. Air and soil radioactivity levels have also increased because of fallout from nuclear testing during the 1950s and 1960s.

- Lead 210, a decay product or "daughter" of radium 226, has a strong tendency to attach to the tips of the fine hairs on tobacco leaves. As the tobacco leaves burn, lead 210 lodges in the lung tissue. Because lead 210 is not water-soluble, it does not wash quickly out of the smoker's body. As it decays, it exposes the body to carcinogenic alpha particles.

- During its half-life of 21.5 years, lead 210 further decays into another toxic isotope, polonium 210.[19] Polonium 210 becomes volatile and dangerous at temperatures above 500 degrees centigrade, well below the temperature of a burning cigarette. It bonds strongly and rapidly to smoke particles. Polonium 210 has a half-life of 138 days, ample time to shoot cancer-causing alpha radiation bullets at and into the bronchi and lungs. Researchers have confirmed that low doses of alpha radiation from polonium 210 can induce lung cancer in animals.[20]

- Not surprisingly, the lung tissue, lymph nodes, and tumors of smokers contain unusual concentrations of the 210 radioisotopes.

Harvard School of Public Health. Their evidence, presented in the *New England Journal of Medicine, Science, American Scientist,* and other publications, has never been refuted.[21] Scientists with whom I spoke at the National Academy of Sciences lamented that the important link among tobacco, radioactivity, and cancer has been tragically "passed over." Some researchers suggested a cover-up that might be economically motivated. If the general public became aware of the risks of low-dose radiation, the safe radiation exposure threshold might have to be lowered. Smokers who have cancer would have concrete proof of the mechanism that causes cancer, further establishing the tobacco industry's culpability. In other words, both the nuclear and tobacco industries would be more clearly liable for the damage to American health.

POWERFUL MEDICINE SHOULD BE USED CAUTIOUSLY

Each year, more than four hundred thousand Americans die of cancer and heart and lung diseases attributable to smoking. Smoking is responsible for 90 percent of all lung cancers, 92 percent of all mouth cancers, and approximately 50 percent of heart disease and cerebrovascular disease between the ages of thirty-five and sixty-four. Native Americans, like other races, are addicted to commercial tobacco and are being destroyed by the same herb that once promoted their health. In 1995, the U.S. Department of Health and Human Services reported that more Native American pregnant women smoked cigarettes than any other ethnic group (20.9 percent compared to 10.6 percent African-Americans and 15 percent whites). Although moderate ceremonial use of organic tobaccos does not appear to be harmful, I am certainly not advising that more people should smoke cigarettes. On the contrary, a clear understanding of the sacredness of tobacco and its proper cultivation and usage can encourage a drastic reduction in smoking and cancer.

14

— PLANT PEOPLE —
The Healing Power of Herbs

N'Tsukw, an Innu elder from northeastern Canada, sat across from me on the mountaintop. Beneath us stretched a shifting panorama of green foothills dotted with lakes and rivers. The constant, unobstructed breeze made the late-summer midday heat tolerable and kept the buzzing mosquitoes at bay among the nearby black spruce trees. N'Tsukw described the ancient landscape. He showed me where glaciers had left their marks, where rivers had been diverted by the white man, leaving dried-up riverbeds, and where Native people had once camped or fished.

"This is a good place to begin our lesson," N'Tsukw said, as he picked up a small stone and placed it between us. "We teach our children like this."

"Once, a long time ago, snow and ice covered the earth. Life was hidden until the warm, life-giving winds of the South melted the snows and revealed the sleeping Stone People."

N'Tsukw touched the stone.

"The stones were created first. They are the elders, the First People."

N'Tsukw removed a small red cloth from his pouch and placed it on the stone. Then he took out a pinch of tobacco and sprinkled it on the cloth.

"This represents moss and lichens, the first plants to grow on the rock. The Plant People were the second creation. As acids from the lichens ate away at the rock, minerals were carried down the mountain with the melting snow. These rich waters nurtured the growth of other plants. Soon, the earth was ready for the third creation, the animals. Just as the plants depend on the stone, so the first animals depended on the plants for nourishment. Finally, we come to the last creation, the world of the two-leggeds. The two-leggeds are the most dependent, the least able to survive and fend for themselves. They need the animals, the plants, and the stone."

Native people define intelligence as the accumulated wisdom that comes with age and experience and the ability to adapt to natural environments in order to survive. Thus, we two-leggeds are both the youngest and the least intelligent of the Four Realms—Stone, Plant, Animal, and Human. To better understand this philosophy, imagine a modern camper who carries in his backpack a camp stove, matches, a down sleeping bag, a portable fishing pole, a water-purification filter, and all the necessities for spending a week in the woods. Now let's imagine an Athabaskan hunter who walks in the woods for an equal length of time but who takes with him only a caribou-hide blanket slung over his shoulder, knowing that he will find or create all of the other necessities during the journey. Each is capable of surviving for a week, but how would the modern camper fare if he were lost and had no camping supplies, only his own natural abilities and wits, on which to depend? Could the hunter, who feels at home in nature, ever even be considered "lost"? In this story, the camper represents the plight of modern people: we have forgotten how to live on what nature provides. The hunter represents the wisdom of the natural world and the people who live in harmony with her.

The Four Realms represent two different types of teachers—stones and animals on the one hand, and plants on the other—from whom humans can learn either directly or through visions and dreams. It requires a great deal of patience to learn from a stone or a wild animal. To understand the ancient teachings of the stone, the human mind must become as still as a mountain. Mountains change, move, grow, age, and flow with the elements. They speak, though it may take millennia for a mountain to form one recognizable sentence. Only in ceremonies such as the Sweat Lodge can the voice of the stone be easily heard, as its life-rhythm is stimulated and accelerated by fire. The glowing, red-hot Sweat Lodge stones communicate spiritual messages to participants. We must also be patient to learn from wild animals, keeping a respectful distance from them and observing their behavior. To interact with them—feeding or attempting to play with them, for example—is to interfere with their ability to hunt, forage, and fend for themselves.

In the natural world, human beings feel a special kinship with plants. Plants neither remain absolutely still, like stones, nor do they run away, like animals. Their processes and rhythms closely resemble our own. They eat, drink, breathe, and grow, and credible research suggests that they also feel and communicate.[1] The life cycle of plants' birth, death, and rebirth mirrors the seasons of our own lives. We can interact with plants in a deep and meaningful way by nurturing their growth. "Plants," says Grandmother Twylah Nitsch, "symbolize nurturing. People who have plant spirit helpers tend to be sociable and extroverted, whereas those who feel closer to stones and animals are more aloof and introverted."

Grandmother Twylah teaches a simple way to find out if you have a stronger affinity with the personal medicine of plants or with the more aloof medicine of animals and stones. Ask yourself which color you like more: green or brown? Which one seems to be more expressive of who you are? Close your eyes for a moment and let the answer or image come to you. If your answer is green, then you have an affinity for "the green," the realm of plants. If your answer is brown, then you are likely to feel more drawn to animals and stones and to have them as helping spirits. This does not mean that a "green person" cannot understand stones and animals or that a brown person cannot become an herbalist. The green and brown test only suggests tendencies and talents. Some people may feel equally drawn to both, though in my experience with students, I find that this is rare. It is possible, however, that a person may change from one to the other at a different stage in life. There is no law that says that one's spiritual helpers or even the type of spiritual helpers is permanent.

ANCIENT MEDICINE

Plant medicine is probably the most ancient and widespread healing tradition on the planet. According to archaeologists, the first herbalist was a sixty-thousand-year-old Neanderthal who was found buried in a cave in the Zagros Mountains of Iraq with trace amounts of pollen from seven flowers that are now known to be medicinal: yarrow, cornflower, Saint Barnaby's thistle, groundsel or ragwort, grape hyacinth, woody horsetail, and hollyhock.[2] The world's first known herbal handbook is a Sumerian clay tablet from 4000 B.C. written in wedge-shaped letters, or "cuneiform."[3] By 2500 B.C., the Egyptian authors of the Ebers papyri and other medical texts were familiar with about one-third of the botanicals listed in modern pharmacopoeias. Pharaoh's physicians ordered the workers on the Giza Pyramid to eat daily portions of garlic, onions, and radishes to prevent the dysentery common in crowded working and living conditions. (Modern science verifies the logic of such a diet. Garlic, onions, and radishes help prevent viral and bacterial infections and improve digestion.) Native Americans and other ancient people knew the properties of natural plant antibiotics long before the discovery of penicillin.[4] They reasoned that plants that protect themselves from disease, fungi, and insect predators should also be able to protect people.

Native Americans freely shared their knowledge of healing plants with the colonists. In 1535, French explorer Jacques Cartier, on his second voyage up Canada's Saint Lawrence River, recorded for Europeans the first example of Native American healing north of Mexico. It was November, and as Cartier's three ships reached the site of present-day Montreal, they were caught in four feet of snow and frozen in deep ice. From November until March, Cartier and his 110 men subsisted on the meager rations stored in the ships' holds. Twenty-five men died of scurvy, "and all the rest were so sicke, that wee thought they should never recover againe, only three or foure excepted," Cartier wrote in an English translation of his journal published in 1580.[5]

Cartier had maintained friendly relations with the Indians since his previous voyage, a year earlier. One day, while visiting the nearby Huron village of Hochelaga, Cartier saw that the chief, Domagaia, seemed to be suffering from the same disease as his sailors. He was emaciated, with rotting gums and swelling in his knees. Ten days later, when Cartier was walking on the frozen river ice, he met Domagaia again. Miraculously, the chief now appeared "whole and sound." When Cartier asked him how he had cured himself, Domagaia replied that he had drunk a tea made from the leaves of the *annedda* tree, Huron for "white pine."

Domagaia asked two women from his tribe to teach Cartier and his men how to treat their disease. The healers taught the sailors to make the tea and how to use a juice pressed from the leaves and bark as a soothing rinse for their swollen limbs. The sailors began to feel better almost immediately, and within a week, they were cured. We now know that white pine is high in vitamin C (31.5 milligrams per 100 grams of pine needles). In the eighteenth century, British naval surgeon James Lind (1716–1794), inspired by Cartier's account, performed the experiments that demonstrated that lemon juice could prevent scurvy.[6]

It can be said without exaggeration that the invaders owed their survival in North America to the generosity of their hosts. Native Americans taught Europeans to treat malaria with quinine, stimulate the heart with foxglove, and treat constipation with cascara sagrada ("sacred bark," *Rhamnus purshiana*), an ingredient in many over-the-counter laxatives. Today, numerous herbal remedies used by Native Americans—such as ginger, ginseng, echinacea, yarrow, nettle, mint, slippery elm, and hawthorn—are routinely prescribed by naturopaths and, increasingly, by physicians. Popular Western herbal formulas for cancer, including the Hoxsey formula and Essiac tea, created by the gifted healers John Hoxsey (circa 1840) and Rene M. Caisse (1888–1978), respectively, were also influenced by Native American medicine.[7]

Many Native American herbs have been distilled or refined into pharmaceuticals. According to Virgil J. Vogel, author of the classic *American Indian Medicine,* "About 170 drugs which have been or still are official in the *Pharmacopeia of the United States of America* or the *National Formulary* were used by North American Indians north of Mexico, and about fifty more were used by Indians of the West Indies, Mexico, and Central and South America."[8] If we include plant- and mold-derived antibiotics, as well as synthetic imitations of plant substances, it is likely that 60 to 70 percent of drugs in modern medicine are derived from plants, many of whose healing properties were recognized by Native Americans.

— A BATH A DAY KEEPS THE DOCTORS AWAY —

Many of the diseases that the colonists learned to treat with plants could have been prevented if they had been willing to practice the most basic Indian medicine of all: good hygiene. Native Americans understood that noxious forces or substances can be transmitted from one person to another and that contagion is less likely to occur if the body is kept clean. Native Americans bathed every morning. Among some tribes, at break of dawn, everyone would plunge in the river, cracking open the winter ice if necessary. Many Native Americans washed their body and hair every day with natural soap, such as the mixture of yucca root shavings and water used by the Apache. The practice of going to the Sweat Lodge, rinsing the hands in a stream, or dipping them in a warm herbal tea before massage or minor surgery, such as bone setting or removing an arrow, all preceded modern ideas about the importance of antisepsis. Native Americans also drank water to cleanse the body internally and as a sacrament during ceremonies.

These practices contrast sharply with the habits of fifth- through late-nineteenth-century Europeans, whether in the Old World or the New. Although ancient Romans and Greeks were famous for their great bath-houses, and Scandinavians enjoyed saunas, most Europeans considered bathing an incomprehensible abomination.[9] Until the twentieth century, Christians denounced cleanliness as being far from godliness. It was equated with pride, sensuality, and love of luxury. In the fifth century, Saint Benedict declared the unwashed body to be a temple of holiness, and his followers called lice "pearls of God." In the Middle Ages, saintly people boasted that, unless they had to cross a river, their feet never touched water. Queen Isabella of Castile (1451–1504), patron of Christopher Columbus, bragged that she had only two baths in her life: one at her baptism and one before her wedding.

Author Alev Lytle Croutier writes in *Taking the Waters: Spirit, Art, Sensuality,* "Prerevolutionary French aristocrats used perfume instead of soap, their teeth rotted because they never cleaned them, and their fingers smelled of stale food. . . . Cleanliness was undesirable, and natural human smell was in vogue."[10] French noblemen were in the habit of urinating against the marble walls of the Versailles Palace. They drank wine, not water, which was often contaminated with human or animal waste. In the United States, the first bathtub was installed in the White House in 1851, after some initial opposition. Private bathrooms were not common in the United States until after the First World War, but local governments often had to enforce their use, with jail sentences for those who avoided baths for more than a week.

Hygiene was no better in medical practice. In the mid-1800s, Ignaz Semmelweis, a Hungarian physician practicing in Vienna, tried unsuccessfully to convince his colleagues to wash their hands before delivering babies. Although he was able to demonstrate a 1,000 percent reduction in infant mortality in wards where physicians and midwives washed their hands, the evidence was rejected and he was branded a troublemaker. Disheartened, Semmelweis returned to Hungary and committed suicide. Until the twentieth century, European and American hospitals were considered pestholes, and, as social critic Ivan Illich points out in his book *Medical Nemesis: The Expropriation of Health,* no one expected to get well by visiting them."[11] Rather, hospitals were a last resort, like a prison, where people on whom society had given up went to die. Physicians saw hospitals as museums for the study of the diseased and dying. And although today there is no question that hospitals can save lives, there is ample evidence that the general health of the American population has improved not because of them but because of better nutrition and hygiene.[12]

When Native Americans were forced onto reservations during the nineteenth century, filthy living conditions coupled with overcrowding and spoiled, tainted, or insufficient rations created the perfect breeding ground for deadly diseases, such as smallpox, tuberculosis, influenza, and trachoma, a disease of the eyes that can lead to blindness. And because Native people no longer had access to their healing herbs or sacred pools for cleansing— indeed, their religion and healing practices were forbidden by law[13]—they were left with no way to heal or to cope.[14]

Children who were taken away to the white-run boarding schools fared even worse: "[T]he boarding school itself was a major contributor to the spread of disease," writes Professor David Wallace Adams in *Education for Extinction: American Indians and the Boarding School Experience, 1875–1928*. "Institutions where no measures were taken to disinfect tubercular sputum, where infected hand towels, drinking cups, schoolbooks, and the mouthpieces of musical instruments passed freely among children . . . were hotbeds of contagion."[15] Unsanitary conditions were especially deadly because the children's disease resistance was severely weakened by the loneliness of being far from family, friends, lands, and culture and because of the fear, anxiety, depression, and feelings of worthlessness that resulted from regular beatings by the teachers.

THE MEDICINE IS EVERYWHERE

The Cherokee healer Keetoowah was fond of saying that medicine and visions seek out the person who is ready. He gave me an example from his own life. When he was middle-aged, he developed prostate cancer. Deciding against conventional medical therapy, he instead treated himself with various herbs, including red clover flowers, which scientists recognize as having the anticancer compound *genistein*. Although the treatment seemed to slow the cancer's progress, it did not arrest or cure it. Keetoowah called his grandfather, then a very old man.

Grandfather said, "You know what to do, Grandson. Smudge yourself, take a bath, put on your best clothing, then take a walk and pray that the medicine shows itself."

"But, Grandfather, I live in the city."

"It doesn't matter. The medicine is everywhere."

Keetoowah followed Grandfather's instructions. After walking a few blocks, he saw a neighbor standing in her open doorway. She waved to Keetoowah and asked him if he would like to see the new pond in her backyard. He followed her around the house, where he saw a small pond with a giant lotus flower floating on the surface. Keetoowah knew that this was the medicine.

"This is going to sound very strange, but I wonder if you would consider giving me that lotus? I need the root to make medicine."

The woman agreed to his request, and Keetoowah took the flower home, boiled the root, and prayed over the liquid. He drank a glass of the tea every day for the next seven days. Within a few weeks, his symptoms disappeared, and tests showed that the cancer was gone. It never returned.

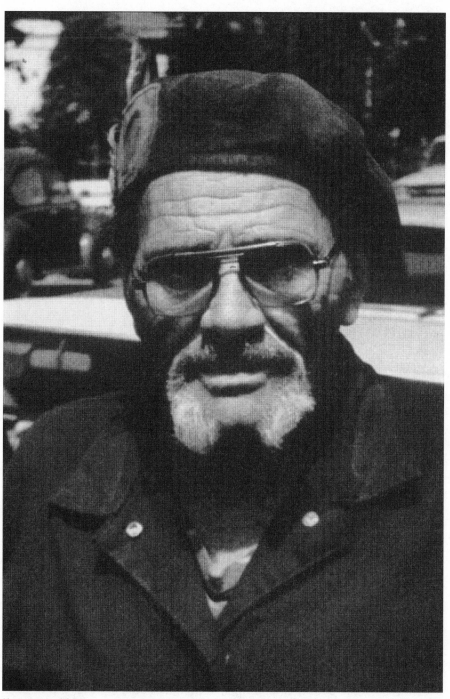

Keetoowah, 1984.

THE ORIGIN OF DISEASE AND MEDICINE

Keetoowah's story is a modern version of a traditional teaching: not only is the medicine everywhere, but it is probably in your own backyard. One Cherokee legend teaches that the Creator placed on Mother Earth all of the plants that can cure diseases that naturally occur in a specific geographic region. My version of the Cherokee Origin of Medicine story is based both on the version made famous by James Mooney in *Myths of the Cherokee* and on one told to me by Keetoowah.

In the ancient times, all of the animals, fish, birds, insects, and plants could communicate with one another. They spoke the common language of peace, harmony, and friendship. People hunted only what they needed and never forgot to express their respect and gratitude.

As time went on, the two-leggeds began to multiply. Their intellects gave them the ability to plan for the future. They cultivated the land to manipulate nature's harvest and set up fences and boundaries. The animals were forced into smaller and more crowded spaces. Soon, the two-leggeds invented bows, knives, blowguns, hooks, and other technologies that gave them an unfair advantage. Their heads swelled with unrealistic images of their own superiority. They trod the ants, worms, and other small creatures—at first, without thought, and later, with contempt. They slaughtered the large animals for flesh, skin, or sport or simply to prove their elevated status. The two-leggeds forgot that they were children of the same Creator. Only a few could still understand the language of nature. The majority of humans babbled a language that only they could understand, or so they believed.

The animals resolved to hold meetings to determine what could be done. The powerful *Yonah,* Bear People, were the first to hold council. It was quickly decided that war was inevitable. "What if every time a human shoots at us, we shoot back?" asked the old Chief White Bear. The Bears decided to use Man's principal weapon—the bow and arrow—against him. One Bear shaped a piece of wood into a bow. Another sacrificed himself so that his sinew could be made into a bowstring. But when they tried to shoot the bow, the Bears' claws got caught on the string. If a Bear trimmed his claws, he could shoot straight, but then how could the Bear climb trees or dig up roots for food? "This will never do," chided the chief. "We will die and starve just to shoot arrows! It is better to trust the natural weapons that Creator has given us." The Bear People are powerful but sometimes slow-thinking.

The wise *Ahwi,* Deer People, were the next to hold council. Under the leadership of their chief, Little Deer, they came upon an ingenious strategy for their protection and to help restore nature's balance. Every time a hunter killed a Deer without asking her pardon, the spirit of the Deer would follow the trail of blood to the hunter's home and there cripple him with rheumatism.

Next, the Fish and Reptiles held council. They decided to make ungrateful two-leggeds dream of slimy snakes and decaying fish. The two-leggeds would lose their appetites and die. And so it went. Each of the creatures, in turn, held councils, complained of Man's cruelty and injustice, and devised a disease of retribution.

Then the Plant People, who were friendly to the two-leggeds, held their own council. "For every disease that an animal inflicts, one of us will be present to cure it, *if* the two-leggeds call upon us with prayer." Thus, every herb, grass, shrub, weed, and tree became a remedy. The spirit of the plants agreed to speak to the two-leggeds in their dreams.

As we have seen many times in this book, harmony with nature is the source of health and good fortune. Conversely, disease and misfortune are caused or augmented by ingratitude to nature, including, as in the story above, our animal relations—for example, not praying before hunting or eating. The importance of respecting nature is dramatically illustrated by a true story I heard from a Cree friend about a modern Christian missionary who wanted to prove that traditional Indian beliefs are false and evil. An Anglican priest from a small reservation in Manitoba was fed up with the medicine man. Although most of the men in the community were impoverished trappers, they refused to continue trapping or hunting deer because the medicine man, after communing with the Deer Spirit, told the people that they had taken their maximum harvest of deer for the season. He warned them to stop hunting deer until the following year and that misfortune might visit anyone who disobeyed. The dubious priest knew that government-set quotas had not been met and convinced a young Cree convert, whom I will call "Brian," to go hunting with him to prove that the elder's advice was based on superstition. "How could hunting, providing for your family, be harmful? It is only dangerous to the deer," he told Brian. "And we can prove it."

One day, Brian and the priest went hiking in the bush, each with a rifle slung over his shoulder. After a short while, they came to a meadow, where they saw a large buck grazing on some grass. The priest told Brian to take the shot. Brian hesitated at first, then braced the rifle against his shoulder, aimed, and fired. He hit the deer in the heart. It immediately keeled over, and at the same moment, Brian screamed and also dropped to the ground, gripping his knee with both hands. Luckily, they were not far from the church. The shocked priest ran back and called an ambulance. A half hour later, the ambulance arrived at the church, and the priest accompanied the emergency medical team along the trail. They loaded Brian on a stretcher, carried him to the ambulance, and drove to the hospital. In the emergency room, a doctor examined Brian and found that his knee was fractured. Even stranger, the skin was not broken, and there were several deer hairs embedded in the cartilage of Brian's kneecap, which had to be surgically removed! Yet as the priest could attest, the rifle had not misfired, nor had any object hit Brian's knee.

When we are disrespectful to the powers, gifts, and teachings that animals represent, we become ill in mind, body, and spirit. If you climb too high, too quickly— the power of the goat—you are likely to fall. Success always requires patience. If you dig up information with the intent of causing embarrassment, you disrespect the power of the badger, a powerful excavator (resulting in diseases that mostly afflict politicians and journalists). The Rabbit Spirit, say the Seminoles, causes kidney stones. Perhaps because this gentle creature does not tolerate obstinacy, she produces them as a sign that she has been offended. As an example of *taach,* the consequences of violating a sacred object, a Piman man from Arizona tells the story of a neighboring Maricopa Indian who killed a rattlesnake for no reason. His wife was pregnant at the time. They had a son, and when he learned to walk, he moved like a snake.[16]

Both the Cherokee and Cree stories remind us that we can lessen the likelihood of disease by always being grateful to the forces that nourish us. We should remember, however, that in today's world, not all disease can be considered a sign of personal wrongdoing. Industries that pollute the land, water, and air or that promote selfishness, greed, or dishonesty misuse the animal powers. We may be suffering for the misdeeds of organizations over which we have too little control.

HOW TO FIND, GATHER, AND PREPARE HEALING PLANTS

Discovering the location of healing plants requires a great deal of patience. You learn to look at the land for the subtlest details and clues. Plants hide under bushes and in rocky crevasses; they fade from view in glaring light and disappear in forest shadows. You may need to climb, crawl, or trudge through mud and swamp for hours. Plants such as the puffball mushroom come up in a day and disappear the next. Some plants, like ginseng and valerian, are known to hide deliberately; they show themselves only when you and they are ready.

As you learn to recognize plant habitats, areas that had seemed uniform and monotone are suddenly filled with variety and color. Even in a seemingly barren desert, the proximity of a spring or the slightest change in soil moisture, mineral content, sunlight, or the insect population causes an entirely different community of plants to flourish.

Native American herbalists teach their apprentices how to recognize and gather plants by taking them on herb walks. I once led a group of my students on a hillside walk to gather mullein root for a Cherokee elder who sometimes prescribes it as a medicinal smoke to heal tobacco addiction. (This usage is uncommon. Native and Western herbalists generally use mullein root, leaf, or flower tea to treat respiratory disorders.) It was springtime, the proper time for gathering roots. Earth-power rises through the root in the spring, into the stem by summer, and the leaves by autumn.

Early morning is the right time to gather most plants, when the air and energy are fresh. Some plants only reveal themselves in moon- or starlight, however.

We walked through the woods and up a rocky hillside covered with low-lying shrubs until we came to a group of mullein plants—green, velvety leaves rising from a hard, rodlike stem, topped with a tall cone of yellow flowers. I offered a pinch of tobacco to the largest and most beautiful mullein plant, representing the species that I would be picking. This Grandfather would not, itself, be picked. I prayed to thank the plant for its beauty and healing power and for allowing me to find it. In the prayer, I explained why I would be picking other members of its tribe—because it was needed as medicine to cure addiction—and promised that I would take only what was needed and use it in a respectful way. Then we began to dig the roots of neighboring mullein plants with garden tools—some Native herbalists still use the more traditional pointed digging stick—careful not to deplete any area. When we had gathered about a dozen roots and placed them in a straw basket, we filled the holes back up. I brought the roots to the elder, who dried them in the sun and then stored the plants in natural containers, such as handmade baskets or cloth bags.

Throughout North America, the most common method of gathering herbs is to pray while offering tobacco or, in the Southwest, cornmeal to the plant. There are numerous tribal and personal variations of plant-gathering rituals. James W. Herrick, author of *Iroquois Medical Botany,* writes that on the Saint Regis Reservation, Kanien'kehaka Nation, there are as many as two hundred ways to gather plant medicines.[17] In some tribes, every aspect of the harvest is prescribed or ritualized. As we have seen, there are times of day and year to gather the root, stem, or leaves of plants. Flowers are usually picked when they first open, fruits when they mature, seeds when they are available, and bark when it can be easily stripped— generally, in the spring or winter. To ensure optimal effectiveness, healers may peel bark from only a certain side of a tree, generally from the east side, where the tree has been bathed by the potent rays of the rising sun. Some healers gather herbs in specific quantities, perhaps in even or odd numbers or in groups of four or seven roots, leaves, or entire plants. In accord with various tribal customs, healers may offer cornmeal, pollen, beads, shells, or other substances to a plant instead of to-bacco. They may thank or speak to the plant in an ancient form of their language, usually reserved for ritual.

Methods of herbal use are equally detailed and varied. Native herbalists use any or all parts of a plant—root, stem, twigs, leaves, buds, fruits, flowers, seeds, and bark—to make infusions, decoctions, juices (pressed or squeezed), tinctures, lotions, salves, poultices, enemas, and smoking mixtures. Some herbs are dried; others are used fresh—eaten, chewed, or held in the mouth. For instance, the Kashaya Pomo of California hold angelica root in the mouth to prevent sore throats and bad breath.[18] I like to chew on sweet flag root (*Acorus calamus,* the American species only, as the Asian and European varieties may be toxic) to strengthen my voice and prevent hoarseness before singing and to prevent fatigue while hiking. Many Native Americans call this plant "bitter root" or "drummer's root." To the Cree, it is "muskrat root" (*wacaskwatapih*) or "rat root," and I must admit that I was once frightened away from gathering it by the hordes of Saskatchewan mosquitoes that hovered around the swamp in which it grew.

Herbs may be used by themselves or in combination with other herbs. A formula is generally made up of three or four herbs, but it may contain a dozen or more.[19] Some Leni-Lenape herbalists specify that herbs must be crushed or ground with stone or wood mortars. If touched by metal, the herbs lose potency. The water used in herbal teas is also important. Perhaps the water must come from a spring or stream or be gathered only with or against the current. Water scooped against the current honors the source of the water; water scooped with the current honors the nourishment water carries as it flows away. Some herbalists mix them together. Tap water and distilled water are never used, except in an emergency, because they do not contain the pure Water Spirit. Having been filtered and chemically cleansed, perhaps of human and industrial waste, they may still bear the energetic imprint of their contaminants.

In his monumental book *Native American Ethnobotany*, distinguished anthropology professor Daniel E. Moerman writes that North American Indians (including Greenland tribes and Native Hawaiians) used at least 3,923 plants and 106 mosses, fungi, and lichens for various purposes such as food, fibers, and dyes. Among these, 2,874 species were used as medicines. How many plants does an individual Native herbalist know? An herbalist may learn hundreds of herbs as she reads the landscape and learns from other herbalists both within and outside her tribe. Her pharmacopoeia thus grows throughout her lifetime. One of the most clinically successful and respected Native herbalists in North America, Kwi-tsi-tsa-las (Norma Myers), from the Kwakiutl village of Alert Bay, British Columbia, had a repertoire of approximately 300 herbs.[20] The well-known Cherokee medicine man Amoneeta Sequoyah knew 642 medicinal plants.[21] The number of available herbs diminishes as we move from the humid and lush Northwest or Southeast to the more arid plains and prairies. Investigators among the Blackfoot of Montana and Alberta documented knowledge of about 185 different species of plants.[22]

As we have seen, many medicine people pray or dream to find herbs. "When the [Cherokee] doctor does not know what medicine to use for a sick man," James Mooney writes, "the spirit of the plant tells him."[23] Healers use their minds, their spirits, and their spirit helpers to empower herbs to cure virtually any specific problem. They will dedicate and re-form the herbs' properties in prayer and ceremony. An herb ordinarily used to cure sore throat may be "doctored up" to treat depression. Even a glass of water can become powerful medicine if infused with spirit. The holy person's herbal repertoire may be smaller than that of the herbal specialist, but not for that reason any less effective. Some healers believe that knowing too many herbs or attempting to treat too many diseases may, in fact, dilute the power of the herb or herbalist. In *How Indians Use Wild Plants for Food, Medicine and Crafts*, Frances Densmore quotes a Lakota healer:

> A medicine man would not try to dream of all herbs and treat all diseases, for then he could not expect to succeed in all nor to fulfill properly the dream of any one herb or animal. He would depend on too many and fail in all. That is one reason why our medicine men lost their power when so many diseases came among us with the advent of the white man.[24]

Whether you learn about plant medicines through elders or dreams, it is ultimately the plant itself that is the greatest teacher. The spirit of the plant teaches its uses. Native healers, like Western herbalists, also experiment *with nontoxic plants* to discover, through trial and error, new uses and properties. Many healers like to experiment on themselves before recommending a new formula or plant usage to patients. Effects can sometimes be predicted based on previous knowledge and on new information received from dreams, other herbalists, or even books. Herbalists who have keen body awareness, however, do not need a book to know how an herb affects the heart, liver, spleen, nervous system, or any other aspect of human functioning. They can, very importantly, *feel* the physiological effects of a plant in their own bodies. I believe that long ago, such sensitivities were common.

THE BEAR'S MEDICINE CHEST

Once, when I was visiting the Six Nations Indian Museum near Onchiota, New York, Kanien'kehaka elder and museum founder Tehanetorens (Ray Fadden) shared a beautiful "message," as he calls his teachings. "Now sit down on the bench, children," he said. To this great cultural historian, in his seventies, I and the other museum guests were children. "I'm going to tell you a story." It was the story of the Origin of Plant Medicines from the Haudenosaunee perspective, and like the Cherokee tale, it contains teachings that are valued by all Native Americans.[25] Which story is true, you ask? Every tribe has teachings about plants, and they are all true! I will paraphrase Grandfather's teaching.

One day, long ago, an old man appeared in the village. He was hungry and weary from his journey. He went to a home that had a turtle shell hung over the doorway, a sign that this was the lodge of Turtle Clan members, to ask for food and a place to rest. His request was denied, and he was told to move on. Next, he went to homes of the other clans—Snipe, Wolf, Beaver, Deer, Eel, Heron, and Eagle—and at each, he was turned away. Finally, he came to the Bear Clan home, where an old woman welcomed him. Although the home was small and her provisions few, she was willing to share what she had. She gave the old man food and a soft deerskin mat on which to rest and sleep.

The next day, the old man woke up feeling ill and feverish. He asked the woman to go into the forest to look for a certain plant. When she returned with the plant, he taught her how to prepare it, and it cured his illness. But the next day, he was ill again, this time with a different sickness. Again, he described a plant to the woman and told her where to find it. She prepared a remedy according to his instructions, and again, after taking the remedy, he recovered. This went on day after day; each time, the man had a different disease and required a different herbal cure. Then, one day, as the woman returned from the woods and was about to enter her home, she saw that it was illuminated by a great light. When she entered, she saw that the old man had been transformed into a handsome young man who was shining like the sun. The young man told her not to be afraid. "I am the Creator," he said. To thank her for her hospitality, he told her that henceforth, Bear Clan members would be the guardians of the Medicine, and that medicine men and women would always belong to the Bear Clan.

Many North American mammals eat the above-ground portions of plants, but only the bear, like humans, has a rotating forearm, giving it the dexterity to dig up healing roots. The bear is the plant gatherer and herbalist of the animals. Medicine people of many tribes say that you can learn about healing plants by watching the bear and remembering what it eats. Bears seem especially fond of osha root (*Ligusticum porteri*), yarrow (*Achillea millefolium*), and bearberry (*Arctostaphylos uva-ursi*).

Osha, an aromatic member of the parsley family, is called "bear food" or "bear root" by many tribes and is used medicinally wherever it grows. The root is brown and "furry," like a brown bear. Zoologists have observed Alaskan Kodiak bears digging the root, chewing it, and rubbing the maceration on their fur. The activity seems to calm them, and the chewed root may protect them against external parasites. Native Americans chew on osha root for sore throats, coughs, headaches, and stomachaches; apply an osha-root poultice for swellings; and burn the root on Sweat Lodge stones or in the Sacred Pipe as a healing and purifying smoke. When "lowlanders" visit my home high in the Rocky Mountains, I usually recommend that they chew osha root or take osha-root tincture each day for the first few days. It helps them adjust more quickly to the altitude. I wouldn't be surprised if Colorado's original Ute and Arapaho tribes used osha to adjust to their high-elevation summer camps and for endurance while hunting or traveling in the mountains.

By observing grizzly and black bears, Tsistsistas people learned that it is good to eat yarrow plants, a member of the daisy and dandelion family with tiny white flowers and feathery leaves. Northern Plains tribes make a tea from the leaves to treat colds and diabetes and from the flowers for coughs, liver problems, and as a spring tonic. In Cree, one of the names for yarrow is *mistigonimaskigah*, "head medicine." For headaches, including migraines, a poultice of all of the above-ground parts of the plant is applied to the head. The Cree also call yarrow *osgunimasgigah*, "bone medicine," because it relieves arthritis pain: the whole plant may be added to hot bathwater, and the above-ground parts may be used as a poultice. The chewed leaves of this versatile plant are applied to cuts to stop bleeding and speed healing. The Lakota call yarrow *taopi pejuta*, "wound medicine." Scientific research confirms that yarrow is anti-inflammatory and has broad-spectrum antibacterial properties.

Bears love to eat the berries of the bearberry plant, a common ground cover with bright evergreen leaves, pinkish white flowers, and red berries related to cranberries and blueberries. The Anishinabe call the plant *Mukwa-Miskomin*, "Bear, his red berries." Interestingly, the Latin name also refers to the bear. *Arctostaphylos uva-ursi* means "bear's cluster of grapes." Frequently, both Native American and Western herbalists incorrectly refer to bearberry as *kinnickinnick*, an Algonquian term that means "mixture" and is not originally a word for the plant at all. The term became associated with bearberry because bearberry leaves are a very common ingredient in Pipe Ceremony smoking mixtures. Tribes as widely separated as the Cherokee of Georgia and the Okanagon of British Columbia use bearberry leaf tea as a tonic or treatment for the kidneys and bladder. The Anishinabe use the tea as a douche for urethritis. The Cree make a tea from a mixture of bearberry stems and leaves and blueberry leaves to help women heal after childbirth. (Chemical analysis shows that bearberry leaves contain arbutin, an excellent antibiotic and diuretic used to treat urinary tract infections.)

Following the bear's example, many Native people also use the berries as an ingredient in foods. Anishinabe herbalist Keewaydinoquay remembers her grandmother's recipe for a food to use during times of famine: bearberries fried in fat, then cracked and mixed with diced dried apples to make a sauce, flavored with wild garlic, wild onion, yarrow, and wild basil.[26] The Cree cook the berries in fat, then pound and mix them with raw fish eggs to make a delicious "caviar." Many northwest coast peoples enjoy eating the berries after soaking them in water or seal oil. In the past, Nuxalk chiefs from the Pacific Northwest coast were served a mixture of the berries with mountain goat grease, which they ate by the spoonful at feasts.

LISTENING TO PLANTS

Flower in the crannied wall,
I pluck you out of the crannies,
I hold you here, root and all, in my hand,
Little flower—but *if* I could understand
What you are, root and all, and all in all,
I should know what God and man is.

—Alfred, Lord Tennyson, "Flower in the Crannied Wall"

Westerners like to pick flowers. From the indigenous perspective, *we have a responsibility toward flowers and plants not to pick them randomly or unnecessarily.* They are not here primarily for *our* enjoyment but for the enjoyment of all creatures. We should enjoy plants in their natural environments and pick them only when necessary for food or healing. Once the flower has been plucked and removed from its surroundings, neither it nor God can be understood.

There are many ways to study plant medicine. You can train with herbalists or read about herbal medicine in the books listed in the "Native American Resources" section of this book. The most important way to learn about plants, however, is by seeking to understand your similarities with them. Human beings and plants breathe; reproduce; react to environmental stimuli such as light, heat, and physical stress; and share the same recycled water, air, and nutrients. Both eventually turn into compost. The more you sense your unity with plants, the more you can "hear" them with your spirit and communicate with them. I have found the following four exercises helpful to develop these abilities:

1. Ask permission to approach the plant. I like to turn my palms outward and walk slowly and respectfully toward the plant as I mentally ask, "May I visit you?"

2. If permission is granted (if not, try another plant or another day), sit next to the plant, close your eyes, and imagine that you *are* the plant. What can you see, hear, and feel? Do you feel the sun shining, the cool moonlight, the shade of a neighboring tree, the breeze? Can you sense insects and running water or water in your roots? What is your relationship to Mother Earth? How do you experience animals' brushing past you and perhaps eating your leaves? Can you hear the birds singing? If you are a tree, do you enjoy a squirrel running up your trunk?

   Imagine the stages of your life, your growth from a seed to an elder. How long is your life span? How do you feel during the spring, during the winter? What do you dream? How do other plants or other members of your species help your development? Imagine a discussion with other plants and with animals in your community.

What are your values? From the perspective of a plant, how do you feel about human behavior? What would you say to a human being who admires you or to a human about to pick you? What do you feel when a human offers tobacco or cornmeal to you or sings to you? Do you have a song? What is your medicine, your gift of healing? How should you be prepared or used for medicine?

3. Now "imagine" yourself again as a human being. Speak to the plant. Sing to it, praising its beauty. If you feel that it is appropriate to pick a member of the species, make a tobacco offering. Before using the plant, consult with an experienced herbalist to make sure that the plant is nontoxic and appropriate for your state of health and that it doesn't interact negatively with any medications you are taking.

4. Place the plant under your pillow before going to sleep. It may speak to you in your dreams. Remember to thank the plant for any messages it gives you.

HOW HERBS WORK

Plant medicines work because they have healing power. From the perspective of Western medicine, this healing potential exists only in chemicals, *active agents,* that have measurable effects on pathogens, diseased cells, immunity, the balance of brain chemicals, or other aspects of human biology. Native Americans say that the active agent, although important, is not the whole story. Plants have intelligence, energy, and spirit, and they may, if they choose, accelerate healing, reduce pain, or cure disease. Sometimes, the appearance of the plant indicates its healing capabilities. Wild bergamont (*Monarda fistulosa*), for instance, has purple flowers, a color that to the Muskogee (also called Creek) Indians, originally from Alabama and Georgia, symbolizes the nerves and the heart. In his *Native Plants, Native Healing: Traditional Muskogee Way,* Native herbalist Tis Mal Crow says that wild bergamont flower tea is used to treat depression and anxiety.[27] Generally, a plant's healing power must be awakened and invited through ceremonial actions, such as prayers and offerings.

– THE ACTIVE AGENT –

The active agent is a chemical constituent of a plant that accounts scientifically for its biological effects. This is the aspect of Native American herbalism that is being investigated by medical science and that can be readily accepted by non-Natives.

For example, many tribes chew willow bark or make a tea of it for headaches, fevers, and as a wash for swellings. Willow bark contains a significant amount of salicin, the same chemical that is artificially synthesized to create aspirin. The

Tsistsistas, Kiowa, Ponca, Pawnee, and other tribes chew the purple coneflower (echinacea) root for sore throats, colds, toothaches, and viruses such as mumps. Echinacea has powerful antiviral compounds, including caffeic acid, chicoric acid, and echinacin. In *The Green Pharmacy,* James A. Duke, Ph.D., writes, "Root extracts of echinacea have also been shown to act like interferon, the body's own antiviral compound."[28] One of the most powerful anticancer chemotherapy compounds is taxol, originally isolated from the bark of the Pacific yew tree and now produced synthetically. Tribes in California and the Pacific Northwest have traditionally used a decoction of Pacific yew bark as a blood purifier, a general healing panacea, and a specific treatment for cancer.

Unlike Western scientists, Native healers consider the entire plant to be the active agent rather than any extracted or refined chemical component. Whole plants, compared to isolated drugs, generally have fewer side effects or less toxicity and longer-lasting benefits. The potential benefits of plant medicines compared to drugs are clearly explained in Dr. Andrew Weil's *Health and Healing.* Plant medicines enter the bloodstream more slowly than drugs and thus do not cause rapid rise in blood levels that may lead to overdose and toxic effects. Because they are administered orally rather than by injection, they are also less subject to abuse. Dr. Weil illustrates this point when he describes the invention of the hypodermic syringe in 1853 by Scottish physician Alexander Wood. "His wife became the world's first morphine addict. That delicious irony says all one needs to know about the relative risks of oral administration of crude drugs versus intravenous administration of refined ones."[29]

— THE APPEARANCE OR NAME —

Some plants work because they resemble the name or appearance of a disease or body part. The idea is that *like treats like,* sometimes called "the Doctrine of Signatures" in Western herbalism, because the appearance of the plant is considered a divine sign of its usage. For instance, *Rudbeckia,* the black-eyed Susan, is called "Deer-Eye," *Ahwi Akata,* in Cherokee because of the flower's appearance. A decoction of the root is used for swellings, snakebites, and weak or inflamed eyes. The maidenhair fern, *Adiantum pedatum (Kaga Skutagi,* "Crow Shin," in Cherokee), unrolls and straightens as it grows. It is used as a poultice to relax and lengthen contracted muscles of rheumatic patients. Many tribes consider American ginseng (*Panax quinquefolius*) to be a powerful general tonic because the root resembles a human being. The Leni-Lenape call the plant "man and woman," because it grows in pairs and appears to be one gender or the other. (It is always used to treat the gender it resembles.) The color of a plant may also be important. For example, yellow-root (*Xanthorrhiza simplicissima*) can treat nausea that produces yellow bile.

Red-colored plants, such as bloodroot (*Sanguinaria canadensis*), are good for the blood.[30] (Interestingly, dentists use compounds found in bloodroot to fight oral bacteria and periodontal disease.)

— CEREMONIAL EMPOWERMENT —

As I described earlier, a plant's power is activated and augmented when it is gathered or used in ceremony or in connection with dream instructions. It is important to remember this principle even when using Western medications. Pray over your aspirin, smudge your antiseptic cream, and they will be more effective. Some plants, such as those which have hallucinogenic properties, are dangerous to use outside of ceremonies. For example, peyote and datura are never used by traditional Native Americans to "get high." They are sacramental herbs that must be gathered and ingested with prayer. Some Native American tribes have drunk wine since precontact times. For example, the Tohono O'Odham make a wine out of the saguaro cactus fruit and drink it amid ritualized songs and speeches designed to attract rain clouds.[31]

I am not saying that plants are ineffective when used in a mundane way, without prayer. Milkweed root (*Asclepias tuberosa*, or *kiu makan*, "wound medicine," in Ponca) can help heal wounds, sores, rashes, and warts whether we believe in its spirit or not. Without an offering of gratitude, however, an herb treats only symptoms and does not reach the emotions and spirit or the deeper causes of illness.

A HEALING STORY

I would like to share with you a healing story that was a turning point in my life. Although it was, in many ways, the beginning of my healing work among Native people, I have saved it for the end of this book because it contains themes that are best understood when one has some familiarity with Native American culture. Ann's healing illustrates the way various healing methods may complement one another. It starts and ends with a dream.

I was invited to present a series of lectures on spirituality and health at a university in western Canada. A few days after my arrival, I had a powerful dream in which I saw the face of an elderly Native woman. The face appeared without background or context. I didn't know where she was or who she was. She just stared at me with an expression that communicated a need to contact me, like a spirit that was reaching out across the dream world. The image seemed so "real" that when I woke up, I called a friend, who was house-sitting at my cabin, to ask if I had received any phone calls or mail from Native Americans. There were none.

I had no way of knowing that the same day as my dream, Ann, a sixty-year-old First Nations political activist who lived a few hours north of the university, came across my name in the university catalog. The catalog listed my guest lecture in "holistic medicine" and did not contain any biographical information about me. When Ann saw my name, a spirit appeared to her in a waking dream and told her that I was a pipe carrier and "medicine man" (her term: I would not presume to call myself one). It was Ann's husband, Michael, who phoned me a few days later to ask for help. He described Ann's waking dream, which I took matter-of-factly, not yet connecting it with my own dream of the Native woman. I was preoccupied with the urgency of Ann's condition. Michael said that Ann had been experiencing abdominal pain for months, and a few days earlier, the pain had worsened. It seemed to radiate throughout her body. She refused to go to the hospital but wanted me to doctor her.

The phone call came on Monday. When Michael suggested that he bring her to see me on Wednesday, I interjected and told them to come immediately. I somehow knew that Ann's condition was critical, and Wednesday would be too late.

Two hours later, they arrived at the guest house where I was staying. I went out to greet the car as it pulled up the driveway. Ann was lying down in the back seat under a blanket, barely conscious. She looked like a ghost. Her skin was deathly pale. As I helped her out of the car, she groaned with pain. I recognized her from my dream. There was no mistake.

I helped Michael carry his wife into the house and to the sofa. They sat next to each other, and I sat close by, across from them on a chair. Ann grasped my hand, an unusual gesture of confidence among people of her tribe, who are innately shy and modest. We were, after all, old friends: we had been introduced in the dream world.

As I smudged her with sweetgrass, I could see that something was broken in her gut. I got an image of blood and fecal matter leaking out and infecting her organs. Ann whispered, "I've been feeling ill for months and got much worse a few days ago. The pain became unbearable."

"My sister," I said gently, "you have waited too long to rely only on Indian doctoring. I'm going to give you some medicine to stop the pain, and I will join you at the hospital." I called an ambulance, and while we were waiting, I prayed over a glass of water to turn it into a tea of invisible spirit herbs. As Ann drank it, her breath deepened and slowed down to a normal pace. She did her best to smile and whispered, "Thank you."

The ambulance arrived fifteen minutes later. Ann was placed on a stretcher, and her husband accompanied her in the ambulance. I grabbed my medicine bag and pipe bundle and followed by taxi. When I arrived at the hospital, Michael was sitting in the waiting room. He explained that Ann had been wheeled into the emergency room and then almost immediately taken into another room for surgery. I took out my sacred pipe, and we did a ceremony right there. I seem to have a talent for not being thrown out of hospitals for smoking.

A surgeon came into the waiting room about five hours later, around one in the morning. He explained that Ann's large intestine had burst from a cancerous tumor in her colon, causing fecal matter to infect all of her internal organs. He could also see that the cancer had spread to her lymph nodes and liver. He had cleaned out the infected matter, excised lymph and intestinal tumors, and created a colostomy, an artificial external pouch for excretion. But he explained that Ann was basically beyond medical help. "There is no way to remove all of the cancer, and she will probably die of the infection even before the cancer can kill her. I believe that she will be gone within twenty-four hours." "Your best prognosis?" I asked. "One month, all of it in the intensive care unit, where she will receive intravenous antibiotics to combat the infection and morphine for the pain."

I returned to the guest house to get some rest. Ann spent all day in a coma. That evening, about seven o'clock, I heard a knock on the door of my room. The chief of Ann's tribe had come to formally request a healing ritual. He presented me with a pouch of tobacco. We prayed and chanted for more than an hour. When we finished, the wind began to swirl and howl like a whirlwind around the house. On a hunch, I called the hospital to inquire about Ann's condition. A nurse told me that Ann had just awakened from her coma and yelled for help. She had a "crazy notion" that the windows were open and wind was blowing around her bed. The windows are never opened in the intensive care unit.

I felt encouraged by the wind. The wind is life. It refreshes the spirit and blows away disease. I was certain that my intervention was for Ann's highest good. I returned to the hospital that evening and explained to the physicians and nurses that I was going to work with them. I would be Ann's traditional healer. I would not tell them how to administer their medicines, nor should they interfere with my work. I doctored Ann for an hour each day for the next few days. I prayed, sang, and brushed her body with unlit sweetgrass, circled my hand counterclockwise over her tumors, to shrink them, and clockwise to send light and energy into the tissues that needed to mend. I pulled out the pain and cancer. She was released from the ICU a total of four days after her surgery. Three days later, she was released from the hospital. In spite of Ann's miraculous recovery from infection and her total freedom from pain, the doctors probably thought that she was going home to die. She was intent on living.

The cancer probably did not go away. Her remission was a subjective one, not verified on laboratory tests, and perhaps for that very reason more inspiring of the hope and happiness that can make one's remaining life, however brief, satisfying. On my recommendation, Ann and Michael attended a healing Sweat Lodge conducted by one of my elders. The elder retrieved a message: Ann would be with her family that spring.

Six months later, peacefully and without pain, she rejoined her ancestors and the great dreaming mind of the Creator.

LAND AND LIFE

As scientists search the North American and Amazon rain forests for herbal cures for cancer, AIDS, and drug-resistant infectious disease, the land that supports these herbs is being rapidly destroyed. Unless worldwide priorities change, soon the only place where we may find healing herbs is on the World Wide Web or in the pages of a book. In 1998, *Earth Island Journal* reported that a twenty-year assessment by world botanists documented that at least one-eighth of the world's plant species were threatened with extinction.[32] That number has not improved today. The United States ranks worst in conservation among the world's nations: 29 percent of our 16,108 plant species—a total of 4,669 species—may soon be extinct. The Worldwatch Institute reports that international commerce has endangered 29,000 plant and animal species. American plants are in high demand. The state of Montana is full of potholes because of overcollection and depletion of wild echinacea to supply the herb industry. Wild American ginseng is endangered and may become extinct within decades. It is used extensively in Chinese medicine, where wild American ginseng roots fetch three times the price of the cultivated variety, the oldest roots selling for as much as $30,000.

The Hopi speak of the importance of "land and life." This is because *land is life.* Each step on the ladder of biological complexity—from stone to plant to animal to human—is dependent on the step that precedes it. From the indigenous point of view, simpler life-forms are our source; they are like older and wiser parents. Simplicity also means increased sensitivity to environmental changes and an inability to absorb, buffer, or adapt to disturbances in the balance of life. This is why plants are especially at risk. A complex system will not suffer a total breakdown if one of its components ceases to function. If a section of your computer's hard drive doesn't work, your computer can store information in another area or "block" of the drive. A person can function and have a fulfilling life even if both feet are amputated. But cut off the roots of a plant and it dies. There are no extra "parts" to compensate for the loss of a limb.

To put it simply, plants are the first and quickest to register the effects of environmental contamination and destruction. In the Sierra Nevada de Santa Marta mountains of Colombia, South America, the Kogi tribe believe that they are witnessing the beginning of the end of life. Snow no longer covers the nineteen-thousand-foot peaks that have always been their home. The waters are evaporating, lakes are shrinking, grasses and delicate tundra plants are shriveling and dying. If it is happening above, where the rivers have their source, it will soon happen down below. The "Elder Brothers," as the Kogi call themselves, are one of the last fully intact pre-Columbian civilizations. In Alan Ereira's excellent book *The Elder Brothers,* the Kogi warn the Europeans:

Younger Brother, stop doing it. You have already taken so much. We need water to live. Without water we die of thirst. We need water to live. The mother told us how to live properly and how to think well. We're still here and we haven't forgotten anything.[33]

Will we listen? The fight to regain and preserve indigenous lands and the indigenous attitude of respect and frugality toward all land is more than a fight to preserve biodiversity or healing plants; it is a necessity for the survival of the human race.

~ APPENDIXES ~

~ APPENDIX A ~

A COMPARISON OF
WESTERN AND NATIVE AMERICAN MEDICINE

WESTERN MEDICINE	NATIVE AMERICAN MEDICINE
Focus on pathology and curing disease.	Focus on health, and healing the person and community.
Reductionistic: Diseases are fundamentally biological, and treatment should produce measurable outcomes.	Complex: Diseases do not have a simple explanation, and outcomes are not always measurable.
Adversarial medicine: "How can I destroy the disease?"	Teleological medicine: "What can the disease teach the patient? Is there a message or story in the disease?"
Investigates disease with a "divide-and-conquer" strategy, looking for microscopic causes.	Looks at the "big picture": the causes and effects of disease in the physical, emotional, environmental, social, and spiritual realms.
Intellect is primary. Medical practice is based on scientific theory found in books.	Intuition is primary. Healing is based on spiritual truths learned from nature, elders, and spiritual vision.
Physician is an authority who may attempt to coerce the patient into compliance.	Healer is a health counselor and adviser.
Fosters dependence on medication, technology, and other aspects of the medical system.	Empowers patients with confidence, awareness, and tools to help them take charge of their own health.

Emphasizes expertise of individual physician.	Therapy frequently involves participation of family and community.
Health history focuses on patient and family: "Did your mother have cancer?"	Health history includes the environment: "Are the salmon in your rivers ill?"
Therapy is unrelated to local physical or spiritual geography.	Therapy is rooted in the North American landscape.
Promotes standard and uniform methods of therapy.	Is diverse, situational, and individualized.
Subject to review, regulation, and sanctions by licensing boards and the state.	Based on patient's right of access to healing; healers accountable to Native American communities.
High medical costs.	Healer achieves status through generosity; no fixed fee for services.
Dangerous and invasive medicine, adverse effects common.	Safe, promotes harmony and balance, adverse effects rare.
Intervention should result in rapid cure or management of disease.	Patience is paramount. Healing occurs when the time is right.
Malpractice defined and litigated in a system of hierarchical justice that punishes offenders.	Healers accountable to Native communities and their consensual justice systems, designed to restore harmony rather than to punish.
Physician's lifestyle is not considered a significant factor in his or her efficacy. Legitimacy based on credentials (academic degrees and license).	Healer is expected to model healthy behavior; efficacy depends on healer's insight, spiritual power, and grace of the Creator. Legitimacy based on behavior and reputation.

— APPENDIX B —

MEETINGS WITH REMARKABLE ELDERS

And in the morning, when they arose, I used to hear the elders; just as the singing of birds sounds beautiful in the morning, at day-break, so it was with the elders who could be heard all over as they sang—they would even sing in response with their wives—they took such pride in themselves, and their journey through life was very beautiful.
—Cree elder Peter Vandall, from
Stories of the House People, translated by Freda Ahenakew

I have studied with indigenous elders—including North American Indian, Hawaiian, African, and Filipino—for more than thirty years. They were not "teachers" in the conventional sense. They were mentors, spiritual guides, and treasured fellow pilgrims along what Cherokee call *Duyukta,* or "the Way," the harmonious, meaningful, and moral life path. Although they inspired me with their experience and wisdom and provided me with a verbal map of the promises and pitfalls of the journey, they were more concerned with pointing out a direction than with transmitting information. It was ultimately up to me to walk the terrain, learning directly from nature and spirit.

I did not seek the elders out; it would have been inappropriate to do so, but when the time was right, somehow we found each other. Once they had tested me or just decided that I was trustworthy and not a spiritual thrill-seeker, they generously shared their wisdom. And I like to think that I may have enriched their understanding by sharing my experiences with them.

Several of the elders became dear friends whom I visited regularly for many years. Most have passed into the spirit, and I miss them. I have written these vignettes to convey the essence of what we shared and to pay tribute to their wisdom.

N'TSUKW: WISDOM FROM THE BUSH

In anthropologist Keith H. Basso's *Portraits of the Whiteman,* an important work on Western Apache humor and culture, there is a cartoon by artist Vincent Craig in which a white man is speaking to a Native American. As the white man is saying, "In essence . . . communication is an irrevocable essentiality," the Native American is thinking. "Someone should teach him to speak Indian." Native Americans prize directness: say what you mean, don't beat around the bush or try to impress people with fancy vocabulary. For me, this quality is exemplified by N'Tsukw ("Otter"), an elder of the Innu Nation.

The Innu are an Algonquian-speaking people from Québec and Labrador. About ten thousand strong, they are culturally and linguistically related to the Cree. They were the first Native people the ancient Viking explorers encountered and the first to successfully resist the colonial invasion. They have never ceded their land to a white man's government. But like other First Nations peoples, they have had to contend with its theft and destruction. Despite the loss of original hunting grounds, the Innu, like their heroes the muskrat and the wolverine, remain close to the earth and protective of their Earth Mother.

I met N'Tsukw in 1976 in Montreal, where I was living for six months to help co-found the Montreal Center for the Healing Arts. A mutual Kanien'kehaka (Mohawk) friend introduced us. Grandfather was living in the city rather than in *the bush* (Indian for "wilderness"), as he preferred, to take care of his beloved ninety-year-old mother. We met at a Greek restaurant.

N'Tsukw arrived at the restaurant wearing jeans and a loosely fitting flannel shirt. He had a wide, angular face and penetrating, observant eyes, the result, I imagined, of years of hunting. He looked out on the world but, as I discovered later, did not let anyone look in at his spirit unless he had earned that right. He was broadly built and moved with strength, confidence, and *rootedness* like a bear. His long black hair, streaked with gray, was tied back in a ponytail. I knew he was in his early fifties, although the vitality of his movements and voice suggested a man at least twenty years younger.

Although Grandfather looks like a bear, he is also like the otter, able to move gracefully between different realities, the land and the water, the ordinary and spiritual realms. Grandfather is a coincidence of opposites. He has a deep knowledge of the ancient ways. I have no doubt that he could survive in the winter woods with only a woolen blanket. Yet he is also extremely well educated, not in universities but through his curiosity and love of learning, which have led him to educate himself by every means possible. He is fluent in three languages—Innu, French, and English—and I still have a hard time finding a book he hasn't read. Unlike so many modern Native Americans, he is vehemently antitechnological, objecting strongly to the intrusions of industry and technology into aboriginal consciousness and lifestyle. Yet, like many Native Americans, he has had to compromise his ideals in order to get by in the modern world. When I met him, he earned his living teaching driver's education, even though he personally walked or bicycled whenever possible. He bicycled the ten-mile journey from his mother's house to the restaurant.

As we sat at the table, his first words to me were "What is the origin of evil?" That was all, no greeting or superficial chitchat. "Greed" was my immediate answer. "No, it's farming," he replied, at which point, Grandfather began a concise and lucid description of humankind's transition from hunter-gatherer to agriculturist. A transcription of his words might easily have been taken for a lecture to a graduate anthropology class. But his speech was pure Native American oratory: strong words spoken from the heart and backed up by experience.

"Hunters," he explained, "have no concept of ownership or class distinction. When a hunter kills a deer, he does not own that deer. The deer belongs to the forest. The hunter is also of the woods. He brings the deer back to his people, and all have a right to it. Choice meat is given to those who are weak or disabled, to the elders, to pregnant women, and to children. Survival of the fittest is never the rule in a hunting culture. Rather, people live together compassionately or not at all. Some ten thousand years ago, humans began to cultivate fields and guard their surplus harvest, creating the hierarchical workforce we know today, consisting of laborers at the bottom, managers above them, and at the top, owners who reap most of the profits. Fields and fences are the source of greed and warfare."

The peace-loving hunter lives a nomadic existence. Unlike the farmer, he has no need to defend private territory. His land rights are based on use rather than ownership, a concept, Grandfather said, that the white man's government never understood. The hunter is a communalist, not a capitalist. Grandfather explained, "The word *capital* comes from the Latin word *caput,* 'the head.' Capitalism means 'getting ahead of someone,' usually for economic advantage." How can you get ahead of Brother Wolf, Sister Moon, Grandfather Mountain? "We are all relatives. People who take advantage of others act as though they have no families."

I felt comfortable with Grandfather. Our conversation was not the beginning of a friendship but a renewal of an ancient and mysterious connection. From N'Tsukw, I learned the rugged spirituality of living close to nature. Yet N'Tsukw also taught me that book learning was not in conflict with Native spirituality. Reading could refine my ability to translate experience into words; books provide vocabulary, but they are not the source of knowledge—the direct and raw experience of life.

Grandfather is fiercely independent and expects the same of his friends. "Be dependent on the Great Creator, *Kitchi Manitou.* Don't be dependent on society or its twisted priorities, such as money and prestige" was his philosophy. Once, early in our association, I asked Grandfather if he ever taught anyone his Native songs. He replied, "In my language, anyone who sings someone else's song is called a liar." Songs received during dreams and visions are personal and rarely shared. Even tribal ceremonial songs must be made one's own before they can be sung truthfully. (As an example of this principle, I once learned an earth-honoring song from a Cree elder, but I didn't really feel right about singing it until I hiked alone one spring day to a beautiful waterfall, where I sang and danced it.)

When I asked Grandfather how the Innu people get in touch with helping spirits, he quoted one of *his* elders: "Be careful. I *warn* you of the spirits." Then he explained that since we do not eat the spirits and they do not eat us, they are not, like the plants and animals, bonded to us in the web of life, the kinship created through mutual dependence. Thus, one must approach spirits with respect and caution. "Learn who the spirits are, whether they are good, messengers from the Great Spirit, or spirits that are out of harmony, ungrateful to the Manitou. But if you encounter a disease-causing negative spirit, never send it back to the one who may have sent it." Instead, he advised, be humble and say, "Creator, I release this [negative spirit] to you. I don't have the wisdom to know what to do with this spirit. You know what is best."

Native Americans value humility, but it is not the Native way to make a show of it. The conscious self-denial practiced among Christian monastics is quite alien to them. Although Native Americans commonly pray, "Great Spirit, pity me," they do not walk with heads lowered, as though *deserving* pity. "There is an *assumption of power*," N'Tsukw once told me, "of one's place in Creation. It's a kind of spiritual bluff, like playing poker. If you walk with dignity, the Creator says, 'This person must be worthy of assistance. I will help him.'"

Grandfather gained much knowledge growing up in the bush of northern Québec. Information "read" in the bush is important to survival and can improve quality of life. A trapper who can see a white ptarmigan camouflaged in the snow or who can recognize the footprint of a badger feels at home in his environment. (Book knowledge, on the other hand, can be deceptive. You may understand the words *ptarmigan* and *badger* yet be unable to recognize or appreciate them.) A simple lifestyle, as close to self-sufficiency as possible, requires sensitivity, skill, intuition, and reasoning. Imagine being able to find a salmon run from a feeling in the ocean air, to locate a caribou herd from a wolf's howl three miles away, or to predict the weather more accurately than a weatherman. Primitive decisions are neither simple nor one-sided; they take into account the effect of human actions not only on other humans but on the balance and survival of life as a whole. Environmental impact is a chief consideration in all indigenous decision making. Native people carefully observe such things as the health of the land, the behavior of wildlife, and changes in the weather to determine how many trees to chop for firewood, how many seals to hunt, and when to gather hawthorn berries, the powerful heart tonic that still grows wild in Québec. By contrast, profit and personal gain motivate decision making in the modern world. "Didn't you know," Grandfather asked me, "that *civilization* comes from the French *si vile-ization,* 'making so vile?'" I never tired of such playful etymologies.

Grandfather likes to reminisce about his childhood canoe trips. Once, while his father was navigating a spring rapid, N'Tsukw noticed that his family seemed nervous and edgy. Then, above the sound of the river, he heard a thunderous roar that kept growing louder. Suddenly, his father raised the paddle high over his head and drove it straight down into the water. As it hit bottom, the canoe twirled in a semicircle around this "lever" and beached on a sandy shallow. The family climbed ashore and ported the boat along a narrow, tree-lined trail that dropped sharply through a pile of boulders. Next to the trail ran a magnificent waterfall. N'Tsukw's father explained that only at one spot in the river was there a cleavage in the shale on the river bottom that allowed that maneuver. Many other Native American travelers had missed the spot and careened over the waterfall a hundred yards farther on and were never seen again.

This was one of N'Tsukw's last childhood experiences in the bush. Shortly afterward, government officials removed him, like other Indian children, from his family and friends to the sterile and abusive environment of the boarding school. In many respects, Grandfather can never return to those original forests and rivers. The trees are being cut down; the rivers polluted with acid rain; and the animals killed by greedy sport hunters, new diseases, and mercury-laced food. His nomadic people can no longer follow the seasons or the moose, elk, beaver, and salmon past the fences and private lands. Original tribal hunting grounds are flooded by hydroelectric dams and disturbed by low-flying military aircraft on training flights. Perhaps most devastating of all, the caribou are disappearing. Once the caribou are gone, the Innu lose the major natural source for waterproof boots. This is not a small matter. A hunter will then have to earn money to buy rubber boots at the white man's market. Self-sufficiency seems impossible. Yet Grandfather continues to offer tobacco to nature wherever he finds it, even to trees in the city park. He remembers, in the words of Cherokee elder Andrew Dreadfulwater (1908–1984),

> This is no world that education can change. This is a God given world. It is not a world that can be changed just because a man decides to. No white man's education has yet made trees grow upside down. No white man's money will get red-birds to share their nest with an eagle. That's the power we see today.[1]

KEETOOWAH: ORNERINESS IS NEXT TO GODLINESS

I'll never forget my first encounter with the Cherokee medicine man Keetoowah. It took place just a few months after I met N'Tsukw, in Berkeley, California, where I lived from 1976 to 1981. I was taking graduate courses in classical Chinese at the university and teaching Taiji Quan ("T'ai Chi") and other Chinese healing and martial arts in weekly outdoor classes in a park. One of my students was a young woman who for the past ten summers had lived with Hopi people, helping to tend their sacred cornfields and developing close ties with traditional elders. When she learned of my interest in Native American culture, she suggested that I meet one of the local

Native American elders, a Cherokee medicine man named Keetoowah. "He's been dubbed 'the crystal godfather' because of his knowledge of quartz crystals," she said. I readily agreed, and Keetoowah and I arranged to meet in the park, where we could talk awhile, then eat lunch in a nearby restaurant.

When I saw a man walking across the grass in the distance in a slow, measured way, I knew immediately it was Keetoowah. Although he was only sixty at the time, he looked much older. His face was weathered by what I sensed were difficult or painful life experiences. He was wearing dirty overalls and a head covering shaped like a turban, made of bright, multicolored cloth. A large eagle feather stood upright from a fold in the material. I later learned that it was the traditional hat of the Cherokee, Seminole, and other southeastern Indians.

As Keetoowah approached me, rather than extending his hand, he stopped, squinted at me, and exclaimed in a heavy Oklahoma accent, "You have the second-biggest aura of anybody I've ever seen. But if I didn't know better, I would say you were pregnant!" I was surprised and impressed. How could he know that I had for years practiced Chinese exercises designed to create a reservoir of healing energy in the lower abdomen? Moreover, ancient Chinese texts described health as being "pregnant" with energy. Keetoowah was a seer, able to perceive energies or spiritual dimensions that were hidden from most people, and he did not hesitate to talk about what he saw. I liked this wild and unpredictable man.

Keetoowah invited me to visit him the next week at his home, an ordinary suburban house on a quiet residential street in Santa Rosa, California. There was a small trailer parked in front and a small, unkempt backyard. Inside, his house was like a crystal cave. There were clear and smoky quartz crystals of every size and shape covering every surface—on tables, chairs, shelves, in the kitchen, and by his bed. The rear of his house contained the workshop, where he faceted stones and made jewelry. Keetoowah loved stones, especially semiprecious crystals: amethyst, citrine, topaz, beryl, and of course, clear quartz. He used them in rituals and crafts and held them over patients or placed them on patients' bodies for healing. But he was not a "professional" jeweler; he rarely sold a piece—that would be like selling a friend.

During my first visit, Keetoowah invited me to sit on a comfortable chair and offered me a cup of coffee. We chatted for about an hour as he asked me about my background, interests, and university studies, puffing all the while on a cigarette. Occasionally, he would rest his cigarette in an ashtray and lean forward, apparently to listen more intensely. I sensed that he was listening to far more than my words. He was listening to my being.

At one point, Keetoowah said, matter-of-factly, "So I hear you're interested in crystals. Let's see if they are interested in you. Hold out your palm." He placed a small, clear quartz stone in one hand and told me to cover it with the other. "Now close your eyes." Twenty minutes later, he told me to open them. "Well, what did you learn?" I described several dreamlike images—shapes and colors, nothing concrete—and a physical sense that the crystal had entered my bloodstream and was flowing through me. Keetoowah puffed on his cigarette in silence, then spoke as if delivering a verdict. "Yes," he said, "I can teach you, because the crystal can teach you." For the next ten years, until the day of his passing, I visited Keetoowah as often as possible, always enjoying several hours of conversation, song, and ceremony, generally followed by a meal at his favorite seafood restaurant. He visited me twice in Colorado, where I was his guide to mountains and rivers and arranged meetings with local Native elders.

Keetoowah was born on Halloween, October 31, 1917, in the Western Cherokee Nation, near Tahlequah, Oklahoma. He believed himself to be a reincarnation of his great-grandfather, Ned Christie (1852–1892), the renowned Cherokee warrior who fought fiercely to defend his people against the encroachment of white civilization. Keetoowah claimed to have all of his great-grandfather's memories, and when, as a young man, he met a United States marshal who had been a member of the posse that shot his grandfather, "The S.O.B. tried to shoot me, too. He thought I was him!" Keetoowah felt that it was more than coincidence that I was born exactly one hundred years, to the day, after the birth of Ned Christie. He said that it was a sign that I had a spiritual connection with his family.

Once, a young New Ager visited Keetoowah's home and asked about becoming "a medicine man." He told him, "I wouldn't wish that curse on anyone!" Keetoowah's life had been marked by illness, alcoholism, poverty, and injury. Keetoowah liked to say that he had done just about everything in his life "except scalp a white man," though he admitted that he came close to that when he fought as a mercenary soldier during the Spanish Civil War. Keetoowah had been born with typhoid fever. After "thirty years without a sober day," he developed cirrhosis of the liver. His relatives in Oklahoma still remember him as "Doc," the town drunk. For all the years I knew him, he had heart disease, severe bronchitis, and emphysema. He believed that faceting stones had damaged his lungs. "Nobody ever told me to wear a mask," he explained, adding wryly, "My lungs might be worth something—they're probably filled with diamond dust." And I'm sure that his cigarette smoking didn't help. During his fifties, he had had cancer of the prostate, which he cured with herbal medicine and prayer. His spine was so twisted from arthritis and injuries that, looking at his X rays, doctors assumed that he was in a wheelchair. Yet he moved freely and walked without aid, claiming that he was supported by spiritual powers.

Keetoowah exemplified a great truth—that a person who endures great hardship need not become resentful or vindictive. It is not easy to remain free of bitterness when you suffer or watch people you love suffer—common experiences on Indian reservations, where poverty, alcoholism, and violence are facts of life. Painful experiences test a person's fortitude, resilience, and compassion for human suffering. In addition, a person whom spirits have chosen to become a medicine man or woman endures additional "tests." They are different for each person. One might be tested by disease, another by attacks from evil spirits. The challenge is to remain strong without sacrificing sensitivity and appropriate vulnerability. A hard-hearted person cannot be a medicine person. Keetoowah said that he used to hate his enemies, "but then I decided I was going to love them to death."

Like his personality, his teachings about culture, history, crystals, or healing ranged from the strictly traditional to the outrageous and wild. He told me that the ancient Cherokee called themselves the Clan of the Keetoowah, *Ani Keetoowah,* a term that is untranslatable, and how they had once lived on an island before making their perilous journey to North America. He recounted legends of the *uktena,* the mysterious Cherokee dragon that long ago lived in the lakes of North Carolina, whose scales became the quartz crystal. Years later, I corroborated these teachings in writings by Cherokee scholars. But Keetoowah also told me that he was really from the giant red star in Orion and that the original inhabitants of the earth were "blue globes in the Gobi Desert." Given Keetoowah's propensity for straight-faced humor, perhaps these were simply jokes that I didn't get.

Keetoowah was not afraid of death; he had experienced it twice, during heart attacks: "One time, I floated up to the ceiling and watched the doctors trying frantically to revive me. I was ready to pass on, but I didn't want those doctors to feel bad about wasting so much effort. So I came back." Word got around that he had died, but not that he had come back. A few months after his after-death experience, he walked into a family reunion in Oklahoma. "My family thought I was a ghost, and they nearly died of fright." Although Keetoowah didn't fear death, he worried about disability. He had watched his wife slowly waste away from Lou Gehrig's disease (amyotrophic lateral sclerosis, ALS). Keetoowah hoped to go out with a bang, not a whimper. He got his wish.

In 1987, I had a vivid dream that Keetoowah was about to die and decided to fly out to California the next day and spend a week visiting him. In reality, he was fine. We had a wonderful time together and felt closer than we had ever been. It seemed that all of our old friends were in town. Ingwe, the Zulu shaman, had recently moved into a house not far from Santa Rosa. Rolling Thunder was visiting the San Francisco Bay area, his first public appearance since the passing of his beloved wife, Spotted Fawn. A steady stream of visitors came to Keetoowah's house, most of them seeking healing or counseling.

Keetoowah was inspired by all of this activity. Never one to follow his medical doctor's advice, now he vowed to take better care of himself. He would watch his diet and be diligent about taking his medications. But the day after I left California, alone in the house and without the counsel of those who loved him, Keetoowah decided to drive his car to a hot springs a few hours north, to purify himself in the healing waters, even though he was under doctor's orders not to drive farther than the corner grocery. About an hour into the trip, his car spun out of control, skidded across the pavement, and flipped on the side of the road. He died instantly.

Keetoowah was a medicine man. Like most medicine men, however, he considered the title a goal toward which one should always strive and that can never be fully attained. Keetoowah said, "I am a pipe carrier. I pray for people and for the Earth." It was from him that I received my Indian name, *Bear Hawk,* as well as the sacred pipe. I can still see him blessing my pipe, blowing smoke along the foot-long stem and red stone bowl, asking the Creator to guide me. I remember his kind words when he saw in my facial expression that I felt unworthy. "If you're not qualified to carry the pipe, I don't know who is!" he exclaimed. Poor teachers act with an authority that makes students feel less than who they are. Keetoowah was the kind of teacher who made you feel more than you are, or perhaps who you really are. I try to be worthy of his trust.

ROLLING THUNDER:
DREAMS AND TESTS FROM THE SPIRIT WORLD

Rolling Thunder was my friend and mentor. He continued the training I had begun with Keetoowah. Most important, Rolling Thunder provided me with a second home in the Nevada desert, where I learned to live in harmony with the land.

I dreamed of this great healer three years before I met him. In the early 1970s, I spent a summer hitchhiking across the United States, from New York to California, on a journey with no particular destination. One evening, asleep in my sleeping bag in a southern California desert, I dreamed that I was lying on a ceremonial blanket. A medicine man was standing over me. Although my eyes were closed in the dream, I could nevertheless see the medicine man's face and actions clearly. He was holding an eagle feather and shaking it at me. Lightning flashed from the tip and struck my body. Instantly, I was an eagle, soaring over a great desert.

Three years later, again in California, a friend told me that a medicine man and Indian-rights activist named "Rolling Thunder" was offering a public lecture at a large auditorium in San Francisco. I had heard the name before, as had many young people. Rolling Thunder had toured with Bob Dylan's "Rolling Thunder Review," and he was the subject of a recently published book. Beyond this, however, I knew nothing about him.

On stage, Rolling Thunder was accompanied by a troop of warriors, drummers, and singers. His "lectures"—really Native American cultural events—included prayer, songs, and emotionally charged discussions of Native American rights, social and legal struggles, and values, particularly respect for and love of the land. I recognized him from my dream as soon as he walked onto the stage. Every feature was exactly the same. But I am convinced that even if he had been wearing a mask, I would have recognized him from his eyes—they were wise yet seemed to belong to another realm, beyond interpretation or understanding, more like the eyes of a wild animal than those of a human being. Although I wouldn't meet Rolling Thunder personally for several years, I knew there was some destiny between us.

The feather in my dream also played a role in that first encounter. Rolling Thunder was standing on the stage, slightly in front of several seated singers and drummers. When the audience quieted down, anticipating the beginning of Rolling Thunder's talk, he announced that his lead singer had a sore throat and was too hoarse to perform. Rolling Thunder would have to doctor him right then and there. Rolling Thunder lifted a large spotted-eagle tail feather resting on a side table and held it in front of his chest for a few moments, becoming introspective and tranquil, as though in a deep state of prayer. Suddenly, with rapid flicks of the wrist, he shook the feather two or three times in the singer's direction. A lightning bolt flashed from the feather to the man's throat, which prompted the startled man sitting next to me to lean over and exclaim, "Did you see that?" The lecture continued, and the singer's voice was strong and clear for the rest of the evening.

"Rolling Thunder" is a fitting name for this charismatic spiritual warrior. Lightning was his ally; he projected it from his hands or feathers when he healed. Rolling Thunder's penetrating eyes always saw beyond the surface. He was aware not only of people's feelings but of their reality, the private world that most of us believe we inhabit alone. And he was, at times, painfully candid when sharing his insights about that reality. His words shook people up like thunder, sometimes for the better, sometimes for the worse. Rolling Thunder once told me that if at least a few people did not become uncomfortable enough to walk out of his talks, he knew that he was not doing his job. Some people are so stuck in their view of life that a spiritual message is too threatening to handle. Rolling Thunder wanted to wake them up.

Rolling Thunder was a strict and demanding teacher. In many ways, he was the most traditional of all the medicine people I have known. Not content to speak about Native American tradition or only to practice it, he *lived* it. He was never tempted by money, power, or fame. He and his Shoshone wife, Spotted Fawn, raised six children in a simple house near the railroad tracks in Carlin, Nevada. Someone was always out front working on Rolling Thunder's old white van. I repaired flat tires more than once. "You'll never see a medicine person in a Cadillac," he used to say.

Simplicity was practiced at Meta Tantay, Shoshone for "Go in Peace," the name of the 262-acre spiritual community Rolling Thunder founded in the desert, not far from his home. Meta Tantay was like a Native American *kibbutz:* residents and visitors worked together planting and harvesting, cooking, caring for and milking the goats—that was my main job—and doing the many other tasks needed to keep a household or farm running. The day always began with a Native American Sunrise Prayer Ceremony, and the evenings often included group songs around a campfire or a talk by Rolling Thunder or a visiting elder.

There were about forty residents when I lived at Meta Tantay—two or three months a year in the early 1980s—and generally a dozen or so visitors. People of any ethnicity, Native American tribe, or nationality were welcome. We lived in large, dome-shaped lodges—Native American wickiups, a flexible wooden frame made with branches and covered by some form of insulation; the favorite at Meta Tantay, for both price and utility, was government-surplus parachutes—some as wide as twenty feet in diameter. Heated by woodstoves and lit, when necessary, by kerosene lanterns, the white domes always had an eerie beauty as they flapped in a spring breeze or glistened under the winter moonlight. Couples and their children and longtime residents had their own wickiups. Single people lived in gender-specific communal wickiups or in the various trailers scattered about the land. A generator could provide electricity, but we generally went without it. What is the good of living in the desert if you cannot see the stars because of electric lights or cannot hear the coyotes because of television! We weren't totally self-sufficient, however. There were groceries, tools, and other materials to buy and property taxes to pay. Guests contributed what they could. If a guest couldn't contribute toward the cost of food and other necessities, then he or she just contributed extra work. Generosity was always voluntary: at Meta Tantay, people kept their own property and bank accounts, unlike residents at some non-Native communes.

Until his retirement in the mid-1980s, Rolling Thunder worked full-time as a brakeman for the Southern Pacific Railroad and generously donated much of his salary to Meta Tantay or to any individuals or groups that were in need. I tried unsuccessfully to refuse his gifts of "traveling money" on several occasions. Some might wonder why an Indian doctor needed to have other employment. Doctoring is a spiritual gift, and Rolling Thunder refused to put a price tag on it. He never charged money for healing; the only offering he required was a pouch of tobacco.

Rolling Thunder was often a target of malicious gossip by Native Americans jealous of his knowledge, power, and popularity. I got quite upset once when a young Native American, whom I met at a powwow, ranted that Rolling Thunder was a "sellout, teaching secret traditions to whites for a price." It was clear that he had not met Rolling Thunder. Rolling Thunder never gave away details of Native American traditions. A person seeking knowledge had to earn sacred information the old way, the hard way, through sacrifice and demonstration of character over a long period of time. Rolling Thunder's favorite topic of conversation was neither secret traditions nor ceremonies, but *Meta Tantay*. At his public lectures, he explained the importance of working on the land, of caring for the garden and animals. He decried the destruction of original Native lands by logging and overgrazing and railed against social injustices still perpetrated against his Shoshone neighbors. People who visited Meta Tantay were greeted by the sweat of hard work, not sweat lodges. They could stay if they were respectful, willing to work and abide by the rules: "No drugs, no alcohol, no violence, and no foreign religions." Rolling Thunder did not want to hear any Sanskrit chanting or Christian praying. "This is *Indian land*. We're not joining you [white people] anymore; while you're here, you're joining us!"

Born in Stamps, Arkansas, on September 10, 1916, to Cherokee and Cajun parents, Rolling Thunder was raised in the Kiamichi Mountains of eastern Oklahoma. At age fifteen, he built a hut there and lived alone in the forest for several years. This period of solitude and silent listening to nature shaped Rolling Thunder's character and spirit. He called it his Vision Quest. Because he learned from medicine people of many tribes, Rolling Thunder was called an "intertribal medicine man." Among his close friends and mentors were the Tuscarora medicine man Mad Bear Anderson and Grandfather David Monogye of the Hopi. "Some people call me a medicine man," Rolling Thunder would say. "I don't claim anything." But to me, Rolling Thunder was a true medicine man and wise Grandfather. Did he have faults? He sure did. He flirted too much, and no one wanted to be around him when his anger stormed. Yet I admire the fact that he made no attempts to deny or hide his faults. He detested gurus.

I was fortunate to be able to meet with Rolling Thunder privately during my first visit to Meta Tantay. Normally, a private meeting with the great man could have taken weeks to arrange—people came to "the land," Meta Tantay, to experience a spiritual way of life, not to meet a "master." Those looking for the exotic were quickly disappointed and searched elsewhere. My early introduction to Rolling Thunder was arranged by his childhood friend Keetoowah. When Keetoowah found out that I was planning to visit Meta Tantay, he said, "Let me call R.T. first."

I was somewhat nervous about meeting Rolling Thunder for the first time. We were to meet in the dining area, "the cook-shack," that afternoon. On the way, I stopped at the outhouse. While I was doing my business, a sudden gust of wind came up and blew the outside latch shut. Trapped, I started banging on the door, hoping that someone would hear and rescue me. No one did. Trying to maintain perspective, I told myself that there must be a hidden reason for this ridiculous predicament—being locked in an outhouse in the middle of the sweltering Nevada desert. I had no choice but to continue banging and waiting until, after about half an hour, I quit making noise. Suddenly, another gust of wind came up and blew open the latch. As I stepped out into the bright sun, who should I see passing by the outhouse on his way to the cook-shack but Rolling Thunder! Smiling, he said, "You must be Ken." We walked together to the cook-shack. Evidently, the spirits at Meta Tantay had used humor to teach me an important lesson—it might be necessary for me to deal with my own "shit" before I could learn anything new. And if I refused to face my problems, the universe, the Great Mystery, would see to it that I did. Once you are committed to "the Red Road" of Native American spirituality, lessons are not a matter of choice.

When you have found a compatible spiritual teacher, you will probably dream of him or her either before or during your training. The dream is a sign that the connection is meant to be and that the learning will go deeper than the conscious mind. About a year later, another dream confirmed my relationship with Rolling Thunder.

I dreamed that we were Apache brothers, living in what is now the state of Arizona, long before the arrival of the white man. I was soon to leave on a pilgrimage to the North. "We will never meet again in this life," my brother told me. "But in the future, you will see me again. I will be older and will look different. You will remember this parting in a dream, but know that it is not a dream. It is real. I will now teach you some words in our ancient language. When you see me again, say them to me and I will remember you from the past." When I awoke, I remembered the words, and when I told the dream to Rolling Thunder, he nodded and exclaimed, "Ho!" an acknowledgment of the dream's truth. Rolling Thunder said that he had always felt a deep spiritual connection with the Apache and with their great warrior and holy man Gokhlayeh (Geronimo). I had also long admired Gokhlayeh and had once received a gift of Apache jewelry from a descendant of his band. Perhaps Rolling Thunder and I were both members of Gokhlayeh's band in other lifetimes. Many Native Americans believe in reincarnation. Yet even if the dream was symbolic of a spiritual rather than a blood relationship, the underlying message was clear. He and I were on the same path; we were thus "relatives" in the Native sense.

The dream seemed proof to Rolling Thunder that I was destined to learn Native American medicine. Like an older brother, he warned me of the dangers and pitfalls of the journey. "I will test you. Evil spirits will also test you. They will try to influence you, because if they can control you, they can harm many others." One of my tests, he said, would mean life or death. Either I would learn the medicine or I would die. Though he said, "It's not too late to back out," we both knew that it was too late. I could sense the Great Spirit's love, light, and wisdom at the end of the trail. Even if I never reached him, no other journey could satisfy me.

— FACING THE SHADOW AND OTHER TESTS —

I would like to share with you a few of these tests. I cannot share every one because some were given with explicit instructions from the Spirit World to keep them private. Some experiences grow more sacred through sharing; others retain their meaning and power only with respectful silence.

Rolling Thunder and I spent many hours under an arbor of willows. We smoked our corncob pipes, talked about spirit and healing, and listened to the silence. In these meetings, Rolling Thunder tested my character and determined that I could take further steps.

Once, after walking for miles in the desert, away from any roads, I came across Rolling Thunder's van. The side doors were open, and R.T. was sitting in the back across from an empty chair. With his prophetic gifts, Rolling Thunder somehow knew that I would appear. He motioned to me to come in and sit. "One thing I can't figure out is why a young man, talented and intelligent, would want to come and work with us poor Indians," he said, in a slow, measured fashion, as if to make sure I caught the meaning of each word. He continued, "You're not going to make any money." I was well aware that Rolling Thunder was trying to find out if I had an ulterior motive for living at Meta Tantay, like so many do-gooders in Indian Country. Was I really a real estate agent looking for a way to buy the land, a journalist, or perhaps a movie producer looking for a new angle on Native American life? Was I truly content to live according to Indian values, always basing my decisions on what is right rather than on money? Rolling Thunder knew the answer to these questions, but he needed to hear it from me.

Speaking from my heart, I talked at length of my love of the ancient ways and my desire to help out at Meta Tantay. When I was finished, Rolling Thunder asked me if I had my corncob pipe with me. I took it from my pocket, and he motioned for me to pass it to him; then he filled it with some of his own herbal smoking mixture. After we smoked together, he taught me his way of gathering and preparing natural herbs for smoking in a corncob pipe and in the Sacred Pipe.

My next test began one night when I was asleep in my wickiup, having a frightening dream in which a malevolent presence was shining a spotlight down the center of my body, stopping on various "energy centers," which are similar to the *chakras* of Indian Yoga. It was looking for a weak place to attack me. Wakening in a cold sweat from this nightmare, I sat up in bed only to see an even more terrifying image: a glowing grayish-white shadow was advancing toward me from the door flap. This was a real evil spirit, perhaps the same one I had seen in my dream, alive in both realities.

If the "shadow" had not been blocking the door, I would have bolted. If I had had a knife, I would have cut a hole in the back of the lodge and run. I tried every spiritual trick in the book to protect myself from harm or to energetically repel malevolent forces. I imagined that I was encased in a quartz crystal. I recited a sacred chant. I projected a mirror in front of me. Nothing worked. My heart was pounding. The spirit kept advancing, and I knew that my end was imminent.

Then I had a near-death experience. During what I assumed were my last seconds on earth, linear time ceased to function, and various life experiences and thoughts occurred in a moment. I realized that I could not protect myself from what I feared, because *I* was the problem. The sense of separation, of being a subjective "I" distinct from objects, is what allows evil to exist. A person who is at one with all of life is free of fear because there is literally nothing to fear. The Buddhist philosopher Alan Watts used to say that good and evil are two sides of the same coin. Now I realized that I was the coin. Simultaneously, I saw as though in a waking dream—but believe me, I was fully awake—the circle of residents at Meta Tantay saying their prayers around a fire during the daily Sunrise Ceremony. I understood the great web of connection with all of life and knew *this was protection*. As if to prove the truth of this, the shadow suddenly exploded, shattering into fragments of light that dissolved into the air. I felt an embracing sense of peace.

I did not share my experience with Rolling Thunder immediately. I wanted the lesson to settle and mature. The very next evening, Rolling Thunder called all of the residents together for a community meeting and discussion. As people were gathering, I felt an odd, unfamiliar tingling sensation in the back of my head. Suddenly, Rolling Thunder silenced the group with a loud exclamation of "Ho!" He explained that I had passed some difficult tests and should now be treated as a teacher. When the meeting was over, Rolling Thunder asked if I had felt anything strange that evening. I told him of the tingling, and he explained that he had launched a psychic attack. No permanent harm would be done; he wanted to see how I handled an attack from behind. The power, he said, came back to him as peace and love. "That's the way to handle an aggressive spirit," he said. "If you battle it, it gets stronger."

After this, Rolling Thunder began to teach me his medicine ways. I learned how to start a ceremonial fire and conduct a Sunrise Ceremony; how to use hands, breath, and imagery to doctor a patient; how to sing and drum medicine songs and social songs; how to make a pilgrimage and gather power. The land and animals were the greatest teachers of all. I learned lessons from nature while hiking in the Ruby Mountains, holy ground of the Shoshone. I practiced traditional dances around a campfire in the desert—seeing the sparks dancing and blending with the shooting stars. I harvested turnips, zucchini, carrots, and cabbages from the garden while watching the magpies swooping and playing across the sandy streambed. I observed eagles circling serenely overhead and listened to coyotes as they wandered freely through the camp at night. (The coyotes never attacked the sheep, goats, or rabbits. Rolling Thunder had made a treaty with them. "You can make a treaty with a wild animal but not with a domesticated one," he said. "We once had dogs here, and *they* attacked our animals.")

Rolling Thunder said, "I can teach you because I know you won't steal my medicine." I wouldn't imitate him but would seek my own connection with the Great Spirit. I am deeply grateful that Rolling Thunder accepted my tobacco. On several occasions, I heard Rolling Thunder remark, "I know my enemies won't forget me, so I sure hope my friends won't." Rolling Thunder passed on in 1997. I will never forget my great friend and teacher.

TWYLAH NITSCH:
EARN WHAT YOU LEARN

"Sparkle your eyes," Seneca Wolf Clan Grandmother Twylah Nitsch would always say when she began a lesson. It was her ingenious way of reminding her students to be joyful, curious, and less preoccupied with themselves. I wish our educational institutions would learn this simple lesson: without a sparkle, it is impossible to learn or remember anything important! Gram's eyes started sparkling when she was born on December 5, 1912, and they were still sparkling in 2001. I remember the first dozen or so times I spoke to her on the phone. I always thought this seventy-plus-year-old woman was a teenager. "Hello. Is Gram there?" "That's me. Who is this?"

Gram was born and lived most of her life on the Seneca Nation, Cattaraugus Reservation, near Buffalo, New York. As a young woman, Twylah was different from the crowd. She was a deep thinker, who felt that life was too important and too short to waste time with gossip or suitors. Young men found her aloof and unapproachable and wryly joked that her name was an acronym for *To Win Your Love Appears Hopeless*. One young man did succeed, and today, she tells the story of how he won her heart by playing a trick on her that she never regretted. Since she had just rebutted his invitation to the local dance, he decided to "go over her head" and court her parents. One day, she came home and found him sitting at the dinner table, a sign that her parents had already accepted him into the family. Here was a man as stubborn and persistent as she was. She decided to give him a chance. Theirs was a long and happy marriage.

I love this story because it reminds me of some of Grandmother's gifts. The lifetime of love Gram shared with her husband and four children helped shape her character and spirit. She is an openhearted teacher who offers a warm, welcoming hug to everyone who walks through her door. You immediately want to adopt her as a surrogate grandmother for your children. It is hard to believe that she ever seemed aloof or inaccessible.

Today, Grandmother advises and oversees the two organizations she founded, the Wolf Clan Teaching Lodge and the Seneca Indian Historical Society (SIHS), a nonprofit organization chartered by the New York State Department of Education. The Seneca Indian Historical Society sponsors research, education, and cultural activities related to traditional Seneca wisdom. The heart of the SIHS is the Wolf Clan Teaching Lodge. Both organizations are currently directed by Grandmother's son, Bob Nitsch, and based in Florida.[2]

The Wolf Clan Teaching Lodge is really a school without "walls"; it springs up where there are authorized teachers to share their knowledge. Students of any background or ethnicity are welcome. Gram starts them off with a teaching she learned from her grandfather, the Seneca medicine man Moses Shongo. He made a circle of twelve stones on the ground, each representing a spiritual gift, a stepping-stone on the sacred path through life. In her version, Gram uses paper and pens rather than stones, but the message is the same. The most fundamental gift is harmony. As a child, Twylah spent a great deal of time listening to the sounds of nature, especially the birds. Each bird has its own song, yet, like all sounds in nature, each song blends harmoniously with the others. People, too, have "songs," and the secret to a life of purpose and happiness is to discover these gifts and to express them, thus giving them to others.

Grandmother *initiates* students into the lodge in a beautiful ceremony in which she, along with four members who represent the Four Winds, blesses the initiate. (It is *not* an adoption or a license to represent the Seneca Nation.) In effect, Grandmother is saying, "You are a child of the Great Mystery. Wake up to this fact!" Without explaining what it means, she gives the initiate a new name and says simply, "Your mission now is to find out the meaning of your name." Thus, the initiation is not an end point but a beginning.

My name was *Ongwe Okdea,* "Man Root," a reference to *Ipomoea pandurata,* a sacred plant used in Seneca purification ceremonies. Interestingly, Grandmother was unaware that my surname *Cohen* comes from a Hebrew root that means grounded or "rooted." Receiving this name was a confirmation of an aspect of my mission of which I have long been aware: to find the common root among spiritual traditions and to build respectful communication among them.

I met Grandmother in 1984 at a multitribal spiritual gathering in New York's Catskill Mountains. One of the directors of the gathering, a Native American from the Midwest, had asked me to open the event by blessing the ceremonial ground. This was an unusual, and not entirely appropriate, request because traditional etiquette required that he ask a local elder. I declined, and when he demanded an explanation, I said, "Where are we now?" He said, "New York State." "And whose land is this?" He said, "Iroquois." I reminded him, "There is a white-haired Haudenosaunee elder standing over there. I don't know her, but I heard that she is Seneca. Ask her to open the gathering. If *she* asks me, I will comply."

Grandma Twylah performed a traditional Seneca blessing, using prayer and song to bless the ground and the gathering. She walked over to me afterward and said, "I overheard your conversation earlier and am glad that you were paying attention. Come visit me in my cabin this afternoon." Later, over a cup of herbal tea, Grandmother invited me to visit her at her home on the Cattaraugus Reservation, Seneca Nation. I eagerly accepted. I felt a close affinity with Seneca teachings because of the seven years I'd spent as an apprentice to Keetoowah. I have heard both Seneca and Cherokee elders say that they are cousin tribes, having left an original ancient island, the sacred land, called *Elohi* in Cherokee, at the same time.

A week later, I took Grandmother up on her offer. Arriving for what I thought would be a personal retreat, I found her living room packed with thirty or forty Indians and non-Indians waiting to hear me lecture. To my astonishment, Gram introduced me as "the crystal man" and announced that my topic would be quartz crystals. Somehow, Gram intuitively knew that I had studied the Native American lore and uses of quartz crystal, even though I had never publicized this fact nor mentioned it during conversation. Nor did she know my teacher, Keetoowah.

I understood that the lecture was a test of my character and training. Discretion is a virtue among Native Americans. Would I make a show of my knowledge of crystal work, revealing its mysteries and, in effect, turning it into an over-the-counter medicine? Knowledge of crystals comes to one only in dreams. Even a teacher's guidance must be validated through dreams before it can be considered one's own. Gram would be watching her students, too. Were they aware of the distinction between a public lecture and the more secretive and selective transmission of spiritual knowledge?

Right away, the students began asking questions. They wanted to know how to heal with quartz, how to purify the stone, where to buy it. I answered them indirectly. I shared the legend of the Cherokee *uktena,* the dragonlike creature whose scales became quartz in the Cherokee homelands. I asked them if they knew that the ancient Chinese word for quartz is also the word for the moon. Did they know how to purify their minds so that whatever medicine they used would work properly? Quartz is a paradox, I explained; it seems to be pure light, yet it is visible and tangible. Perhaps people are the same, a reflection of the Great Spirit, alive in both waking and dreaming realities. By telling stories or asking questions, I was guiding students to find their own meaning, to learn through introspection. The meeting lasted two hours. I went to bed not knowing whether I had passed the test.

At about six o'clock the next morning, Gram stormed through the house, knocking on bedroom doors and saying, "Get to the Teaching Lodge, right now!" There were about five students living in her house and several people who had stayed the night and were in sleeping bags on the living room floor. Once we were seated on benches in the simple wooden shack behind her home, Gram told us how the original homeland of the People was destroyed because of the misuse of sacred powers, including both their own helping spirits and powerful gifts of nature, like the quartz. "The floods came. The great tree fell over, and from the hole, water fountained up and pierced the sky dome. Waters came down from above as well. Some of the People escaped by boat to Turtle Island."

After this powerful teaching, Gram told me that I had handled the situation of the previous evening in the proper way. Clearly, she was not so happy with some of her students. "Truth is found by listening," she said, "not by talking or expecting truth to be handed to you on a platter. I am glad you steered clear of techniques. No *technique* can bring you closer to the Great Mystery!" Then she asked me if I would like to share with her some of the medicine songs that I had learned from other elders; she would teach me her own. I began commuting to the reservation as often as possible, sometimes teaching there myself, but always continuing to learn from Gram. Three years later, Gram initiated me into the Wolf Clan Teaching Lodge. Shortly thereafter, I received a teaching certificate from the Seneca Indian Historical Society. I take these gifts as a serious responsibility—a commitment to continue learning and never to assume that I know. I share with my own students the important lesson that Gram shared with me. A good life is based on the values of kindness, respect, gratitude, and humor.

WAR EAGLE: DON'T JUDGE A BOOK BY ITS COVER

The Chinese saying "The sage wears clothes of patchwork cotton but in his bosom hides the precious jade" expresses how I felt about War Eagle, a Lumbee-Cherokee gourd dancer, stone healer, herbalist, jeweler, pipe carrier, and healer. I used to visit a small town in Arkansas during the 1980s, where the locals were generally quite interested in Native American culture, but they seemed to ignore the local Cherokee elder, War Eagle. War Eagle just didn't fit the medicine man stereotype. He didn't have long hair or wear feathers. He didn't live in a tipi but in a beat-up old trailer. He prided himself on having the largest collection of historic barbed wire in the United States, from old ranches and ghost towns, and dozens of boxes filled with ancient arrowheads, found during his barbed-wire hunts. "Go ahead and visit him," some locals told me. "All he does is tell dirty jokes."

Sure enough, when I paid him a visit, I had to sit through an hour or so of very raunchy jokes. It was the strangest "test" of a visitor's character and intent of any elder I had known. War Eagle liked poking fun at people: white and red, men and women, especially himself. If a student seemed to be putting him up on a pedestal, War Eagle might allow him to hear his audiocassette of "sacred and secret Indian music"—sung by Alvin and the Chipmunks.

From that first meeting, I felt that I had known War Eagle all my life. There were no barriers to work through. I listened to his jokes, and I told him some of my own. He especially enjoyed the Jewish jokes, since when he tried to tell them, he could never get the Yiddish accent right (although he could speak Cherokee with a British accent). Humor helped War Eagle cope with personal hardship. He had congestive heart failure, diabetes, a prosthetic foot (from complications due to diabetes), and chronic pain. When I knew him, his health had deteriorated to the point at which he had to cut back on work.

There wasn't a mean bone in War Eagle's body. "Guide your children with love and understanding," War Eagle recommended. "Never whip them. Nurture their hearts with love, and then love will overflow from them to others." He was very much in love with his wife, Helen, a descendant of the Comanche leader Quanah Parker. I remember once seeing War Eagle give Helen a peck on the cheek, saying, "I'll always be with my wife, because she's just too ugly to kiss good-bye." In truth, Helen was a beautiful person inside and out, and War Eagle doted on her. Both War Eagle and Helen were generous to a fault. Every time I visited their home, they took out a bag of "goodies," beautiful turquoise nuggets and cabochons, and insisted that I take my pick. I felt as if I were a child back in my grandparents' home in Forest Hills, New York. War Eagle was a good example to me of love, kindness, humility, and humor.

In 1987, War Eagle had a vision that transformed his life. One evening, he lay in bed, just falling off into sleep, when he suddenly bolted upright, walked over to a bedroom chair, and sat down. Helen called to him to ask what was wrong. No response. He just sat there, motionless. After about an hour, he got up, walked back over to the bed, and lay down, not sleeping, moving, or talking, as though in a trance. The next morning, War Eagle said that he had visited the Spirit World, where ancient spirits and ancestors taught him their secrets. Among other things, he had learned how to charge quartz crystals in sunlight to use them for healing. He also learned how to return to the Spirit World at will in order to find answers to people's problems. Most extraordinary of all, after this vision, his spoken Cherokee went from a few words to near fluency.[3] One year later, he founded "The Eagle Tribe Medicine Society," open by invitation to anyone committed to learning what he called "the Ways," the way of life and the values of indigenous peoples. For the next two years before he died, War Eagle sent members a small newsletter with his poems and stories and his teachings about spirituality, herbs, and stones. Sometimes, the newsletter would come with a tiny packet of herbs and instructions: "Boil the sassafras in a cup of water to make a delicious spring tonic."

It was just a few months after his great vision that War Eagle and I met. The vision had turned him into an elder overnight. Yet War Eagle seemed unwilling to fully assume his new role. He was bedridden at the time and filled with self-pity. He told me that his painful prosthetic foot made him feel like an eagle with clipped wings. He had loved powwow dancing; for years, the Eagle Spirit had made his heart soar and his feet move lightly to the drumbeat. Now he could hardly move at all. I asked War Eagle, "Where is your sacred pipe?" It was locked away in a suitcase in the bedroom closet. Helen rummaged through messy piles of boxes and papers until she found it. She placed it on the foot of the bed, and War Eagle motioned with his chin for me to open it. I carefully removed his pipe bundle: a twelve-inch ashwood pipe-stem and small pipestone bowl, wrapped in red cloth. War Eagle asked if I would pray for him with his pipe. I sang and prayed and blew smoke over War Eagle's body. I told him that the spirits did not want him to dwell in negative thinking and that each day he should go outside to greet the sun proudly. At the end of the ceremony, War Eagle seemed to have renewed hope and energy. He stood up, steadied himself on the bedpost with one hand, raised the other hand toward the sky, and prayed in Cherokee. His pain was significantly diminished, and by the next day, he was walking slowly, and proudly, without his walker.

War Eagle passed into spirit at age sixty-two on December 29, 1990, the hundredth anniversary of the massacre of Native Americans at Wounded Knee. After his funeral, Helen asked me to lead a Native American passing-on rite for him in one year's time. A year is the traditional waiting period before a person's soul can be released to the Spirit World. Until then, the soul of the departed remains earthbound, sometimes visiting people in dreams.

War Eagle kept busy as the time approached. Shortly after he died, some friends, unaware of his passing, visited the winter home War Eagle and Helen kept in Arizona. They knocked on the trailer door, whereupon War Eagle appeared at the door and invited them in for a cup of coffee. A few weeks later, the friends were driving through Arkansas and heard that War Eagle's wife, but not War Eagle, was back. Helen was sitting in a lawn chair outside the white trailer when they drove up. They exchanged greetings. Then the friends excitedly told Helen about their recent visit with War Eagle, saying how happy they'd been to see how much better he was doing. Laughing, Helen exclaimed, "That must have been his spirit. He's been dead for weeks!" Incredulous, the friends protested that War Eagle had looked great and that he told them that all his pain was gone. He was also walking normally.

Not long afterward, Helen was listening to a tape of some favorite country music she had recorded from the radio for her daughter. When the music ended, she was about to turn off the cassette player when she heard a familiar voice on the tape saying, "Thank you. War Eagle." There was no mistaking it—it was War Eagle's voice. (The tape was new and had been purchased after War Eagle died. The cassette player only had a slot for one tape, and thus Helen could not have mistakenly dubbed in a portion of another tape.) War Eagle continued to surprise his friends and relatives in their waking and nighttime dreams, sometimes teaching, sometimes teasing or joking, but always making it clear that he was happy and free, for the rest of that year. Then, according to the custom, I sent him on his way, releasing his spirit with the smoke of the Sacred Pipe. When the ceremony ended, the wind whirled about the cabin, and several small chickadees appeared, chirping on the windowsill. Chickadees, though small and humble, share the same spirit as the great golden eagle, which many Native Americans call the "war eagle." At the close of the ceremony, I read a poem that War Eagle had given me shortly before his passing:

The Great Spirit chose me from His heap of stones
A dull rock—not shining

Against His great wheel he polishes me
In sparks of pain to smoothness
Gentle that I might not ignore those
Who touch me
Smooth that I might reflect His Light
His Color
The Great Spirit wears me on His Hand

I cannot see the seeds of corn
I planted deep within the earth
Yet I know they will grow
And stand tall in the sun
When their summer comes

I cannot see the seeds of love
I planted deep within your mind
Yet I know they will grow
And stand tall in your heart
when your winter comes[4]

OUT OF AFRICA:
INGWE, THE LEOPARD MAN

During one of my early visits to Meta Tantay, Rolling Thunder introduced me to another guest, *Ingwe,* or "Leopard," an African-American healer who had recently returned to the United States from several years' training with the high Zulu *Sanusi* ("Holy Man") and *Umlando* ("Keeper of Tribal Lore"), Vusamazulu Credo Mutwa, in South Africa. Ingwe had intended to stay in South Africa for the rest of his life. But *Baba* ("Respected Elder") Mutwa, as people call him, insisted that Ingwe first return to the land of his birth to learn about North America's indigenous tradition.

Baba Mutwa knew about Rolling Thunder, perhaps through Doug Boyd's biography of him, *Rolling Thunder,* or perhaps because medicine people just know one another. Indigenous elders around the world speak the same spiritual language, and their thoughts can be sent or received across any distance. Baba Mutwa recorded an audiotape that served as a spoken letter of introduction for Ingwe to play for Rolling Thunder. I listened to the tape in Rolling Thunder's home. Baba's voice carried such power and love that we could truly feel his presence as he said, "This is my son, Ingwe, one of the AmaZulu, the children of light . . ."

Ingwe and I became friends. In spite of very different backgrounds, we found ourselves walking a very similar trail: we were two Americans, of different race, close in age, each searching for roots in the land of his birth.

Each morning, shortly after sunrise, the work leaders at Meta Tantay would assign the residents various jobs: gardening, feeding the animals, milking the goats, repairing leaking roofs, gathering winter wood, child care and cooking, and so on. Ingwe and I would always convince the work leader to allow us to work at least part of the day together. We were usually assigned "the water truck." That meant driving an old black truck with a water tank in the back. We picked it up each day after lunch and drove it through the camp, stopping at each wickiup to fill the residents' barrels with water for drinking and washing. We also watered hundreds of newly planted mahogany trees, once native to this region but cut down by the early ranchers. The only roads through the desert were the tire ruts from our previous trips. As we bumped along, Ingwe and I spoke of many things: life in Africa, Zulu massage therapy and divination, warrior training, Jewish Cabala—it was a fascination of his—and prayer.

One summer afternoon, after our work was done, we drove the truck a few hundred yards out into the desert, until the wickiups and other buildings disappeared from view behind a sandy hillside. As we stood in the shade of the truck, Ingwe took out a corncob pipe, filled it with tobacco, and lit it with a match. He drew the pungent smoke into his mouth and puffed it out a few times. Then he prayed, "Great Master, Great Master, thank you for this beautiful desert . . ." Between puffs of smoke, he continued, "May our minds and hearts be open to this beauty, inspired by it, deepened by it." In the still desert air, the smoke rose from his pipe like dark, wispy clouds. It was just an ordinary pipe, but in Ingwe's hands, it became a sacred pipe, and through it, he communed with the Creator. Ingwe's words were a litany of pure poetry. He was thankful for *everything:* the air, the water, the sand, the distant mountains, the sun, the moon, the snakes, the coyotes and eagles, the ants and mosquitoes. As I listened, tears ran down my face, my mind wiped clean of selfishness. There was *only* the Creator and Creation. To this day, I feel that Ingwe, more than any other holy person, opened my heart to the meaning of prayer.

I remember one morning when it was our job to try to get the billy goats to eat their hay. The goats were kept in a large fenced enclosure divided into two sections—four or five billies on one side and twice as many nannies on the other. We loaded hay into the billies' feeding bin. Then, closing the gate and leaning over the fence, I tried to coax the billies. "Ble-e-e-e-e," I said, imitating their sounds. "Come and get it." The billies were in heat and insisted on hugging the opposite fence, close to the nannies; they were not interested in food, and some had been losing weight because of their lovesick starvation diet. To make themselves more appealing to the nannies, they would urinate on themselves and utter strange warbling sounds. I tried calling them again, but again, they ignored my entreaties. Ingwe watched, amused, until, taking pity on me, he said, "Ken, this is not how to do it. Watch." He took a little bit of hay and held it outstretched over the fence, then said softly, in Zulu, "Father, come here. Father, come here." One billy turned and walked over to the fence, until his face was only a foot from Ingwe's. Ingwe kept talking with the billy in Zulu, and the billy seemed to answer, in billy-goat language, whenever Ingwe paused. Then the billy began to eat the hay in Ingwe's hand. And when it was gone, he moved over to the hay bales, followed by the other goats. I looked on in wonder. Ingwe explained that goats, like other animals, respond only to their relatives. If I wished them to respond, I needed to let them know that I was one of their family. It was not enough to imitate the billy-goat sounds or even to address them as "Father." You had to *feel* your connection with them, to realize that animals are older relatives; they have been on earth longer than humans. Yet both are children of the same Great Creator.

During the few years of his life that remained, Ingwe never returned to South Africa. He moved to East Oakland, California, rented a small apartment, and supported himself with a variety of part-time jobs, while trying to readapt to the American lifestyle. He had expected to meet African-Americans interested in studying Zulu culture. Instead, he encountered intolerance, prejudice, and jealousy. His Christian neighbors called him "the witch doctor" and accused him of practicing "black magic." Some African-Americans interested in tribal religions were jealous of Ingwe's wisdom and power. Others were confused by him. Ingwe looked and spoke like a black American, yet he was culturally Zulu.

I believe that Ingwe might have found a very different reception had he known how to contact any of several groups sincerely studying and practicing African religion, particularly Nigerian Yoruba, in the Bay Area. Unfortunately, these groups were so carefully hidden that they were as invisible to Ingwe as they were to most white Americans. I learned about them years after Ingwe's passing.[5]

Ingwe died tragically. He was murdered, his body left on a bank of the Russian River in northern California. As far as I know, his killer was never captured. It is strange that I, a white man, should have been the only one to receive Ingwe's art. I learned his methods of healing, divination, and vision-seeking. After five years of traveling back and forth between Oakland and Colorado, staying a few weeks each time, I became a keeper of the sacred Zulu bones. I learned how to cast and interpret them or, rather, how to listen to the voices of the ancestors and spirits who guided their casting. I keep my bones with a strand of Baba Mutwa's own prayer necklace, a precious gift that I received from Ingwe.

FILIPINO SHAMANISM:
UNDOING THE SORCERER'S CURSE

"Oh, my God my God, you were hit by *barang* and *paktul* [two kinds of hexes; see page 184], but you are still alive!" These were the first words Nonoy, an extraordinary Filipino healer, spoke to me when we were introduced. It was an intuitive knowing; no one had told him of my recent psychic battle with sorcerers who wanted to kill me, my life-threatening heart infection, and subsequent recovery.

When we met, Nonoy was in his forties and living in Canada. As a younger man, he had for many years directed a psychic healing research society in Manila. It was dedicated to the study and practice of indigenous Filipino and other healing traditions, with a particular interest in looking at scientific research on healing phenomena. With humor and a bit of self-deprecation, Nonoy describes himself as a "scrounger" and "spongeologist," to distinguish his unique combination of experiential and academic learning from what a mere archivist does. When he learns of a healing or martial arts technique that is in danger of being lost, he travels any distance to "sponge" it. In the Philippines, this often means traveling to small islands by canoe, perhaps to meet a reclusive master who knows a prayer for healing cancer or a way of using *panagagaw*, "boxing techniques," to defeat a swordsman.

Nonoy is a master of the powerful Filipino martial arts *Eskrima-Kali* and *Sibat* and recounts fascinating, frightening accounts of duels with rivals jealous of his martial abilities. To him, healing and martial arts are closely related. The knowledge that kills is also the knowledge that heals. A person who knows where to strike an opponent and how to move internal energy for maximum power also knows how to use that energy to heal. The Philippine martial arts *guro*, or "teacher," must be able to heal students in case they are injured during training.

Filipino healing emphasizes prayer (*oración* in Tagalog) and psychic surgery. Specific prayers and incantations are used to treat specific conditions and must be transmitted from teacher to student ceremonially. Psychic surgery includes the transfer of life energy to a patient and the removal of intrusive, invisible pathogens or their physical "manifestations" in bones, insects, human or animal tissue, or other objects. The healer may elect to personally perform the surgery or may call on a spirit to perform it in an invisible realm.

Nonoy tells enthusiastic tales of healings he has witnessed. In one, he watched as a female healer rubbed her fingers along the arm of a child sick from an infected, almost gangrenous wound. When she lifted her hand, a red spider could be seen emerging from a small cut in the child's skin. The wound was entirely healed by the next day. A psychic surgeon healed another child's migraine by pulling a large worm from his scalp. Although the spirit of a disease may also be removed with prayer, without such displays, Nonoy and other practitioners of psychic surgery believe that intrusive objects may spontaneously manifest on the surface of the body. "The objects reflect the low and sickly vibration of the disease," Nonoy says. Many Filipino healers specialize: there are psychic dentists, cataract surgeons, brain tumor specialists, and so on. Nonoy is a general practitioner, a prayer doctor.

Like Native Americans, Filipino healers regard place as an important element of healing. Nonoy told me of one elderly healer who could often be seen acting strangely: he would bend over, touch the ground with his fingertips, roll his hands like a waterwheel up toward his body, and then drum his fingers on his abdomen. Then he would bend over and repeat these movements again and again, becoming more and more animated and joyous. The local villagers considered him "loco," though they respected his great healing power. One day, while taking a walk in the jungle, Nonoy happened upon the elder performing his mysterious ritual and decided to ask him what he was doing—something no one had bothered to do before. The old man smiled and explained, "I am gathering the *mana,* the life energy of the land, and storing it in my body. This is what I use for healing." The old man was a *baba-lan,* a Filipino shaman. *Babay-lan* enter an altered state of consciousness to retrieve power or information that can be of service to their community. Nonoy described the *babay-lan* in a letter he sent to me in 1988:

> *Babay-lan practice fire walking, distance healing, trance healing, spirit healing to neutralize attacks by malevolent nature spirits or voodoo type psychic attacks. They do psychic dances to communicate with the spirits. One of their more interesting practices is called "calling of the light" or calling of the original inborn energy. They believe that when a person is born a "string of energy" connects him to the sky, the world of the spirits. As the person matures, the "energy strings" or energy field becomes weak and scattered. The modern lifestyle uproots him from his source; he loses his primeval self, and sickness is the result. To cure sickness, babay-lan perform a ceremony where they do shamanic dances with all their power paraphernalia and together with the proper oracion or power words, call back the "scattered strings" [bands of energy]. The energy is brought back to the center of the head. The ill person is reconnected to spiritual and Divine forces and healed at least in mind and spirit, and, often, in body.*

After our first meeting, I filled in the details of my heart infection and cure. Repeating a familiar theme, Nonoy commented, "Never seek revenge. Never send negativity to anyone." He continued, "Yet you must learn how to produce these hexes yourself, so you can undo them in others. Once you understand how the psychic knot is tied, you will have no trouble unraveling it in your patients." In order to learn sorcery and healing, he said that I needed to first be initiated into his spiritual church in Manila. This would protect me from harm by formalizing my connection to God's love, wisdom, and power. The initiation could be performed whether or not I was physically present.

I wrote a formal request for initiation to Nonoy's own *guro,* the director of the church, explaining my spiritual goals and ideals and my healing philosophy. A few weeks later, he telephoned Nonoy from Manila to tell him that my request had been granted. I had been initiated, and Nonoy was given permission to give me a *libretta,* a book of *oración,* the secret power words and prayers of the psychic healers.

Not long thereafter, I met Nonoy at a friend's studio. As we sat cross-legged, across from each other on the hardwood floor, Nonoy explained the principles of *oración* training:

"The art is passed on only to the most trusted and dedicated students. It is divided into two broad categories: psychic defense and psychic healing. Psychic offense is seldom taught, although it exists. The system utilizes secret power words, like mantras; secret rituals; power-feeding [using intent and prayer to spiritually charge an object]; power objects, such as thorns of bamboo, certain seeds, rocks, leaves, ashes, animal parts such as claws, crocodile teeth, etc.; and meditations to help the student break through to another level of consciousness or reality. This generates tremendous cosmic and psychic force. The practitioner learns the secrets of developing both earth and cosmic force for psychic defense and healing.

"*Oración* is the link to the healer's power. Without it, the patient's body will not open up, and the healer is unable to see or remove the intrusion. You can use *oración* by itself as a healing method or in conjunction with laying on of hands, psychic surgery, or other methods."

Nonoy then removed from his briefcase a small, diary-sized book wrapped in white silk. Before unwrapping it, he made the sign of the cross, closed his eyes, and prayed. I also took out a small book filled with blank pages. I made the sign of the cross, as I had been instructed, and prayed in silence. Nonoy handed me his *libretta* and asked me to copy in my book the lengthy *oración* contained on the first five pages. After I finished, we practiced reciting the prayers several times so Nonoy could be sure that I had the proper pronunciation and rhythm. After each prayer, I blew a puff of air from my mouth to send the prayer out. "If the prayer is not sent with the breath, the power gets stuck in the mouth. Stagnant power causes sickness and rots the teeth." Nonoy advised me to bring my *libretta* to church, so I could dedicate my practice to God:

"Go to church every Sunday and bless your *libretta* with holy water. On all other days of the week, bless your *libretta* at home by lighting candles, putting on your

Santo Niño necklace ["the Baby Christ," a talismanic representation of Christ as a child, sometimes with an erect phallus, a symbol of his potency and power], burning frankincense and myrrh, and reciting the *oración* you have just received. Do this 'power-feeding ritual,' at church and at home, without fail for the next six months. It will empower you *and* your *libretta*. After six months, I can begin transmitting to you the specific *oración* for healing various illnesses."[6]

Filipino *oración* are incantationlike mixtures of Latin, Hebrew, and Tagalog. My power-feeding *oración* also included multiple Hail Marys and the Lord's Prayer. Healing power flows from Jesus Christ, who, for Nonoy, represents the patron and archetype of healing. Filipino healing traditions are, like Mexican *curanderismo,* a blending of Catholic and indigenous traditions. In fact, over the years since I completed my training, Mexican-Americans have been my most frequent Filipino-healing clients.

I reminded Nonoy of my Jewish ethnicity. "I am Jewish, you know, and unbaptized." I had been to church before and saw no conflict between the teachings of Christianity and Judaism. I was, however, curious about how Nonoy, a Catholic, rationalized my participation in church rituals. He said, "What does it matter? Go to church, bless yourself with holy water, pray to God. Call him Jesus if you wish, or Adonai, or Great Spirit. God doesn't care what name you use!"

BRIEF ENCOUNTERS ON THE HEALING JOURNEY

It takes time to become wise, but wisdom is not a product of time. A person who has walked the Red Road for ten years is not necessarily wiser than a person who has just set off on the journey. The former has the benefit of experience, the novice, relative freedom from preconceptions and formulas, the mental ruts that form over time. In the late 1980s, I studied at the New Seminary, an interfaith seminary that taught all of the world's religions. It's a two- to three-year program. I remember Rabbi Joseph Gelberman's response when a student asked him, "Isn't three years far too little time to understand even one of the world's religions?" The rabbi replied, "How long do *you* think it takes to understand God?" His point was clear: would a ten-year program be better? Even a lifetime is not enough. The commitment to the journey is what's important. I believe that we can never understand the Great Spirit, but we can learn, sometimes through education, sometimes through patience and silence, to trust more in the unknown.

The meetings that I describe in this section were brief encounters, from a few days to a few weeks, yet of such depth and power that they transformed my life. I continue to nurture the seeds that these elders planted in my mind.

— MOSOM —
A CREE MESSENGER FROM THE FOUR WINDS

The great Cree medicine man Paskwaw Mostos Awasis ("Buffalo Child"), more commonly known as *Mosom* ("Grandfather") Albert Lightning, was born in 1900 and lived most of his life at his ranch on the Ermineskin Reserve in Alberta, Canada. One spring day in 1985, while I was visiting my Cree brother, Joseph, in Saskatoon, he and I were suddenly inspired to pay a visit to the elder at his home in Alberta. Joseph phoned Mosom first to ask permission to visit. It was granted, so we climbed into Joseph's blue pickup truck and sang our way across the province.

Although Joseph knew Mosom quite well, this was my first visit. When we arrived at his house, I made the traditional offering of a pouch of tobacco. Then we shook hands and turned to sit down in the room's comfortable chairs. We sat in absolute silence for about twenty or thirty minutes. Mosom was perfectly still, yet I knew that he was alert and "seeing," perhaps testing my ability to be comfortable with the silence. People are born with two ears but one mouth because they are supposed to listen more than they speak. If I couldn't hear the silence, how could I hear his words?

Suddenly, something prompted me to whisper to Joseph, "Could you please ask Mosom in Cree if I may bring my drum in from the car and sing a song for him?" I knew that Mosom spoke fluent English, but asking the question in Cree seemed the proper thing to do. (I can sing in Cree but have a very limited vocabulary.) When Mosom nodded, I went outside and brought back a single-headed deerskin drum. Asking Joseph to stand with me, I announced that I wished to sing a "Chief's Honoring Song."

When the song was over, Mosom became quite animated. He took an ordinary book of matches from his pocket, handed it to Joseph, and said, "Read this." Joseph could barely make out the small print. "Two spirit people coming to visit you today. Cancel other appointments." Then Mosom glanced in my direction and explained, "As we were sitting, I thought you two were the people the spirits referred to, but I was only certain after Bear Hawk sang that song. You see, about three hours before you called, I got this message and wrote it down. I was originally supposed to speak at a powwow tonight, but I canceled it. You're the ones I'm supposed to speak with."

We listened to Mosom's wise words until the early morning hours. His voice filled the room; it seemed not to be coming from his body but to surround us from the Four Directions. He had no need to speak about unity with nature: his very being demonstrated it. His voice was a wind blowing from the mountaintop or through the trees. He talked of the Shaking Tent Ceremony, of the Sweat, of Cree prophecies, his views of death and the Afterlife. Mosom encouraged me to continue praying with the sacred pipe. He was pleased that I had performed a pipe-blessing of the Meewasin Medicine Wheel, an ancient ceremonial site in Saskatchewan, and agreed that Keewaytin, the spirit of the North Wind, dwelled there.

I saw Grandfather only one more time before his passing. Joseph and I were again driving through Alberta, this time on our way to a powwow. We stopped by Mosom's house and were directed to a nearby Sweat Lodge. The sweat had just ended when we arrived, and Mosom was relaxing on a lawn chair outside of the lodge. He was wrapped in a large towel, which was still steaming from his body heat. The three of us sat together for a while, and Joseph and I gave some gifts to Mosom before leaving him to continue on our journey. It seems a fitting last image of this great man: his mind alert, his eyes twinkling, body and spirit purified and ready to leave this world as he had entered. Mosom joined his ancestors a year later, in April of 1991.

— ELDERS AT BIG COVE —

Although I didn't know any Cherokee people before I was in my twenties, I honestly feel that they helped to raise me. Keetoowah, Rolling Thunder, and War Eagle were like parents who taught me many of the values by which I live and who encouraged me, through example and words, to walk the Red Road. I seem to meet Cherokee people wherever I travel—Keetoowah in California, Rolling Thunder in Nevada, War Eagle in Arkansas—and I have also visited with elders near Tahlequah, Oklahoma, home of the Western Cherokee (forcibly relocated from their southeastern homelands by the United States government during the Trail of Tears, 1838–1839). But until 1990, I had never been invited to old Cherokee country, to the Cherokee's beloved Smoky Mountains in North Carolina, and I do not feel it is proper to visit another person's home unless invited. Luckily, synchronicity brought such an invitation in the winter of 1990, when a Cherokee-language expert, who was lecturing in Denver, suggested that I visit a friend of his, the minister at the United Methodist Church in Cherokee, North Carolina. "He seems as much involved in Cherokee tradition as Christian," he told me.

I drove to North Carolina that spring; or rather, I drove into spring as I descended from the cold Rockies to the wildflowers on the Plains. My first stop was the Smokies, where I camped, preparing and purifying myself for the days ahead. Hiking in the woods one afternoon, I heard dull, heavy footsteps beating the ground rhythmically; it sounded like drumming. Certain it was a bear hidden in the bushes, I recalled the words of Keetoowah: "We Cherokee have a treaty with Yonah, the Bear. He is our relative, and we always show him respect." I offered some tobacco in the direction of this Grandfather.

The minister at the church was indeed knowledgeable and enthusiastic about

Cherokee tradition. But not everyone in the community was as open-minded. Both Cherokee and non-Cherokee Christians,[7] many from nearby fundamentalist churches, had complained that he shouldn't smudge the church with cedar smoke before services! Such old Indian rituals are from the Devil, they complained. The minister told me, "I have never understood why Middle Eastern frankincense, commonly burned in churches, is from God, but North American cedar is from Satan. I practice smudging because it is a beautiful purification ritual that makes people feel closer to nature, God's Creation." I knew that I had found a kindred spirit. The minister introduced me to a member of his staff, a full-blood Cherokee who offered to take me into the Big Cove community, where many of the full-bloods lived and where the Cherokee language was widely spoken.

We drove first to the home of an elderly herbalist who, it was clear after my host made the introductions, did not quite know what to make of me. Who was this white man? What did he want? Then I presented her with a gift of tobacco, cloth, and groceries and said, *Siyo Elisi, Tohiju. Aya Yonah Tawodih dagwado.* "A respectful greeting to you, Grandmother. How are you? My name is Bear Hawk." She broke into a wide smile and began speaking to me in Cherokee so fast that my translator could barely keep up with her. She led us outside to her garden, where she told me the Cherokee names of each plant, its uses, and how to prepare it. I could see that this grandmother was longing to share her encyclopedic knowledge of Cherokee herbalism. Sadly, often the younger generations of both reservation and urban Indians have relatively little interest in the old ways, though that interest is growing. I left her home sensing the contrast between her physical poverty and the great wealth of her knowledge.

Next, we visited one of the great Eastern Cherokee traditionalists, a very old and frail man who radiated great inner strength, Hayes Lossiah. Grandfather was a master craftsman who still spent his time chipping arrowheads, fletching arrows with turkey feathers, and gathering reeds to make Cherokee blowguns, a traditional Cherokee hunting weapon. We connected immediately. I had brought groceries for Grandfather, but it was respect, friendship, and frequent use of my favorite Cherokee word, *Wado,* "Thank you," that opened the door. He invited me into his home, and his family cooked a delicious meal. Before I departed, Grandfather presented me with one of his beautiful handmade arrows.

The day before I left North Carolina, I offered a "Thank-You Ceremony" in the outdoor arbor and chapel behind the Methodist church. I wanted to thank the Cherokee people and this beautiful land for their teachings. The minister, Grandfather Hayes, and about a dozen others attended. I smudged, prayed, offered a Sacred Pipe Ceremony, and shared many songs. Grandfather asked if he could use my turtle shell rattle so he could rattle along. At one point, Grandfather slapped his thigh, exclaiming, "I haven't heard this kind of singing in many, many years." He was elated. Elders like Grandfather have brought me so much joy; I was glad to see that it was possible for me to return the favor.

— HAWAI'I —
SPIRIT AND FLESH

When I give a workshop, I always try to learn something of the traditions of the place where the workshop is being held. I also ask permission of a local elder before teaching other indigenous traditions on his or her turf. Thus, when I was invited to Honolulu, Hawai'i, to teach a workshop on Taoist healing arts, I asked my Japanese host if she could arrange a meeting with a traditional Hawaiian. A week before my workshop, I arrived in Hawai'i and met with Lahe'ena'ea, a young Hawaiian-rights activist and healer-in-training, descended from the Hawaiian warrior chief Kahekili.[8] We sat on the wooden floor of Lahe'ena'ea's apartment on either side of a ritual mat that had belonged to her illustrious ancestor and discussed our lives and philosophy. My gift to her was a few pieces of rare *chen xiang* (aloeswood), a fragrant incense from Hainan Island, China, which she graciously accepted. She gave me a small piece of handmade *tapa cloth,* made from the bark of the paper mulberry tree, reminding me of the blankets that Native Americans give to honor a person. Lahe'ena'ea sensed that I had a connection with Hawaiian spirituality. When our conversation was over, she offered to speak about me to her elder, a *kahuna* ("master") healer and professor of Polynesian languages, and perhaps arrange a meeting.

She called me the next day: "The elder will meet you after you first consult with the spirit of the land at one of our sacred power spots, *heiau.* He has asked me to accompany you to a *heiau* and teach you its meaning. If the land welcomes you, he will welcome you."

A few days later, we drove to the site, a quarter mile of red earth sloping down to a cliff over the ocean, set off by a ring of lava rocks. Following Hawaiian tradition, we took off our shoes; then each of us picked up a *pohaku,* a special stone—or rather, we let a *pohaku* find us—and wrapped it in a ti leaf (*Cordyline fruticosa*), the sacred plant often found near *heiau.* Holding the stone, we asked permission to enter the site and then began walking through the *heiau* on a trail of soft, red clay. I was told the proper direction to walk and shown the section of the *heiau* that was *kapu,* "forbidden." As soon as we came to a small plateau, my guide stopped and asked me to make myself comfortable for a few minutes. I sat down as she then began a hula chant and dance. Lahe'ena'ea's voice was strong and filled with *ha,* the sacred breath. When she finished, she said, "The hula is a way of praying with the body."

At the far end of the *heiau,* Lahe'ena'ea left me alone to meditate under a tree that she called "the Tree of Life," telling me that I could remain there as long as I wished. She would wait for me by the car.

I lay down in a natural groove in the earth made by the large roots of the tree and closed my eyes. After a few minutes, I could hear sounds—a harmony of gentle ocean waves and the voices of Hawaiian men, as if singing together in a chorus. Although the words were in Hawaiian, I understood their meaning. I was told that many ancient people had meditated in this place and that their spirits were still present, ready to guide anyone who approached them with respect.

After a while, I opened my eyes, silently expressed my gratitude, and continued out of the *heiau*. I left my ti-leaf-wrapped stone as an offering by one of the guardian lava rocks. Before putting on my shoes, I wiped the thick clay off the soles of my feet, wondering if it might be permissible for me to take some of this sacred earth back with me in my medicine pouch. I rolled the clay into a ball, held it under my navel, and asked permission. I heard a voice in my mind: "There is no need to take. We will always be here for you. But as a sign of our friendship, open this sphere and you will find a small gift. You may keep the gift and carry it in your medicine pouch." I opened my eyes and pressed the edges of the ball; it crumbled, revealing a small, pyramid-shaped stone. I carry this stone with me to this day.

The next day, I met with the Hawaiian elder. After presenting some gifts, I explained that I wished to build a bridge of friendship between the medicine of my home and that of Hawai'i. I then recounted my experience at the *heiau*. When I finished, the elder exclaimed, "Aloha, Brother!" He embraced me. From that point, we spoke as friends and relatives. This was also the beginning of my trail of initiation into the sacred teachings of Hawai'i. The people and the spirits opened to me and were extremely generous.

I was invited several times to the islands. On the Big Island, I was fortunate to meet Pua, a spiritual healer and adopted daughter of one of the great Hawaiian kahunas, Emma DeFries, in the lineage of Queen Emma.[9] Pua and her husband, Herb, are individuals of great love, wisdom, and hospitality. For many years, they directed a healing center on the Big Island and graciously offered to sponsor my seminars. During one of my visits, I received a beautiful initiation-transmission. Pua prayed over me and breathed the sacred breath, the *ha,* into my crown. We were, as Native North Americans would say, "made relatives." The Hawaiian spirit was now actually inside me. I felt that Auntie Emma was now a member of my family, not by blood but by something even deeper, by breath. This connection was soon to be confirmed in a mysterious way.

I returned to Colorado. About a month before my next visit to Hawai'i, I began to have a frequent waking vision. Every day at sunset, I would see a beautiful Hawaiian woman standing in the small kitchen of my log cabin. She had long brown hair, a red cloth dress that reached to her ankles, and Hawaiian or Eurasian features. She seemed to be about thirty years old, a few years younger than I was at the time. I had a sense that we were related. I was single at the time and was hoping that this vision was a premonition of my wife-to-be, of a woman I would meet when I returned to the islands.

Unfortunately, my upcoming seminar had such low registration that I would probably not even recover my travel expenses. I decided to return to Hawai'i nevertheless. Teaching was, frankly, not very important at that stage in my life. I was traveling to learn. Of course, now I had an additional motivation. I hoped to meet the Hawaiian spirit woman and melt in her eyes.

I spent four weeks on the Big Island. During the early part of my stay, I combed the island for traces of the mysterious woman, describing her to nearly every friend and colleague, hoping for some lead. I should have remembered that dreams fade when they are pursued with too much vigor; dream spirits reward those who are patient. I soon realized the futility of my search and shifted my priorities to the present.

Wonderful things happened during that visit. My Hawaiian hosts led me on a pilgrimage to an active volcano that is home to the fiery and temperamental goddess Pele. In the lava fields, I ate the sacred berries that grow there to protect Pele's domain. If I had not been meant to visit, I would have been sick to my stomach and forced to turn back. Later that day, I entered the holy of holies: a giant lava cave that forms Pele's womb. Over the next few weeks, I visited many such sacred sites and *heiau*. But the highlight was my visit with the Hawaiian kahuna David "Papa" Bray.

Papa Bray was the son of the famed healer and spiritual teacher David Kaonohiokala Bray, known as "Daddy Bray." When Daddy Bray was dying, he called each of his sons to his bedside. The children knew who was going to inhale their father's last breath and receive his *ha*. It would be the son who had followed and learned from father, the one who was most knowledgeable in Hawaiian language and spirituality. It certainly would *not* be the alcoholic younger son, David.

The children visited Daddy Bray's bedside one at a time. David was the last to enter. As David stood by his father, Daddy Bray took off his amulet necklace and breathed onto it, placing it around David's neck. Papa Bray told me that from that point on, he never touched alcohol again. He learned his father's ways through the transmission of *ha,* through his father's spirit, and later, by studying the notes his father had left behind.

As Papa explained this story, I understood the source of his great humility. He was more than a prodigal son. Papa had been the lowest of the low. He had died and been reborn in the same lifetime. I sat on his couch with a group of Native North American and Hawaiian guests and listened to his beautiful stories and teachings, remaining silent to show respect. I spoke only when spoken to. The conversation was quite animated at times, and I hoped that my silence would not be misconstrued as a lack of interest. When it came time to leave, I was the last guest to put my shoes on and step out the door. Papa Bray gently touched my arm and motioned me back into the house. He whispered, "By the way, we've been having a drought here for weeks. I'd appreciate it if you could help us out." I told Papa that I would try my best. He gave me a hug and a slip of paper before I left: "Share this teaching from my father." The paper contained this message:

— THE SECRET MEANING OF *ALOHA* —

A	*ala,* watchful alertness
L	*lokahi,* working with unity
O	*oiaio,* truthful honesty
H	*haahaa,* humility
A	*ahonui,* patient perseverance

Aloha to the Hawaiian of old is God in us. It means, "Come forward, be in unity and harmony with your real self, God, and mankind. Be honest, truthful, patient, kind to all forms of life, and humble."

I was deeply honored that Papa Bray had asked a "youngster" for help. The next evening, I was at a friend's house, leading a prayer ceremony for a group of about twenty people who were interested in learning about Native American culture. We sat in a circle, cross-legged on the floor, as I passed a shell filled with burning sage and cedar and asked each person to send a prayer of gratitude with the smoke. When, at last, the shell returned to my hands, I held it overhead and said, "*Mahalo,* 'Thank you,' for this beautiful land and water. I pray that the nourishing rains fall soon." At that moment, it began to rain. We could hear it pounding on the roof. But this was no ordinary rain. It was a spirit rain. We could hear and feel it falling around us, although we were sitting comfortably indoors, quite dry. I knew that *I* had not brought the rain, but rather the community of prayers and good minds had sent a successful petition to the Creator, perhaps through his helpers: Ku, the guardian of the nation's welfare; Kane, the spirit of freshwater; Kanaloa, god of the deep ocean; and Lono, patron of agriculture and the fertility of the land.

I never did meet the mysterious Hawaiian woman. On the last day before my return flight, while Pua and I were sitting at her kitchen table, she asked, rather nonchalantly, "Ken, have I ever shown you a picture of Auntie Emma?" When I shook my head, she continued, "I have an old photograph that I'd like you to see. It was taken when Mother was about thirty." Pua disappeared into another room and soon came back and sat next to me. There was no mistaking it! This was the beautiful Hawaiian woman who had appeared in my home! Auntie Emma had enticed me to Hawai'i to lead me through many of the same initiations and sacred places where she had once taken her own daughter. Pua smiled mischievously at me. She said that she had known the identity of the spirit woman all along.

— DR. UMUNAKWE: —
AN IGBO INITIATION

In the summer of 1990, I was teaching a workshop on the Chinese healing art, T'ai Chi (also spelled "Taiji Quan") in Atlanta, Georgia, and staying at the home of a local T'ai Chi teacher. On the morning of my last day in Atlanta, Shabari, a Native American friend who lived nearby, called me with an urgent message: "There is a Nigerian Igbo tribe master shaman staying in my home who says he knows you and wishes to see you before you leave," Shabari explained. The shaman, Dr. Umunakwe, had been touring the United States. As part of his spiritual practice, each morning he would consult the *agbara*, the "spirits," to learn what to do or avoid that day. In New Orleans, his most recent stop, he was told, "Go to Atlanta. There, you will meet a spiritual woman and three others whom you must teach." He was also given the name of an institute that Shabari directs out of her home, which sponsors ecological and spiritual workshops. It took only a phone call for Dr. Umunakwe to find out that the institute existed and another to get directions to it, about an hour outside of the city. A few days later, Dr. Umunakwe arrived in his rental car and knocked at the door. When Shabari answered, she was greeted by a very dark-skinned man dressed in casual Western attire who announced, with only a trace of an accent, that he had come to teach her. Shabari was used to the unpredictable ways of Spirit. She took him in.

About a month later, Shabari happened to mention to Dr. Umunakwe that I was in town. He immediately responded, "I have dreamed of him. I know him," and insisted that I was one of his destined students.

Shabari arranged a dinner and meeting at her home on Sunday evening, after my workshop ended. One of the students in the workshop drove me to the forested estate. Shabari introduced me to Dr. Umunakwe before dinner, and we sat on rocking chairs on the white, unscreened veranda, looking out over a green meadow edged by the lush Georgia forest. Dr. Umunakwe was drinking beer, a custom among his people, and I was smoking my corncob pipe. He was the first to break the silence.

"I will teach you the herbs, remedies, and diagnostic and treatment methods of the Igbo people. This is the last initiation you will need in your lifetime. I *know* about your previous training and experience. The spirits have shown me how deeply you have studied Native American healing. Igbo tradition will complete your education and answer many remaining questions." His words left me somewhat confused for two reasons. On the practical side, I was supposed to fly home the next day, and my ticket was nonchangeable and nonrefundable. Because I was living on below-poverty income, I simply did not have the money to purchase a new ticket. When I told Dr. Umunakwe my concern, he said with a distant look but in a matter-of-fact tone, "The spirits say to call the airline right now. They will change the rules." I called and asked the agent to look at my reservation. Could I take a different flight on another day? "No problem." "And what will the penalty be?" "No penalty, Mr. Cohen, you can fly back whenever you wish." I call this kind of experience "the twi-light zone."

But there was also a spiritual question gnawing at me. I asked Dr. Umunakwe, "I mean no disrespect, but I need to know *why* you are offering me so much power and knowledge. I have always believed that power can be very dangerous. What is your motivation, your purpose in wishing to teach me Igbo tradition?" Dr. Umunakwe offered the only reply that I would have accepted: "I know that you will use spiritual power to serve God and God's Creation."

We went to a stream in the forest that bordered Shabari's land. Dr. Umunakwe asked me to kneel in it and ask the water for guidance and healing. He then placed water on my feet, chest, hands, and head, while praying in his language. He said, "You are a priest of Agbara Miri, the Water Spirit." After this baptism and trans-mission of power, he began to teach me his ways. Unlike Native American elders, Dr. Umunakwe not only permitted but required that I take notes on every tech-nique, every bit of information, so I could refer back to them when needed. We spent a week, seven or eight hours a day, discussing, practicing, sharing, and heal-ing. I learned the use of everyday plants, foods, and animal parts to treat disease, in-cluding cucumber, banana, corn, and turtle shell. I learned how to massage away pain using a sacred stone from Igbo land. Most important, I learned how to com-mune with the *Ndichie,* or ancestors—both my own and those of my clients—and with the major Gods of the Igbo to find the source and cure of an illness and to bless and empower a medicinal food or tea. "You will see that these Gods are not un-known to you. Thunder, Mountain, Water, Earth, Peace . . . These spirits belong as much to America as to Africa, yes? You can use Igbo rituals to call on the spirits of *this* land." I discovered that his rituals were similar to Native American practices with which I was already familiar and based on the same fundamental values and philosophy of life. Dr. Umunakwe also taught me how to identify whether a spirit or spiritual practice conflicts with my medicine and so must be avoided. (For example, a person with a mouse spirit helper should avoid rituals that invoke cats!) I continue to use Dr. Umunakwe's teachings to evaluate the compatibility of other indigenous spiritual practices with my own.

At the end of each day, Dr. Umunakwe would invite me to ask questions, answering each one thoughtfully and precisely. Then he would look at my notes and ask me to explain what I had learned. After just three days of training, I felt that I had absorbed as much as I had in three years with other teachers. In the final stage of the training, I worked as a healer in the clinic Dr. Umunakwe had set up in Shabari's institute. I offered consultations to many people, the majority African-Americans, about their health problems. As I communed with the ancestors and the *agbara,* Dr. Umunakwe entered a trance state to assess if I was receiving information accurately and treating correctly.

The "graduation ceremony," as Dr. Umunakwe called it, followed the clinical "test." Returning to the stream where my initiation took place, I prayed and was prayed over, first in the stream, then in a nearby field, under the midday sun. Using his palms, Dr. Umunakwe placed the power of water and fire in my body and then blew spirit into the crown of my head. "You are now an *ayonohawmo,*" he said, "one whose eyes see the spirit, a master shaman.[10] My people will treat you with respect. You have been initiated at the same level of power and training as myself."

Before I left Dr. Umunakwe, he gave me his address in Imo State, Nigeria, adding an odd caveat. "But do not send anything to me," he told me. "Instead, write your letter, address the envelope, and burn it. I will read it and respond." A few months after I returned home, I learned that Dr. Umunakwe had died of complications from diabetes. Suddenly, I understood his urgency to teach. I believe that he knew his time was coming and that the only way I would be able to contact him again would be through the Spirit World.

Dr. Umunakwe was an unusual man. He lived in what author Carlos Castenada called "the crack between the worlds," simultaneously aware of the ordinary sensual reality and the world of spirit. His personal history seemed of little importance to him; thus, I never knew anything about his childhood, his family, his education—information that normally we would have shared with each other in the course of working together. Or perhaps these facts were just irrelevant, considering the short time we would have together. Dr. Umunakwe was a blend of ancient and modern; he spoke the ancient language of his people and also an elegant and educated English. As I look back to our time together, I realize perhaps the most extraordinary thing of all: I do not believe that he ever noticed the color of my skin. I cannot claim to have the same understanding of Igbo culture as one who grows up Igbo or who drinks from the wells of Nigerian soil. I have not lived in Africa. But I am forever grateful for those brief, magical days when Africa lived in me.

THEY JUST WON'T LET ME BE JEWISH!

I suppose I could have titled this section "Is the author a Shmohawk?" I have a great love for Judaism, the tradition of my ancestors. Although I have never tried to deny my background, I have had some very funny experiences when various associates, Native and non-Native, have pegged me as a born-again Indian and when *they* had a hard time accepting my ancestry. The following stories may suggest that I have a sense of humor. I believe, however, it is more accurate to say that the Creator has a sense of humor. Just look at my Jewish nose and Indian heart! At least I do not have to contend with problems of transference: a patient's assumption that the healer is an exotic and all-powerful guru. I am grateful that in a culture that judges a book by its cover, I don't look the part.

— FIRED AT LAST! —

I may be the only non-Indian teacher of Native American studies who was ever fired from an academic position because he was considered "prejudiced against whites." I cofounded a Native American studies program at an accredited university, which shall remain nameless, during the early 1990s. During her review of new faculty, the academic dean decided to drop in on Bear Hawk's popular class. The subject of the lecture that day was the appropriation and misrepresentation of Native American spirituality by anthropology and the New Age movement. Although students participated enthusiastically in the discussion, the dean's opinion was that I was prejudiced. At the next faculty meeting—one that I was unable to attend—she voiced her opinion, overruled the objections of colleagues in my department, and concluded that I was inappropriate for their institution. Good riddance. I quit.

— ONE OF THE PEOPLE —

In the late 1980s, my Cree brother, Joseph, and I were invited to drum and sing at a powwow on a reservation in Montana. After one of the evening dances, we took a walk outside, followed by a group of Indian children, ranging in age from about eight to thirteen years old. The kids were discussing something among themselves, when one of them remarked, "We know that Joseph is Cree, but we can't figure out what tribe you're from." I asked them, "What's your best guess?" They named several northern Plains tribes with which they were familiar. I said, "All wrong. I'm a full-blood." "Yes, we know that, but full-blood what?" I declared, "Full-blood Russian Jew." At first, they thought I was joking, until Joseph told them it was true. My honesty did not alleviate their confusion. To these children, no matter what I said, I was one of "the People."

— A JEWISH INDIAN —

I had just spent a delightful hour sharing stories and songs with my brother and an elder Cree medicine man. They were fascinated by the melodies, rhythms, and words of my various Salish songs—you know, the "ish" tribes: Swinomish, Snohomish, Suquamish, Skokomish. At one point, Grandfather smiled contentedly and said, "Isn't it wonderful how varied our Indian people are. I am Nakota, Assiniboine, and Cree. Your brother is full-blood Cree. And you are . . . ?" I said, matter-of-factly, "Jewish." "Yes, Jewish," he replied. "Our traditions are so rich." It was not the appropriate time to contradict or possibly disappoint the elder. But Joseph realized what had happened. Later that day, he remarked, "I guess Grandfather thought that Jewish was another 'ish.' " "And I'm now a real Jewish Indian," I chuckled.

~ NOTES ~

INTRODUCTION

1. Christopher Ronwanièn:te Jocks, "Spirituality for Sale: Sacred Knowledge in the Consumer Age," *American Indian Quarterly 20*, nos. 3 and 4 (1996): 418. The reader is referred to all of the essays in this superb volume for a thorough discussion of various contemporary themes in Native American spirituality.

2. Progress in repatriation has been commendable but slow. At the end of the twentieth century, the Smithsonian Institution still had approximately nineteen thousand Native American skeletons.

3. I especially admire the works of Joseph Medicine Crow (Crow), Gregory Cajete (Tewa), Alfonso Ortiz (Tewa), Edward Benton-Benai (Ojibwa), Basil Johnston (Ojibwa), and such collaborative projects as *The Sacred Tree* and *The Sacred: Ways of Knowledge, Sources of Life*.

4. Exceptional examples of such enlightened ethnography can be found in the works of Karl Schlesier, Keith H. Basso, Richard K. Nelson, Frank Waters, Joseph Epes Brown, and Rodney Frey.

5. Bert Kaplan and Dale Johnson, "Navaho Psychopathology," in *Magic, Faith, and Healing: Studies in Primitive Psychiatry Today*, ed. Ari Kiev, M.D. (New York: Macmillan, 1964), 203–29.

6. Daniel C. Noel, *The Soul of Shamanism: Western Fantasies, Imaginal Realities* (New York: Continuum, 1997), 60.

7. From the viewpoint of Jungian psychology, the imagination and the practice of visualization are neither more nor less real than any other dimension of experience. Nevertheless, the terminology and tone of Noel's work clearly imply that to consider visions and images as part of a reality deeper than the imagination is a politically and cognitively incorrect stance for a Westerner—equivalent to "playing Indian." Thus, the Native American disease category of "soul loss" is described as "a loss of imagination . . . and only a psychology of imagining—better still, an imaginal psychology—can offer the necessary shamanic healing" (Noel, *Soul of Shamanism*, 73).

8. Another kind of reductionism occurs when some Native American authors elevate their healing traditions beyond the reach of mere non-Indian mortals. They imply that white people do not have the *ability* or the *right* to be involved in Indian spirituality. The curious thing about these polemics is that by making such an incredibly big deal about "secrets," they attract more attention to them. Don't think of a pink elephant for the next three seconds! Talking excessively about secrets reinforces stereotypes of the mystical and stoic Indian. I acknowledge the dangers of appropriation. I do wonder, however, about which strategy is more effective in guarding cultural treasures: warning people again and again of the dangers of trespassing or just being private and discreet. There is a biblical precedent that makes Euro-Americans fascinated by forbidden fruit.

   Some Native authors recommend that non-Indian scholars be contented with writing descriptions of Native American spirituality but should not attempt interpretation. (See Ronald L. Grimes's "This May Be a Feud, but It Is Not a War: An Electronic, Interdisciplinary Dialogue on Teaching Native Religions," *American Indian Quarterly 20*, nos. 3 and 4 [1996]: 437.) I am fascinated that a prominent Native American lawyer supports this separation of data from interpretation. I had always thought that a lawyer's competence was measured by his ability to select facts that can be woven into impressive and convincing fantasies! Is it really preferable to leave interpretation entirely to the readers? In any case, doesn't description always involve translation and interpretation?

   Native American healing is also put out of reach by authors who demean or romanticize indigenous people with stereotypes of the "primitive brute" or "noble savage." Psychohistorians portray ancient healing systems as part of humanity's infancy, a time before the development of a separate ego. Their myth runs something like this: Thirty or forty thousand years ago, people believed that they were one with nature. They lived by instinct, without discrimination, ethics, or consciousness of a separate self. With the advent of agriculture, approximately ten to fifteen thousand years ago, *Homo sapiens* had matured to a level of neurological complexity that allowed them to understand that they were separate from the trees and mountains. They could now lay claim to, own, and defend property, which included serfs, slaves, and women. The unfortunate result of such an "advanced" belief system was war and environmental destruction. Now, after further evolution, we realize again that man and nature are interdependent. We can reclaim the wisdom of humanity's childhood. Native Americans will lead the way. They will show us how to "walk in balance."

There are several things wrong with this philosophy. Primitive people were more thoroughly individuated than modern people. Survival in nature forced them to rely on their own creativity and resources. Anthropologists have shown that the cranial capacity of primitive humans was larger than that of modern people, and their decision-making processes may have been more complex than our own. Primitive humans considered the effects of their actions on the entire ecosystem on which they depended. The record of postagricultural civilization clearly demonstrates that modern people have generally only paid attention to the effect of their actions on other people. The ecosystem is only given a clear priority when it is damaged to such a degree that it causes famine, illness, or economic hardship.

Modern people are expert at using the rational parts of the brain to manipulate and interpret facts and figures. Original peoples developed the whole brain as they learned the lessons of wind, water, sun, and earth. If you wish to see an example of complex deductive reasoning combined with equally astute sensitivity and intuition, ask a modern Cree hunter how he locates his prey. It seems to me that the "primitive world" was one of greater complexity, a complexity that modern people fear.

Many books that mention or discuss Native American healing make a tacit assumption that healing knowledge and techniques have progressed from infancy to adulthood. There is no logical reason to make such an assumption. Yet it is important to understand that Native Americans realize that we cannot turn back the clock; as much as some may wish to go back to the Old Ways, they also accept the reality of the modern world. Education and mastery of technology are as important to today's Native Americans as they are to any other race.

9. Ken Wilber, *Sex, Ecology, Spirituality: The Spirit of Evolution* (Boston: Shambhala Publications, 1995), 581.

10. One of the most interesting examples of this phenomenon concerns a "Choctaw medicine man" I met about twenty years ago. He gave me a self-published recording of "traditional medicine songs." I was confused by the style of the music: vocables set to melodies that seemed to bear an uncanny resemblance to the songs of my own European Jewish ancestors. I brought the tape to an ethnomusicologist at a Canadian university who confirmed that the music was "definitely Middle Eastern, perhaps Sephardic [Spanish Jewish]." These were indeed "traditional" songs; they were *nigunim*, Jewish songs without words. The next time I saw the medicine man, I confronted him with my discovery. After a moment of hesitation, he asserted with as much confidence as he could muster, "My family escaped forced relocation from our Southeast homelands by hiding with a Jewish family. Their music must have influenced my ancestors." Not long after this conversation, the medicine man corrected another loophole in his story. He realized that his clan belonged to another tribe. He reprinted his promotional literature with a new clan affiliation. (No, it wasn't Levite.)

11. After writing this introduction, I discovered a prior use of the term *integral* as a research methodology in William Braud's excellent essay "Integral Inquiry: Complementary Ways of Knowing, Being, and Expression," in *Transpersonal Research Methods for the Social Sciences: Honoring Human Experience*, ed. William Braud and Rosemarie Anderson (Thousand Oaks, Calif.: Sage Publications, 1998), 35–68.

12. Greg Sarris, *Keeping Slug Woman Alive: A Holistic Approach to American Indian Texts* (Los Angeles: University of California Press, 1993), 45–46.

13. Gregory Cajete, Ph.D., *Look to the Mountain: An Ecology of Indigenous Education* (Durango, Colo.: Kivaki Press, 1994), 195.

14. Everett R. Rhoades, M.D., "Two Paths to Healing: Can Traditional and Western Scientific Medicine Work Together?" *Winds of Change* 11, no. 3 (1996): 51.

15. *Alternative Medicine: Expanding Medical Horizons. A Report to the National Institutes of Health on Alternative Medical Systems and Practices in the United States*, NIH publication 94–066 (Washington, D.C.: U.S. Government Printing Office, 1994), 99.

16. For example, Native American therapies are offered at the Indian Health Service hospital at Chinle, Arizona; the Lander (Wyoming) Valley Medical Center; and the Riverton (Wyoming)

Memorial Hospital. There exists no networking organization or comprehensive listing of these various collaborations. For an excellent summary of developments in cross-cultural health education and healing, see *Tribal College Journal* 5, no. 3 (winter 1994).

17. One of the finest of these cooperative ventures, combining high-quality allopathic medicine with Native American cultural values, is located near Tacoma, Washington: the Puyallup Tribal Health Authority's $8 million Takopid Health Center, which opened in 1993.

18. The most famous community-based health education programs in Indian Country are probably the Zuni Wellness Center in Zuni, New Mexico, and the Four Worlds Development Project, coordinated from the University of Lethbridge, Alberta. For a summary of Native American community-based programs and resources for treating diabetes, see Mary Anne Hill, "The Curse of Frybread—The Diabetes Epidemic in Indian Country," *Winds of Change* 12, no. 3 (summer 1997): 26–31.

19. According to anthropologist James Herrick, indiscriminate sharing of sacred information "constitutes a breach of the established ways and may result in the destruction of the power of the medicine and the administrators of it" (James W. Herrick and Dean R. Snow, eds., *Iroquois Medical Botany* [Syracuse, N.Y.: Syracuse University Press, 1995], 35).

20. There are 554 federally recognized tribes in the United States, with an additional 221 tribes in various stages of the recognition process. See the books and maps of George Russell (Saginaw Chippewa) for excellent and regularly updated information about Native American populations and reservations. Russell Publications, 9027 N. Cobre Drive, Phoenix, AZ 85028. E-mail: russell@nativeamericanonline.com.

21. Russell H. Bernard, "Preserving Language Diversity," *Cultural Survival Quarterly* (fall 1992): 15. Loss of language can also have serious political consequences. As languages are lost, the courts may be less likely to recognize or respect the rights of unique ethnic groups. It is easier to claim someone as a citizen of the dominant nation if he or she speaks only the colonial language.

22. These terms and translations are from an excellent Canadian First Nations' newspaper, *Alberta Native News* 16, no. 4 (April 1999), 8.

23. These examples are from William Bright, *The Karok Language*, University of California Publications in Linguistics, vol. 13 (Berkeley: University of California, 1957), 95.

24. Robert Leavitt, "Language and Cultural Content in Native Education," in *First Nations Education in Canada: The Circle Unfolds*, ed. Marie Battiste and Jean Barman (Vancouver: UBC Press, 1995), 131.

25. I am not the first to note a relationship between Zen Buddhism and Native American spirituality. Zen philosophy has influenced several noted Native American authors, including Frank Waters and Gerald Vizenor.

NATIVE AMERICAN OR AMERICAN INDIAN: CAN YOU BE POLITICALLY CORRECT?

1. Clans are a common and major facet of Native American identity. Clan affiliation may determine suitable marriage partners (one does not marry a person of the same clan), ceremonial responsibilities, hospitality obligations (providing lodging and other hospitality to members of one's own clan), personality traits, and even career. For example, some tribes believe that Bear Clan people are quiet, sensitive, and powerful—traits that make them excellent healers. Tribes may have as few as three clans (for example, the Kanien'kehaka, Mohawk) or as many as sixty (for example, the Diné, Navajo). Some tribes, such as the Nuu'chah'nulth (Nootka) and Kwagiulth (Kawakiutl) of the Pacific Northwest, do not have a clan system.

2. To a psychologist, the various early terms for Native Americans—even those that were derogatory—might symbolize a repressed longing for a life unbound by feudalism, Puritanism, and perhaps civilization in general. It is ironic that Europeans, who learned the custom of daily bathing from the Native Americans, commonly described the indigenous Americans as "filthy, dirty, and degraded."

3. James J. Rawls, *Indians of California: The Changing Image* (Norman: University of Oklahoma Press, 1984), 198.

4. I cannot help wondering about the original connotation of "the chosen people." Might not the

Jewish tribe also have considered themselves "the People"? In any case, "chosen people" need not connote superiority or elite status. As a Jewish friend commented, "Yes, we are chosen. But chosen for what? Perhaps chosen to be a historical example of tenaciously clinging to culture and values in the face of oppression."

5. The concept of blood quantum has racist origins. In 1705, Virginia passed laws that defined Native Americans or people who were half Native American ("half bloods, half breeds, mixed bloods") as legally inferior.

6. Taiaiake Alfred, *Peace, Power, Righteousness: An Indigenous Manifesto* (Don Mills, Ontario: Oxford University Press, 1999), 86.

7. This is seen most clearly in the commonly used Hawaiian word for white person: *haole*. Although many Hawaiians believe that *haole* simply means "pale or colorless," the term originally referred to the missionaries who accompanied Captain Cook to the islands. They were described as without (*ole*) breath or power (*ha*). They did not sing their prayers out loud, as the Hawaiians did, but rather muttered them under their breath, as though weak and ashamed.

8. See Thomas Buckley's "Yurok Doctors and the Concept of Shamanism," in *California Indian Shamanism*, ed. Lowell John Bean (Menlo Park, Calif.: Ballena Press, 1992), 117–55.

9. John (Fire) Lame Deer and Richard Erdoes, *Lame Deer: Seeker of Visions* (New York: Washington Square Press, 1972), 144–45. Interesting definitions can also be found in William S. Lyon's *Encyclopedia of Native American Healing* (New York: Norton, 1996).

10. This connotation is made very clear in the Cheyenne word for holy person, *maheonhetan*, "someone who serves the sacred," contrasted with an ordinary healer, *náetan*, who may not emphasize the use of spiritual powers or helping spirits in his practice. (Karl H. Schleiser, *The Wolves of Heaven: Cheyenne Shamanism, Ceremonies, and Prehistoric Origins* [Norman: University of Oklahoma Press, 1987], 14.)

11. From Lyon, *Encyclopedia of Native American Healing*.

12. Kinship terms are common in traditional Indian communities. Everyone is an aunt, an uncle, a cousin, a brother, a sister, a grandfather, or a grandmother.

13. Floyd Looks for Buffalo Hand, *Learning Journey on the Red Road* (Toronto, Ontario: Learning Journey Communications, 1998), 58.

14. The term *allopathic* was coined by the German physician Samuel Hahnemann (1755–1843) to distinguish it from the medical system he founded: homeopathy, "like disease." Homeopathy is based on the law of similars, or "like cures like." As Dr. Andrew Weil explains, "A substance that produces a certain set of symptoms in a healthy person has the power to cure a sick person manifesting those same symptoms" (Andrew Weil, M.D., *Health and Healing: Understanding Conventional and Alternative Medicine* [Boston: Houghton Mifflin, 1983], 17).

15. World Health Organization, *Research Guidelines for Evaluating the Safety and Efficacy of Herbal Medicines* (Manila: WHO Regional Office for the Western Pacific, 1993).

16. *Declaration on Traditional, Alternative and Complementary Medicine*, 1998 World AIDS Conference, Republic of Geneva.

17. I would love to see statistics comparing suicide rates among conventional physicians with suicide rates among practitioners of various CAM modalities. I believe that the results would be too embarrassing for most Western medical journals to print!

18. Francis La Flesche, *A Dictionary of the Osage Language*, bulletin 59 (Washington, D.C.: Bureau of American Ethnology, 1932), 193.

1: THE POWER OF SILENCE

1. Carl G. Jung, *Symbols of Transformation* (Princeton, N.J.: Bollingen, 1956), 325.

2. John (Fire) Lame Deer and Richard Erdoes, *Lame Deer: Seeker of Visions* (New York: Simon & Schuster, 1972), 145.

3. Knud Rasmussen, *Across Arctic America: Narrative of the Fifth Thule Expedition*, trans. W. E. Calvert (Copenhagen, 1925; New York: Putnam, 1927), 385.

4. Maureen Trudelle Schwarz, *Molded in the Image of Changing Woman: Navajo Views on the Human Body and Personhood* (Tucson: University of Arizona Press, 1997), 9.

5. Basil Johnston, *Ojibway Ceremonies* (Lincoln: University of Nebraska Press, 1990), 162.

6. Keith H. Basso, *Wisdom Sits in Places: Landscape and Language among the Western Apache* (Albuquerque: University of New Mexico Press, 1996), 85.

7. Bernard Lown, M.D., *The Lost Art of Healing* (New York: Houghton Mifflin, 1996), 10. Dr. Lown was cofounder of the International Physicians for the Prevention of Nuclear War. His book is an example of humane, humble, and wise medicine.

8. Rodney Frey, *The World of the Crow Indians: As Driftwood Lodges* (Norman: University of Oklahoma Press, 1987), 164.

9. The link between shamanism (the religion of hunter-gatherers) and the meditative practices of Yoga, Buddhism, and Taoism is well documented in scholarly literature. For example, mythologist Joseph Campbell explains that a number of the disciplines of Yoga "appear to have been derived from shamanism; as, for example, the regulation of the breath and use of dance, rhythmic sounds, drugs, controlled meditations, etc. . . ." (*The Masks of God: Oriental Mythology* [New York: Viking, 1962], 283). Mircea Eliade, in his classic *Yoga: Immortality and Freedom*, also notes that elements of the aboriginal shamanism of India were incorporated into Yoga as well as into the Buddhist Tantras of India, Mongolia, and Tibet ("Yoga and Aboriginal India," in *Yoga: Immortality and Freedom* [Princeton, N.J.: Princeton University Press, 1969], 293–358). Indeed, the Siberian word *shaman* may be derived from *sramana*, the Sanskirt word for a wandering ascetic.

    Cambridge University professor Joseph Needham outlines the two roots of Chinese Taoism: philosophers who meditated upon the Order of Nature (Tao) and "the body of ancient shamans and magicians which had entered Chinese culture at a very early stage . . ." (*Science and Civilisation in China*, vol. 2 [Cambridge, U.K.: Cambridge University Press, 1956], 3). The earliest Taoist monasteries were called *Guan*, which may be translated "a place to observe nature." For the link between shamanism and Taoist healing exercises and meditations, see my book *The Way of Qigong: The Art and Science of Chinese Energy Healing* (New York: Ballantine Books, 1999) and my audio course *Taoism: Essential Teachings of the Way and Its Power* (Boulder, Colo.: Sounds True, 1998).

10. Gary Snyder, *A Place in Space: Ethics, Aesthetics, and Watersheds* (Washington, D.C.: Counterpoint, 1995), 128. Paul Shepard, the visionary elder of the American environmental movement, and Spanish philosopher José Ortega y Gasset both describe the hunter's mystical and meditative union with the animal. "The hunter is the alert man . . . ," writes Shepard (*The Tender Carnivore & the Sacred Game* [Athens, Ga.: University of Georgia Press, 1973], 147). See also José Ortega y Gasset, *Meditations on Hunting*, trans. Howard Wescott (New York: Charles Scribner's Sons, 1972).

11. Tom Brown Jr., *The Tracker: The Story of Tom Brown, Jr., as Told to William Jon Watkins* (New York: Berkley Books, 1978), 114.

12. Gerald Vizenor, *Summer in Spring: Anishinaabe Lyric Poems and Stories*, new ed. (Norman: University of Oklahoma Press, 1993), 12.

13. Bear Heart with Molly Larkin, *The Wind Is My Mother: The Life and Teachings of a Native American Shaman* (New York: Crown, 1996), 243.

14. Twylah Nitsch, *Entering into the Silence: The Seneca Way* (Irving, N.Y.: Seneca Indian Historical Society, 1984), 5.

15. The practice of silence described above is an original synthesis derived from several sources, including instructions from Native American and Chinese Taoist elders, seven-deep-breaths meditation from indigenous Hawaiian teachers, and Native American healing chants that incorporate specific breathing techniques.

16. Norman Hallendy, *Inuksuit: Silent Messengers of the Arctic* (Toronto, Ontario: Douglas & McIntyre, 2000), 84–85.

2: THE FOUR WINDS: GETTING ORIENTED IN THE REALM OF THE SACRED

1. The *cangleska wakan*, "sacred hoop," is sometimes represented in Native American paintings, quillwork, and beadwork and may be worn as a hair or dance ornament.

2. In the Maliseet language, spoken in Maine and New Brunswick, words for shapes do not exist as independent terms. Shape is considered an attribute of concrete objects and is integrated into

nouns or verbs. Thus, a discussion of the abstract notion of "circles" would not be possible in some Native languages. Interestingly, the ancient Chinese considered the circle to be the shape of heaven, the spiritual shape. The square was the shape of the earth and mundane existence, perhaps because it is associated with linearity and the logical structures of human language. In the colloquial English of the 1960s, people who were stuck in rigid modes of thought and behavior were called "squares." I wonder why members of the hippie generation never labeled themselves "rounds"?

3. John G. Neihardt, *Black Elk Speaks: Being the Life Story of a Holy Man of the Oglala Sioux* (1932; reprint, Lincoln: University of Nebraska Press, 1961), 164–65.

4. Theodor Schwenk, *Sensitive Chaos: The Creation of Flowing Forms in Water and Air*, trans. Olive Whicher and Johanna Wrigley (London: Rudolf Steiner Press, 1965), 13.

5. See "Traditions and Culture: The Significance of the Tipi," *Alberta Native News* 13, no. 12 (December 2000): 55.

6. Carl Gustav Jung, M.D., *Psychology and Religion* (New Haven, Conn.: Yale University Press, 1938), 71.

7. The quartered-circle motif is ancient and has worldwide distribution. Iraqi Sammana ware from 4000 B.C. pictures antelope and birds whirling in the four directions. Similar images are found in ancient art throughout North America. An engraved shell dated A.D. 700–1200 found at Spiro Mound, Oklahoma, shows whirling winged rattlesnakes around a circle that encloses an equal-armed cross.

8. Frank Waters, *The Book of the Hopi: The First Revelation of the Hopi's Historical and Religious World-View of Life* (New York: Ballantine Books, 1969), 11.

9. A rich discussion of the quartered-circle motif can be found in Robert L. Hall, *An Archaeology of the Soul: North American Indian Belief and Ritual* (Chicago: University of Illinois Press, 1997), 98–101. I am indebted to Dr. Hall's excellent research for much of the information in this paragraph.

10. There are remarkable parallels between Native American and ancient Egyptian thought. The Egyptians recognized four races—Asians, Nubians, Libyans, and Egyptians—which some Egyptologists believe were once connected with directions and colors. Four gods—Horus, Seth, Thoth, and Anti (a falcon god)—rule the four directions: north, south, west, and east, respectively. The sky rests on four pillars, four legs of a cosmic cow, one in each direction.

11. Lee Irwin, *The Dream Seekers: Native American Visionary Traditions of the Great Plains* (Norman: University of Oklahoma Press, 1994), 58.

12. As I found out later, the standardization of the Four Winds color symbolism among the Lakota is a recent phenomenon, probably dating only from the 1970s. See William K. Powers, *Sacred Language: The Nature of Supernatural Discourse in Lakota* (Norman: University of Oklahoma Press, 1986), 143. Yet it is important to note that some ceremonies, among the Lakota and other tribes, are relatively invariable and do use very specific colors and symbols.

13. Outstanding examples of pan-Indian medicine wheels can be found in the book *The Sacred Tree* (Lethbridge, Alberta: Four Worlds Development Press, 1984). *The Sacred Tree* is based on a council of Native North American elders and spiritual leaders that took place in 1982 at the University of Lethbridge in Alberta, Canada. The purpose of the gathering was to discuss strategies to eliminate alcohol, drug abuse, suicide, and associated problems common in Native communities.

Michael Tlanusta Garrett (Cherokee) and Jane J. Carroll, assistant professors of counseling at Western Carolina University and the University of North Carolina, respectively, discuss Four Direction wheels as counseling tools to help clients find harmony and balance ("Mending the Broken Circle: Treatment of Substance Dependence among Native Americans," *Journal of Counseling & Development* 78, no. 4 [fall 2000]: 379–88). Marg Huber, an intercultural mediation consultant for the Commission on Resources and Environment in British Columbia, Canada, uses the Four Winds to help clients resolve conflicts. For example, when the mediator and clients are symbolically in the East, the climate is set by purifying with cedar smoke and helping people feel at ease. In the South, people discuss their feelings and issues openly. In the West, participants seek and extend understanding and compassion. In the North, mediators help their clients find solutions. (Marg Huber, "Mediation around the Medicine Wheel," *Mediation Quarterly* 10, no. 4 [summer 1993]: 355–65.)

14. Here again, there is great diversity among Native nations. Some tribes have strict rules about the starting direction in ritual and whether to circle clockwise or counterclockwise in group discussions, dancing, or ceremony. For instance Anishinabe, Innu, and Lakota people dance clockwise. The Inuit say that clockwise ritual motions are *Sila maligdlugo*, "according to the Natural Order." Yet Haudenosaunee dances are generally performed in a counterclockwise direction. Lakota generally begin ceremonial offerings to the West; Cherokee, to the East.

15. Jesus Christ and Moses, for example, are widely appreciated among Native American healers. People who follow their example are also Earth People, but to understand the connection among Jesus, Moses, and the Red Road, we need to be willing to venture outside the confines of the Church and religious dogma. The real "Imitation of Christ" is to find what Christ found, to go out into the wilderness, into the silent desert of the soul, where you can better hear "the still, small voice" (1 Kings 19:12). God is not a concept, a "graven image" to be worshiped, but rather a spirit that reveals herself when we practice inner silence. The Christian text *Theologia Mystica*, attributed to Saint Paul's Athenian disciple Dionysius the Areopagite, emphasizes the importance of "agnosia," the *unknowing* of all things in order to know God. Only by giving up our concepts of God can we perceive God's presence around us. In the desert, Jesus discovered that the Kingdom of Heaven is "spread upon the earth and men do not see it" (*The Gospel According to Thomas,* Log. 114).

Similarly, the first words Moses heard on Sinai were an invitation to unknowing: "Take off thy shoes, for thou art on Holy Ground." Shoes come between our feet and the ground. If we could take off our shoes—that is, shed rigid beliefs and identification with social roles—then the ground would be holy everywhere. Like Native healers, we could see that God's sublimity is found in the everyday, even in something as common as a burning bush. (Jewish mystics believe that to see God in a burning bush is to see God in nature. God is in *every* burning bush, and all people are equally capable of seeing her. And in case you are wondering, yes, in Judaism, God may properly be called him or her. I doubt if *he* gave birth to the world!)

16. Knud Rasmussen, *The Intellectual Culture of the Iglulik Eskimos,* vol. 7, no. 1, Report of the Fifth Thule Expedition (Copenhagen, 1929), 119–20.

17. According to *The Sacred Tree,* the South Wind's quality of sensitive and keen perception is symbolized by the Cougar. I want to emphasize, again, that you should not assume that all tribes or individuals interpret the Four Winds in a similar manner. For the Zuni, the Cougar is an animal of the North. I personally associate the sensual quality of the South with the Deer and the sexuality of the South with the Elk. The Makah, of northwest Washington State, have a very different interpretation of the Elk. The Elk, through most of Makah history, has been associated with subsistence. Whale harpoons were made from his antlers.

18. Richard Katz, *Boiling Energy* (Cambridge, Mass.: Harvard University Press, 1982), 235.

19. For a detailed discussion of this discipline and how to do it, see my book *The Way of Qigong: The Art and Science of Chinese Energy Healing* (New York: Ballantine, 1999).

20. See Donald Y. Gilmore and Linda S. McElroy, eds., *Across before Columbus? Evidence for Transoceanic Contact with the Americas prior to 1492* (Edgecomb, Maine: New England Antiquities Research Association, 1998).

21. Cherokee elders Keetoowah and Rolling Thunder both insisted that ancient Native Americans knew about the existence of Chinese people (personal communication, 1980). Gilmore and McElroy's *Across before Columbus?* presents evidence of Chinese characters in American Indian petroglyphs, though I find the documentation unconvincing. There are also interesting linguistic and cultural connections between Hopi and Tibetans and between the Zuni and the Japanese. For the latter, see Nancy Yaw Davis, *The Zuni Enigma: A Native American People's Possible Japanese Connection* (New York: Norton, 2000).

22. When the great psychologist Carl Jung was asked in a television interview whether he believed in God, he replied, "No. Why should I believe? I know!" To know God is to trust God and to be open to her guidance. In Judeo-Christian terms, trust means understanding God as the great I Am, as pure *being* without attribute. Not I am this or I am that, just *I Am.* Moses asks God her name, and God replies, "I AM That I AM." Jesus was a master of paradox and often used paradox to shock his listeners into expanded states of awareness. He recalls God's holiest name and expresses his identity with this name when he says, "Before Abraham ever was, I AM" (John 8:58).

23. Allen Klein, *The Healing Power of Humor* (Los Angeles: Tarcher, 1989), 5.

24. James R. Murie, *Ceremonies of the Pawnee* (Lincoln: University of Nebraska Press, 1989), 31, 38–39.

25. Oh Shinnah Fast Wolf, "Odyssey of a Warrior Woman," in *Profiles in Wisdom,* ed. Steven McFadden (Santa Fe, N.M.: Bear & Company, 1991), 151–152.

26. John G. Neihardt, *Black Elk Speaks: Being the Life Story of a Holy Man of the Oglala Sioux* (1932; reprint, Lincoln: University of Nebraska Press, 1961), 176.

27. Michael Crummett, *Sundance* (Helena, Mont.: Falcon Press, 1993), 40.

28. In the most dramatic form of "waking dreaming," known in Western psychological literature as *lucid dreaming,* the dreamer wakes up in the dream; he knows he is dreaming and consciously directs the dream to provide answers to spiritual questions or solutions to life problems.

29. Black Elk expressed a very similar philosophy of the ubiquity of the center. He told his friend John G. Neihardt that in his vision, he stood on Harney Peak in the Black Hills, the center of "the hoop of the world." "But," he added, "anywhere is the center of the world." (Neihardt, *Black Elk Speaks* [1961], 36.)

30. *The Sacred Tree* (Lethbridge, Alberta: University of Lethbridge Press, 1985), 63.

31. There is a prophecy in Cree country that the Purification will begin in the Northwest, particularly the Puget Sound region of Washington State, home of the Thunderbird and the power of transformation. My own vision is that the Purification is associated with the North and its attributes: the Fire Element, white color, and Caucasian race. To me, these qualities suggest a specific place: Iceland. Iceland, the land of fire (volcanoes) and ice (glaciers), is the most geologically active country in the world and one of the last places on earth where pure air and water can be found. Iceland is also the only country in the world where Europeans were the original inhabitants; they did not displace or colonize other peoples. It is Europe's northern outpost and the last vestige of Europe's ancient shamanic tradition (called *seidr* in Icelandic). In other European countries, there has been a revival of interest in Nordic, Druidic, Pagan, and other indigenous traditions, but no one really knows how these were originally understood or practiced. Iceland's geographic and linguistic isolation allowed the ancient wisdom to be maintained and transmitted to the present.

    At the turn of the millennium, the spirit of the North Wind was focused in Iceland to call attention to the ecological wisdom that lies buried in Europe's past and to remind *all people* to return to their indigenous roots.

32. Twylah Nitsch, *Entering into the Silence: The Seneca Way* (Irving, N.Y.: Seneca Indian Historical Society, 1984), 16.

33. See Huber, "Mediation around the Medicine Wheel," note 11.

34. Michael Tlanusta Garrett, "Reflection by the Riverside: The Traditional Education of Native American Children," *Journal of Humanistic Education and Development* 35, no. 1 (September 1996): 19.

35. Thom Henley, *Rediscovery: Ancient Pathways, New Directions* (Vancouver, B.C.: Lone Pine Publishing, 1996), 19.

3: THE CYCLES OF TRUTH: WISDOM FROM THE WOLF

1. In the words of Rupert Ross, an attorney who works closely with Cree and Anishinabe people.

2. Rupert Ross, *Dancing with a Ghost: Exploring Indian Reality* (Toronto, Ontario: Reed Books Canada, 1992), 62. Although Ross writes primarily about the values that underlie First Nations' jurisprudence, in which teaching and counseling take precedence over blame and punishment, his book applies equally to the ethics of Native American healing.

3. Ibid., 172.

4. Ibid., 170.

5. Deenise Becenti, "A New Life Begins at Sunrise," *American Indian* 1, no. 4 (fall 2000): 1217.

6. Being a member of the Seneca Wolf Clan Teaching Lodge should not be construed as equivalent to being a member of the Seneca Nation Wolf Clan, a designation implying descent from or adoption by a Wolf Clan matriarch. Unfortunately, Grandma Twylah, a teacher I greatly admire and love, has not always made this distinction clear to the many non-Indian students who began to study with her during her seventh and eighth decades of life. Misunderstandings were sometimes com-

pounded by Grandma's mixing authentic Seneca teachings, such as stories of the Peacemaker, the founder of the Haudenosaunee Confederacy, with diverse personal interests in subjects such as UFOs and channeling. This has unfortunately resulted in antagonism from some Native Americans, who believe that Seneca Wolf Clan Teaching Lodge students misrepresent Seneca tradition or represent themselves falsely as Seneca Indians.

Speaking from the heart is an elder's prerogative. Students are responsible, however, for using discrimination and reason—an essential Haudenosaunee value. I trust that my discussion of Grandma's exposition of core Native values helps to clear the air and engender a wider and well-deserved appreciation for Twylah Nitsch's lifetime of service.

7. I was initiated into the Wolf Clan Teaching Lodge in 1986 (Seneca name *Ongwe Okdea,* "Manroot"), received a teaching certificate from Grandma Twylah not long thereafter, and continued to visit and study through the early 1990s.

8. Personal communication (1984) from Grandmother Alloday, wife of the late Eli Gatoga and director of the Good Medicine Society. I am an honorary member of the society and in 1985 was principal singer at a Spring Festival that it hosted in Fayetteville, Arkansas.

9. The Anishinabe Creation Story is beautifully recounted in Edward Benton-Banai's *The Mishomis Book: The Voice of the Ojibway* (Hayward, Wis.: Indian Country Communications, 1988).

10. Barry Holstun Lopez, *Of Wolves and Men* (New York: Charles Scribner's Sons, 1978), 39.

11. Andrew Dreadfulwater, "We'll Have Hats with Feathers in Them . . . But We Won't Be No Indians," *Interculture* (Montreal: Centre Interculturel Monchanin) 17, no. 4, issue 85 (October–December 1984): 23.

12. During the last five hundred years, Americans have treated North America's indigenous people with such disrespect that self-esteem, which means respecting oneself, has become a major psychological challenge. In 1881, Helen Hunt Jackson wrote *A Century of Dishonor*, a classic description of Indian-white relations. Honor is lost when Native Americans are stereotyped as savages or saints. Honor is lost when children are sent to boarding schools where they are punished for looking, speaking, or acting Indian or when teachers demean Native children by denying the validity of indigenous history and science in favor of the official curriculum. Honor is lost when words are empty and treaties are broken.

13. During battle, Plains Indian warriors would demonstrate their bravery by touching their enemies with a coup stick rather than striking them with a weapon.

14. "An attack on America is an attack on Indian Country," said Bureau of Indian Affairs Assistant Secretary Neal McCaleb on the day of the tragedy. In a sense, the World Trade Center was an Indian monument. Kanien'kehaka (Mohawk) Indians, famous for their high-steel construction skills, helped to build the towers in the late 1960s. Statements of grief and condolence poured in from Native American nations. The Prairie Band Potawatomi of Kansas and Tulalip Nation of Washington contributed $100,000 each to relief efforts, and other tribes were equally generous. It is ironic that some terrorist groups believed that their attacks were justified by U.S. colonialism in the Middle East. Let them take a lesson from America's own colonial victims—the American Indians, whose land was taken and sacred sites pillaged; who in the 1800 were subjected to biological warfare from "gifts" of smallpox-infected blankets; whose religion was illegal until the 1970s, and yet who universally condemned the cowardly and horrific attacks on the innocent and on our Mother Earth.

15. Charles Hudson, *The Southeastern Indians* (Knoxville: University of Tennessee Press, 1976), 168–69.

16. Jay Miller, *Tsimshian Culture: A Light through the Ages* (Lincoln: University of Nebraska Press, 1997), 38.

17. Benton-Banai, *Mishomis Book*, 15.

18. Miller, *Tsimshian Culture*, 83.

19. For a passionate and philosophical account of the biology of whales, see Roger Payne's *Among Whales* (New York: Delta Publishing, 1995).

20. Miller, *Tsimshian Culture*, 174.

21. Thomas E. Mails, *Fools Crow: Wisdom and Power* (Tulsa, Okla.: Council Oak Books, 1991), 140.

22. Steve Wall and Harvey Arden, *Wisdomkeepers: Meetings with Native American Spiritual Elders* (Hillsboro, Oreg.: Beyond Words Publishing, 1990), 107.

23. Evan T. Pritchard, *No Word for Time* (Tulsa, Okla.: Council Oak Books, 1997), 195.

24. Gilbert Malcolm Sproat, "Sproat to Macdonald," October 27, 1879, Department of Indian Affairs [Canada], vol. 3,669, file 10,691. Similar reasoning was used in the United States to justify the breakup of tribally held lands. In the 1880s, Senator Henry M. Dawes of Massachusetts visited the Cherokee in Oklahoma. He described the Cherokee as having a nearly perfect society, in which there was "not a pauper in that Nation, and the Nation does not owe a dollar." They held their land in common, had their own schools and hospitals, and each family owned their own home. Dawes nevertheless lamented a society he felt was *based on the wrong economic principles*. He observed that in Cherokee society, "there is no enterprise to make your home any better than that of your neighbors. *There is no selfishness, which is at the bottom of civilization*" (italics added). Thus, in an effort to instill civilized virtues, Senator Dawes sponsored the General Allotment Act, which became federal law on February 8, 1887. Indian land was divided into individual allotments, with any unassigned land available to whites. Through a combination of legal maneuvering, swindling, and fraud by white settlers and government officials, however, most Native Americans never received their land parcels. Whites began a practice of adopting orphaned Indian children in order to receive land allotments. Horses and farm animals were given title to parcels that became the property of their white owners. Within twenty years of the Allotment Act, the Cherokee, like other Indian nations, had lost more than 90 percent of their land. I have heard many of my Cherokee friends say that the old strategy of "divide and conquer" had become "divide Indian land to conquer their spirit."

Federal policy only underscored the tremendous differences in values between white and Indian people. When Lakota Chief Red Cloud (circa 1820–1909) reflected on the white lifestyle, he said, "You must begin anew and put away the wisdom of your fathers. You must lay up food and forget the hungry. When your house is built, your storeroom filled, then look around for a neighbor whom you can take advantage of and seize all he has." (Quoted in Ralph K. Andrist, *The Long Death* [New York: Macmillan, 1964], 134.)

25. Knud Rasmussen, *Observations on the Intellectual Culture of the Caribou Eskimos* (Copenhagen: Report of the Fifth Thule Expedition, 1921–24, 7, no. 2; reprint, New York: AMS Press, 1976), 49.

26. Eli L. Huggins, "Smohalla, the Prophet of Priest Rapids," *Overland Monthly* 17 (1891): 213.

27. Marshall Sahlins, *Stone Age Economics* (Hawthorne, N.Y.: Aldine de Gruyter, 1972), 17.

28. Ibid., 35.

29. Stanley Vestal, *Sitting Bull: Champion of the Sioux* (1932; reprint, Norman: University of Oklahoma Press, 1957), 127. My description is adapted from Vestal's book.

30. Ibid., 128.

31. Cancer researchers and clinicians note that a dynamic, fighting spirit often bodes improved response to therapy and better prognosis than an attitude of passive acceptance. This seems as true among animals as among people. George Solomon, one of the pioneer researchers in psychoneuroimmunology, found that "behavioral differences even among identical (inbred) animals may have immunologic consequences." Aggressive, fighting mice have smaller virus-induced tumors than the nonfighters. (George F. Solomon, "The Emerging Field of Psychoneuroimmunology," *Advances* 2, no. 1 [1985]: 9.)

32. Paul A. W. Wallace, *The White Roots of Peace: The Iroquois Book of Life* (1946; reprint, Santa Fe, N.M.: Clear Light Publishers, 1994), 81. An inspiring version of the Thanksgiving Address is given in English and Mohawk in *Thanksgiving Address: Greetings to the Natural World; Ohén:ton Karihwatéhkwen: Words before All Else*, produced in 1993 as a collaborative project of the Native Self Sufficiency Center, Six Nations Indian Museum, Tracking Project, and Tree of Peace Society.

33. Dorothy Mack, "Thankless Tasks," *Red Cedar Bark* (spring 1997): 6.

4: THE VISION AND VISION QUEST: MESSAGES FROM THE SPIRIT

1. William James, *The Varieties of Religious Experience* (1902; reprint, New York: New American Library, 1958), 298.

2. A. Irving Hallowell, *Culture and Experience* (Philadelphia: University of Pennsylvania Press, 1955), 104.

3. See Karl H. Schleisier's great and inspired work *The Wolves of Heaven: Cheyenne Shamanism, Ceremonies, and Prehistoric Origins* (Norman: University of Oklahoma Press, 1987), 4.

4. "The Seri," Southwest Museum Papers, no. 6 (Los Angeles: Southwest Museum, 1931), 13.

Caves have been used for dreaming and vision-seeking throughout the world. Chinese Taoists dream and meditate in caves in order to commune with deities. Japanese shamans consider caves to be sealed alchemical vessels or wombs in which sacred power grows and gestates. In Sufism, students practice an initiation ritual called "the Blue Death," a period of several days of meditation in the utter silence and darkness of a cave. Sufi teacher Jabrane M. Sebnat describes the Blue Death: "In order to live fully and go beyond the suffering and anguish of death it is necessary 'to die before dying' " (*Blue Death [Little Emotional Death]* [n.p.: Michel Engel Productions, 1983], 6).

5. This spontaneous Vision Quest is not always advisable or safe. The Vision Quest requires a high degree of emotional stability so that the seeker is not overwhelmed by sacred powers. The experience can be so powerful and awe-inspiring that there is a danger of losing rather than gaining orientation and direction. A saying of mythologist Joseph Campbell is worth remembering: "The mystic swims on the waters of the unconscious; a schizophrenic drowns in them" (personal communication, 1980). Native American elders have already traversed the sacred terrain. Their guidance and interpretation provide context and meaning and may help the seeker overcome obstacles to a vision's fulfillment.

6. John G. Neihardt, *Black Elk Speaks: Being the Life Story of a Holy Man of the Oglala Sioux* (1932; reprint, Lincoln: University of Nebraska Press, 1961), 49.

7. For an exceptional discussion of the relationship of prophecy to meditation, see Aryeh Kaplan, *Meditation and the Bible* (New York: Samuel Weiser, 1978).

8. The burning bush is highly respected by many Native Americans. It is represented by the sacred fire in the tipi used for Native American Church ceremonies.

9. Lawrence Kushner, *The River of Light: Spirituality, Judaism, and the Evolution of Consciousness* (San Francisco: Harper & Row, 1981).

10. For information about Handsome Lake, see Arthur C. Parker, *The Code of Handsome Lake, the Seneca Prophet*, New York State Museum Bulletin 163 (Albany: New York State Museum, 1913), and Anthony F. C. Wallace, *The Death and Rebirth of the Seneca* (New York: Random House, 1969). The Ghost Dance movement founded by Wovoka is described in James Mooney's classic *The Ghost-Dance Religion and the Sioux Outbreak of 1890* (1896; reprint, Chicago: University of Chicago Press, 1965). For the Wanapam prophet Smohalla, see the carefully researched work of Robert H. Ruby and John A. Brown, *Dreamer-Prophets of the Columbia Plateau: Smohalla and Skolaskin* (Norman: University of Oklahoma Press, 1989). Various Native American dreamer-prophet traditions are described in Clifford E. Trafzer's *American Indian Prophets* (Newcastle, Calif.: Sierra Oaks Publishing, 1986).

11. For further information or to support the Chief Plenty Coups Peace Park, write to Friends of Chief Plenty Coups Association, P.O. Box 100, Pryor, MT 59066.

12. Rodney Frey, *The World of the Crow Indians: As Driftwood Lodges* (Norman: University of Oklahoma Press, 1987), 80.

13. Robert A. Brightman, *Grateful Prey: Rock Cree Human-Animal Relationships* (Berkeley: University of California Press, 1993), 81. In a similar vein, Lakota people pray, "Pity me that my people may live." This phrase is not an expression of self-abnegation, a *mea culpa*, as some Christians might interpret it. Spirits do not favor people who wallow in guilt or shame—negativity only attracts more negativity. Rather, asking for pity is a kind of spiritual bluff. If, because of your sacrifice and humility, you are *worthy* of being pitied, blessings and grace are more likely to occur.

14. Lee Irwin, *The Dream Seekers: Native American Visionary Traditions of the Great Plains* (Norman: University of Oklahoma Press, 1994), 101.

15. Jay Miller, ed., *Mourning Dove: A Salishan Autobiography* (Lincoln: University of Nebraska Press, 1990), 37.

16. Marilyn Schlitz, "Amazon Dreaming," *Noetic Sciences Review* 45 (spring 1998): 13.

17. Frank B. Linderman, *Plenty-Coups: Chief of the Crows* (Lincoln: University of Nebraska Press, 1930), 300–301.

18. I wonder what effect is produced by seeing images of the Indian killers George Washington and Andrew Jackson day after day in our billfolds? How do these not-so-subtle images affect the self-esteem of Native American people?

Washington is known among the Haudenosaunee as "Town Destroyer." In 1779, he ordered General John Sullivan to march his troops through Haudenosaunee territory and completely destroy all of their towns and farmlands. Sullivan burned homes and fields and chopped down orchards all along the Susquehanna River and its tributaries. Before the American Revolution, the Haudenosaunee lived in approximately thirty villages. By the spring of 1780, only two remained. See Anthony F. C. Wallace, *The Death and Rebirth of the Seneca* (New York: Random House, 1972), 141–44, and Donald A. Grinde Jr., *The Iroquois and the Founding of the American Nation* (San Francisco: Indian Historian Press, 1977), 107–13.

Andrew Jackson's role in the forced removal of the southeastern tribes is well known and need not be repeated here. Jackson did not hesitate to befriend Indians in order to put them on the front lines of battle against other tribes. Nor did he ever miss an opportunity to use bribery, deception, intimidation, thievery, or murder to get Native Americans to part with their land. In 1814, at the famous Battle of Horseshoe Bend, Jackson ordered his men to cut off the tips of the noses of the dead Creeks to get an accurate body count. Several of his white soldiers flayed the dead warriors' skins to make belts or horse reins. See John Ehle, *Trail of Tears: The Rise and Fall of the Cherokee Nation* (New York: Doubleday, 1988), and Charles Hudson, *The Southeastern Indians* (Knoxville: University of Tennessee Press, 1976). My Native friends ask, half-jokingly, "Isn't the motto on U.S. currency 'In Gold We Trust'?"

5: WHERE HEALING DWELLS:
THE IMPORTANCE OF SACRED SPACE

1. I know a single father who visited a similar site to receive a gift of "mothering energy" to help him raise his daughter. According to Cherokee tradition, a man can only understand or heal a woman if he communes with or invokes the Spirit of the Feminine or a feminine power embodied in a place.

2. Alice C. Fletcher, *The Hako: Song, Pipe, and Unity in a Pawnee Calumet Ceremony* (Washington, D.C.: U.S. Government Printing Office, 1904; reprint, Lincoln: University of Nebraska Press, 1996), 73.

3. Yet Indian people accept that such sacred centers do not exclude other sacred centers. When the mind and heart are purified and blessed by vision, then, as Black Elk reminds us, "anywhere is the center of the world." John G. Neihardt, *Black Elk Speaks: Being the Life Story of a Holy Man of the Oglala Sioux* (1932; reprint, Lincoln: University of Nebraska Press, 1961), 43.

4. C. A. Meier, *Healing Dream and Ritual: Ancient Incubation and Modern Psychotherapy* (Einsiedeln, Switzerland: Daimon Verlag, 1989), 29.

5. Sigmund Freud only saw dreams as expressions of repressed emotion, without spiritual origins or components. Swiss psychiatrist Carl G. Jung and those who followed him restored the ancient Greek emphasis on dreams as sources of spiritual advice and growth.

6. According to Rabbi Lawrence Kushner, "God is the bosom in which creation happens day after day, the ground and the source of everything that exists, the very Place of Being itself. And to be awake and present 'in this place' is to encounter God." (*God Was in This Place and I, I Did Not Know* [Woodstock, Vt.: Jewish Lights Publishing, 1991], 31–32.) The Tabernacle in Hebrew is called *mishkan*, which can be accurately translated as "a mutual dwelling place." According to psychotherapist Lakme Batya Elior and Rabbi Gershon Winkler, "It means a mutual honoring of that shared space. . . . And it is that honoring that makes the shared space a sacred place, whether that shared space be a sanctuary for the Divine Presence, or a home, or a relationship, or the environment, or the planet." (*The Place Where You Are Standing Is Holy: A Jewish Theology on Human Relationships* [Northvale, N.J.: Jason Aronson, 1994], 4–5.)

7. In order for the Catholic Church to consider a cure miraculous, it must meet five criteria, established in 1735 by Cardinal Lambertini (later Pope Benedict XIV): (1) The disease must be proved to exist and be incurable or unlikely to respond to treatment. (2) The disease must not have been at a stage at which it would have resolved itself without treatment. (3) The patient must not have had any potentially curative medication or treatment, or the treatment must be demonstrated to have failed. (4) The cure must be sudden or reached over a period of days. (5) The cure must be complete rather than partial. The cure must furthermore be certified by the International Medical Commission at Lourdes, by the Catholic Church, and by a committee set up by the local diocese.

See J. Garner, "Spontaneous Regressions: Scientific Documentation as a Basis for the Declaration of Miracles," *Canadian Medical Association Journal* 111 (December 7, 1974): 1254–64.

8. Stephen F. De Borhegyi, *The Miraculous Shrines of Our Lord of Esquipulas in Guatemala and Chimayo, New Mexico* (Santa Fe, N.M.: Spanish Colonial Arts Society, 1956), 6. (Reprinted from *El Placio* 60, no. 3 [March 1953].)

9. To become a member of the Wanuskewin Circle of Friends or for further information, write to Wanuskewin Circle of Friends, R.R. 4, Saskatoon, Saskatchewan, Canada S7K 3J7.

10. Alice Ware Davidson, Ph.D., R.N., "Healthcare Environments and Their Relationship to Human Well-Being," *Bridges* 5, no. 2 (summer 1994): 15–17.

11. Roger S. Ulrich, "View through a Window May Influence Recovery from Surgery," *Science* 224 (1984): 420–21.

12. The importance of family for hospitalized patients is well recognized in pediatric care. Many children's hospitals provide beds for parents to sleep in the same room as their children. It is a shame that adult needs for family support and participation in the healing process are less acknowledged.

  A study of 586 children admitted to the National Children's Hospital, Dublin, Ireland, over an eight-month period found that those with resident parents had shorter hospital stays than children whose parents slept elsewhere. Surprisingly, although beds were available for all parents, only 30 percent of children aged three and under had a parent who decided to sleep in the hospital. (M. R. H. Taylor, M.D., Ph.D., and P. O'Connor, M.D., "Resident Parents and Shorter Hospital Stay," *Archives of Disease in Childhood* 64 [1989]: 276. Adapted in *Advances: The Journal for Mind-Body Health* 7, no. 1 [1990]: 22–23.)

13. More research is needed before medical science accepts that the healing power of places is more than psychological and that places exert a direct spiritual and energetic influence on health. An easy way to demonstrate the subtle effect of place on the course of disease would be to measure the effectiveness of a standard treatment among patients in different locations. Better yet, a group of hospital patients receiving identical therapy for the same disease could be divided into two groups. The rooms of one group of patients are ritually purified daily (by prayer, visualization, drumming, or some other method); the rooms of the control group are not purified. Two distinct protocols could be followed. In one, patients in the purified group do not know that their rooms were purified. In the other, the purified group knows that their rooms were purified. I hypothesize that healing effects would be strongest with this combination of subtle energy influence and positive expectation (placebo). A third experimental group could be added who believe that their rooms were cleansed when, in fact, nothing was done. The third group would rule out placebo as the sole effective agent. I have been recommending these experiments to scientists for nearly a decade. So far, no one has taken up the challenge.

14. For a more complete view of the Creation story and sacred teachings of the Ojibwa (Anishinabe) people, read Edward Benton-Banai's *The Mishomis Book: The Voice of the Ojibway* (Hayward, Wis.: Indian Country Communications, 1988). Because it is written in the style of a traditional oral teaching, you feel as though you are listening to a wise *mishomis* (grandfather), and you are!

15. Erna Gunther, *Ethnobotany of Western Washington: The Knowledge and Use of Indigenous Plants by Native Americans* (Seattle: University of Washington Publications in Anthropology, 1945), 20.

16. James A. Duke, Ph.D., *The Green Pharmacy* (Emmaus, Pa.: Rodale Press, 1997), 451. This eminently readable and insightful work by one of the world's great experts on herbal medicine is highly recommended to all students of herbal medicine.

17. See Michael Moore, *Medicinal Plants of the Mountain West* (Santa Fe: Museum of New Mexico Press, 1979), 94.

18. Some California Indians do, however, use a variety of true sage, a coastal scrub plant called the California white sage, *Salvia alpine*.

19. See Herbert E. Wright, "Environmental Change and the Origin of Agriculture in the Old and New Worlds," in *Origins of Agriculture*, ed. Charles A. Reed (The Hague: Mouton, 1977). Artemisia was a common medicine in ancient Europe. In ancient Rome, artemisia absinthium tea was drunk during sacred rituals and was used as a medicine for colitis and other digestive disorders. It was even part of the prize, a gift of health, for the winner of the four-horse chariot race, symbol of the power of the Roman Empire. See Wilhelmina Feemster Jashemski, *A Pompeian Herbal: Ancient and Modern Medicinal Plants* (Austin: University of Texas Press, 1999).

20. William W. Dunmire and Gail D. Tierney, *Wild Plants of the Pueblo Province* (Santa Fe: Museum of New Mexico Press, 1995), 152.

21. For a bouquet of olfactory information and resources, contact the Olfactory Research Fund, 145 East Thirty-second St., New York, NY 10016–6002; (212) 725–2755. See its *Compendium of Olfactory Research. Explorations in Aroma-Chology: Investigating the Sense of Smell and Human Response to Odors, 1982–1994.* The reader is also referred to the following excellent works: David Howes, ed., *The Varieties of Sensory Experience: A Sourcebook in the Anthropology of the Senses* (Toronto, Ontario: University of Toronto Press, 1991), and Constance Classen, David Howes, and Anthony Synnott, *Aroma: The Cultural History of Smell* (New York: Routledge, 1994).

22. D. M. Frame, trans., *The Complete Essays of Montaigne* (Stanford, Calif.: Stanford University Press, 1965), 229.

6: ASKING FOR HELP:
FINDING AND PAYING A HEALER

1. Marilyn Schlitz, Ph.D., and William Braud, Ph.D., "Distant Intentionality and Healing: Assessing the Evidence," *Alternative Therapies in Health and Medicine* 3, no. 6 (November 1997): 62–73.

2. Thomas H. Lewis, *The Medicine Men: Oglala Sioux Ceremony and Healing* (Lincoln: University of Nebraska Press, 1990), 182. Thomas writes with rare insight, and his book reflects the integrity, directness, and simplicity with which he approached Lakota healers on the Pine Ridge Reservation. "I am a physician," he said. "Tell me how you approach medical problems." He recognized the medicine men and women as professional colleagues. They could learn from each other.

3. Jerome D. Frank, Ph.D., M.D., and Julia B. Frank, M.D., *Persuasion and Healing: A Comparative Study of Psychotherapy*, 3d ed. (Baltimore: Johns Hopkins University Press, 1991), 260.

4. Several of the studies that I cite in this section are explained in detail in Dr. Dean Ornish's beautiful book *Love and Survival: The Scientific Basis for the Healing Power of Intimacy* (New York: HarperCollins, 1998).

5. D. Spiegel et al., "Effect of Psychosocial Treatment on Survival of Patients with Metastatic Breast Cancer," *Lancet* 2 (1989): 888–91. The implications of this study are explored in Dr. Spiegel's inspiring book *Living beyond Limits* (New York: Ballantine, 1993).

6. James P. Lynch, *The Broken Heart: The Medical Consequences of Loneliness* (New York: Basic Books, 1977). The next two sentences are a sampling of Dr. Lynch's convincing evidence.

7. J. H. Medalie and U. Goldbourt, "Angina Pectoris among 10,000 Men. II. Psychosocial and Other Risk Factors as Evidenced by a Multi-variate Analysis of a Five Year Incidence Study," *American Journal of Medicine* 60, no. 6 (1976): 910–21.

8. W. T. Boyce, C. Schaefer, and C. Uitti, "Permanence and Change: Psychosocial Factors in the Outcome of Adolescent Pregnancy," *Social Science & Medicine* 21, no. 11 (1985): 1279–87.

9. K. Orth-Gomér and J. V. Johnson, "Social Network Interaction and Mortality: A Six Year Follow-up Study of a Random Sample of the Swedish Population," *Journal of Chronic Diseases* 40, no. 10 (1987): 949–57.

10. Ornish, *Love and Survival*, 42.

11. This term appears in Frank and Frank, *Persuasion and Healing*, 7.

12. More than 250 published scientific studies have examined the effect of some aspect of religiosity on morbidity and mortality. The results of all of these studies are remarkably consistent. As researcher Dr. Jeffrey S. Levin explains, "[I]n studies in which at least ordinal-level measures of religiosity are used (e.g., religious attendance, subjective religiosity, and various other behaviors and attitudes), the greater the intensity or degree of religiousness, the better the health and the less of whatever illness is being investigated." (Jeffrey S. Levin, "Investigating the Epidemiologic Effects of Religious Experience: Findings, Explanations, and Barriers," in *Religion in Aging and Health: Theoretical Foundations and Methodological Frontiers*, ed. Jeffrey S. Levin [Thousand Oaks, Calif.: Sage Publications, 1994], 5.) For a thorough study guide and workbook on the effects of religion on health, see David B. Larson, M.D., M.S.P.H., and Susan S. Larson, M.A.T., *The Forgotten Factor in Physical and Mental Health: What Does the Research Show? An Independent Study Seminar* (Arlington, Va.: National Institute for Healthcare Research, 1992).

13. Richard Katz, *Boiling Energy: Community Healing among the Kalahari Kung* (Cambridge, Mass.: Harvard University Press, 1982), 56.

14. Morris Edward Opler, "The Influence of Aboriginal Pattern and White Contact on a Recently Introduced Ceremony, the Mescalero Peyote Rite," *Journal of American Folk-Lore* 49 (1936): 1375.

15. L. Bryce Boyer, "Folk Psychiatry of the Apaches of the Mescalero Indian Reservation," in *Magic, Faith, and Healing: Studies in Primitive Psychiatry Today*, ed. Ari Kiev, M.D. (New York: Macmillan, 1964), 406.

16. James Mooney, *Sacred Formulas of the Cherokees*, Seventh Annual Report of the Bureau of American Ethnology (Washington, D.C.: 1886; reprint, Nashville, Tenn.: Charles and Randy Elder—Booksellers, 1982), 337.

17. Ibid.

18. David E. Jones, *Sanapia: Comanche Medicine Woman* (Prospect Heights, Ill.: Waveland Press, 1972), 73–74.

19. James H. Howard in collaboration with Willie Lena, *Oklahoma Seminoles: Medicines, Magic, and Religion* (Norman: University of Oklahoma Press, 1984), 24.

20. I do not pretend that there is an easy solution to the complex and controversial problem of commercializing the medicine. I have only scratched the surface. I generally disagree with selling any object that is designed specifically for ceremony or that closely imitates such objects. For example, the Haudenosaunee Confederacy has strongly censured the sale of its sacred masks ("faces"). Some Hopi people feel that it is disrespectful to sell "kachina dolls," caricatures of sacred beings.

Yet I feel that there should be exceptions to the prohibition against selling potentially sacred objects. I am not against financial reimbursement for the many Native American pipe makers who sell their sacred pipes at Pipestone National Monument, Minnesota. They mine the red pipestone in the traditional, laborious way, without the benefit of power tools, and spend many long hours sculpting it into beautiful and functional art. As much as I would like to ensure that sacred pipes are purchased only by people who know the traditional and respectful way to use them, I know that this is an impossible goal. The same can be said of drums. At a Native art market, I met a Lakota drum maker who explained that she prays and blesses the drums as she makes them. I was glad they were for sale. I paid with "frogskins" (green U.S. currency), a pouch of tobacco, and a heartfelt *Pilamayelo* (Thank you).

My personal philosophy is that a medicine person should never sell his or her personal spiritual medicine, the medicine received or confirmed by visions and dreams. If your medicine is tobacco, do not sell tobacco. If your medicine is cedarwood or quartz crystals, do not sell them. If your medicine consists of interpreting dreams, never set a rigid price for this service.

7: WHAT IS INVOLVED IN A NATIVE AMERICAN HEALING? TRADITIONS, PROTOCOLS, AND MOONTIME POWER

1. The Apache violin, or *tsii'edo'a'tl* ("wood that sings"), is an ancient instrument played during some social songs, ceremonial songs, and healing rituals. The body of the instrument is made of the century plant (related to agave), common in Arizona. The bow is willow or sumac, and the strings on both the violin and bow are traditionally horsehair or sinew, although today, conventional violin strings are sometimes used. Many Apache medicine people have played the "wood that sings," including Geronimo.

2. Swinomish Tribal Mental Health Project, *A Gathering of Wisdoms—Tribal Mental Health: A Cultural Perspective* (LaConner, Wash.: Swinomish Tribal Community, 1991), 127.

3. The neurophysiology of rhythmic sensory stimulation and auditory driving has been explored since the 1940s. The classics are: V. J. Walter and W. Grey Walter, "The Central Effects of Rhythmic Sensory Stimulation," *Electroencephalographic and Clinical Neurophysiology* 1 (1949): 57–86; William Sargant, *Battle for the Mind* (London: Pan Books, 1959), 92; and especially, the important works of Andrew Neher: "Auditory Driving Observed with Scale Electrodes in Normal Subjects," *Electroencephalographic and Clinical Neurophysiology* 13 (1961): 449–51, and "A Physiological Explanation of Unusual Behavior in Ceremonies Involving Drums," *Human Biology* 34 (1962): 151–60. See also various works on music therapy—notably, James Evans, Ph.D., and Manfred

Clynes, D.Sc., eds., *Rhythm in Psychological, Linguistic and Musical Processes* (Springfield, Ill.: Charles C. Thomas, 1986).

4. Gregory Cajete, ed., *A People's Ecology: Explorations in Sustainable Living* (Santa Fe, N.M.: Clear Light Publishers, 1999), 17.

5. The most immediate effect of sensory saturation is more physical than metaphysical. It blocks the transmission of pain signals. With repeated or long-term exposure, drumming and dancing rhythms can reset or reprogram biological clocks. Many conditions—such as insomnia, chronic fatigue syndrome, cardiac arrhythmia, bipolar disorder, seasonal affective disorder, seizure disorders, and the common disorientation that occurs after jet travel—have dysrhythmia as an essential component. According to James R. Evans, associate professor of psychology at the University of South Carolina (Columbia):

> Some [researchers] perceive the human body as a collection of oscillating subsystems more or less in harmony with each other; and the greater the harmony among the systems the less the "dis-ease," while the greater the dissonance the more severe the "disease." According to some such views, internal order can be increased and hence the quality of the human "body symphony" enhanced by exposure to ordered stimuli such as certain music, poetry and rhythms of nature and/or by participation in rhythmic movement activities as diverse as dancing, jogging, and certain martial arts. One might guess that dancing to music under the stars on a beach would be highly conducive to reestablishment of internal order! ("Dysrhythmia and Disorders of Learning and Behavior," in Evans and Clynes, *Rhythm in Psychological, Linguistic and Musical Processes*, 266–67)

Several studies have also shown the beneficial effects of auditory rhythms on motor control and gait training in Parkinson's, stroke, and brain injury patients. See Michael H. Thaut, Ph.D., "Rhythmic Auditory Stimulation in Rehabilitation of Movement Disorders: A Review of Current Research," in *Music in Human Adaptation*, ed. Daniel J. Schneck and Judith K. Schneck (Blacksburg, Va.: Virginia Polytechnic Institute and State University College of Engineering, 1997), 223–29.

6. Tragically, Native American "spiritual" teachers have sometimes broken the rule of appropriate sexual behavior, and women need to take special precautions when studying with them. There are reports of women who have been seduced or raped by self-proclaimed medicine people, even within the sacred Sweat Lodge or during other ceremonies.

Native Americans have long been victims of political, social, and religious oppression; one common human strategy of avoiding the repressed anger of victimization is to turn other people into victims. This does not, however, justify or excuse misbehavior or the implicit cowardice that makes a person see shadows outside rather than face those within. In all cultures and religions, there are people who seem mature in spiritual matters but are immature emotionally. Do not be misled by promises of power, "secrets," or the charisma of exotic teachers. Do not shift your authority into a teacher's hands or ignore your inner voice. Promiscuous sexual relations are *never* part of Native American medicine training. Spiritual people consider sexuality an expression of love and caring and never use it manipulatively.

The problem of ignoring and trespassing sexual boundaries is well recognized in Indian Country. In May of 1999, a conference was held in Minneapolis entitled "Strengthening the Circle of Trust—1999," described as a "Conference on Sexual Abuse and Exploitation by Native American 'Spiritual Leaders/Medicine Men.' " It was attended by Native American therapists, social workers, legislators, spiritual leaders, victims of sexual abuse, and others involved or interested in these issues.

7. William N. Fenton, *The False Faces of the Iroquois* (Norman: University of Oklahoma Press, 1987), 169.

8. Ibid., 170.

9. James Mooney, *Myths of the Cherokee* (1888; reprint, Nashville, Tenn.: Charles and Randy Elder—Booksellers, 1982), 298.

10. Ibid.

11. Today, many Native Americans have ambivalent feelings about recording traditional songs. While they wish to maintain the vitality of context-based experience and learning, they also recognize the

importance of preserving the linguistic and melodic nuances of songs that may be only rarely sung. I have the same mixed feelings. I do not allow recordings when I conduct a ceremony or offer a medicine teaching (often interspersed with songs). Yet I will occasionally give a student a recording for personal use, as a kind of study aid and to jar memory. My Native friends have done the same for me. On the rare occasions when Indian associates and I make recordings for one another, we are careful to pray beforehand to honor the song, to ask for the ability to sing it properly, and to understand its hidden meanings. We make the act of recording a ceremony, smudging ourselves, the recorder, and the audiocassette.

A healer's effectiveness does not depend on how many songs he knows but on how well and wisely he uses them. A Native healer's song repertoire is similar to an herbalist's pharmacopoeia. I know healers who have memorized as few as three or as many as three thousand songs.

12. "The women have been entrusted with the Water and the men with the Fire. These are two things that sustain life. If you take care of them, they will take care of you" (Eddie Benton-Banai, Three Fires Medewin Society, News from Indian Country [mid-April 1994], 25). The women-moon-water association is widely held by Native American people. As another example, Asatchaq (1891–1980), a Tikigaq storyteller from northwestern Alaska, described the following ritual, remembered from his youth: In the springtime, women sought the help of the moon spirit for success in the whale hunt. As the new moon rose, they stood on their iglus and raised pots of water, taken from a sacred freshwater pond, to the moon. If the woman was spiritually powerful, the moon spirit would magically drop small whale effigies in the water, a prediction of a successful hunt. See Tom Lowenstein and Tukummiq, translator, *The Things That Were Said of Them: Shaman Stories and Oral Histories of the Tikigaq People* (Berkeley: University of California Press, 1992), 16–20.

13. A ceremony honoring fire-water, male-female medicines was performed at the opening of the 12th Annual Indigenous Environmental Network's Protecting Mother Earth Conference, held August 2–5, 2001, on the traditional lands of the Okanagan Nation, British Columbia, Canada. As more than two thousand participants observed, indigenous men from Mexico transferred a symbolic fire of spirituality and life to the firekeepers of the Okanagan Nation. Then indigenous women performed a water ceremony. As reported by journalist Jim Kent in *News from Indian Country* 15, no. 16 (August 2001), 13A, the women "had been asked to bring a sample of water from their homeland—whether it was polluted or not. Those samples were then poured into a common container to symbolize the waters of the Four Directions. Spiritual leaders then blessed the container and asked the Creator to heal all the waters of Mother Earth—including that which is held in each person's body."

14. The widely publicized birth of deformed frogs in the Great Lakes region of the United States and the rapid decline of amphibians worldwide are visible signs that we have upset the delicate balance of life. Scientists believe that frogs are bioindicators, like a miner's canary, that warn that contaminants have passed a critical threshold and are probably already affecting human health. See Christopher Hallowell, "Trouble in the Lily Pads," *Time*, October 28, 1996, 87; and Ashley Mattoon, "Deciphering Amphibian Declines," in the Worldwatch Institute's *State of the World 2001* (New York: Norton, 2001), 63–82. Beginning in 1996, scientists reported that frogs with missing, extra, or withered limbs; smaller sex organs; and shrunken eyes were becoming common in Wisconsin, Minnesota, South Dakota, Vermont, and Québec. Because frogs respond sensitively to their aquatic environment, they are among the first to show the effects of acid rain, heavy metal and pesticide contamination, ozone depletion, and global warming. Amphibians have existed for about 350 million years, surviving three mass extinctions, including that of the dinosaurs. If human beings continue destroying the environment, amphibians may not survive *their* extinction.

Other forms of aquatic life are also showing clear signs of planetary sickness. Alaskan Natives have been reporting unexplained oddities in ocean life for years: darkened fish livers, lesions on fish, and hairless seals. See "Researchers, Scientists to Rely on Alaska Natives in Pollution Studies," *News from Indian Country: The Nations Native Journal* 12, no.18 (late September 1998): 11A.

15. In the Lakota language, the word *isnati*—literally, "to dwell alone"—means both moontime and moontime isolation. Among Native American tribes, the Puberty Ceremony, held during a young woman's first period of isolation, is a cause for celebration. The Lakota call it the Buffalo Ceremony, because it invokes the nurturing and life-sustaining virtues of the Buffalo. See Marla N.

Powers, *Oglala Women: Myth, Ritual, and Reality* (Chicago: University of Chicago Press, 1986), 66–73.

According to the Diné, the first *Kinaalda*, Puberty Ceremony, was created by the Holy Woman Changing Woman, who created the Diné people and whose body became the inner being of the Earth, changing with the seasons. Changing Woman developed the power of reproduction from the dews of various plants that were put into her body. See Charlotte Johnson Frisbie, *Kinaaldá: A Study of the Navaho Girl's Puberty Ceremony* (Salt Lake City: University of Utah Press, 1993), 399 (field notes of David McAllester, 1961).

16. Theda Perdue, *Cherokee Women: Gender and Culture Change, 1700–1835* (Lincoln: University of Nebraska Press, 1998), 30.

17. Dianne Meili, *Those Who Know: Profiles of Alberta's Native Elders* (Edmonton, Alberta: NeWest Press, 1991), 152.

18. The logic of these customs is increasingly acknowledged by Western scientists. Joan Borysenko, Ph.D., describes moontime as a period of "expanded connection with universal energy . . . so powerful that it could effectively short-circuit a ceremony or affect the energy bodies of other people" (*A Woman's Book of Life: The Biology, Psychology, and Spirituality of the Feminine Life Cycle* [New York: Riverhead Books, 1996], 52). Christiane Northrup, M.D., writes, "This society likes action, so we don't appreciate our need for rest and replenishment. . . . I think that the majority of PMS cases would disappear if every modern woman retreated from her duties for three or four days each month and had her meals brought to her by someone else" (*Women's Bodies, Women's Wisdom: Creating Physical and Emotional Health and Healing* [New York: Bantam, 1994], 103).

Some tribes recommend dietary adjustments during moontime. The California Pomo avoid meat and fish because they contain blood, the substance that moontime women are trying to expel. Among the Washo of California and Nevada, the Puyallup of Washington, and the Ho Chunk of Wisconsin, moontime women commonly fasted from food and drink, except water. I believe that these proscriptions may not be advisable, however, for women who are anemic or who feel weak and depleted. Additionally, women who do not have access to a moon lodge or other sacred retreat space and who lack adequate social support may find that complete fasting causes an uncomfortable increase in sensitivity and feelings of fragility or vulnerability. Rebecca D. Cohen, Ph.D., counselor and menstrual researcher, advises, "In today's society, the most important dietary rule for moontime women is to listen to the body and to eat whatever feels most natural and harmonious" (personal communication, 1998).

19. Traditional Jews also consider moontime a spiritual purification, during which women separate from their men for seven days and then rejoin them after a ritual bath called the *mikvah*. Rabbi Aryeh Kaplan explains that the monthly separation prevents relationships from becoming dull and jaded. "A woman's monthly period can therefore be seen as one of God's many gifts to humanity. Rather than something negative, it is a means of preserving the close bond between man and wife. It affords the couple a monthly honeymoon, where their marriage is constantly renewed" (Rabbi Aryeh Kaplan, *Made in Heaven: A Jewish Wedding Guide* [Brooklyn, N.Y.: Moznaim Publishing Corporation, 1983], 75). Rabbi Kaplan describes people who do not follow these natural laws as "cut off from their source."

20. Robert M. Sapolsky, *Why Zebras Don't Get Ulcers: A Guide to Stress, Stress-Related Diseases, and Coping* (New York: Freeman, 1994), 122. I highly recommend this delightful book, full of wisdom and humor. You can reduce your level of stress by just reading it.

21. James H. Howard, *The Ponca Tribe* (Lincoln: University of Nebraska Press, 1995), 146.

22. David E. Jones, *Sanapia: Comanche Medicine Woman* (Prospect Heights, Ill.: Waveland Press, 1984), 48.

23. Rebecca D. Cohen, "Empowering Women through Sacred Menstrual Customs: Effects of Separate Sleeping during Menses on Creativity, Dreaming, Relationships, and Spirituality" (Ph.D. diss., San Francisco: Saybrook Graduate School, July 2001).

24. Robert L. Van de Castle, Ph.D., *Our Dreaming Mind* (New York: Ballantine, 1995), 382. This is a magnificent book. Data about menstrual dreams can be found on pages 376–90.

25. Ibid., 378.

26. Alice B. Kehoe, "Blackfoot Persons," in *Women and Power in Native North America*, ed. Laura F. Klein and Lillian A. Ackerman (Norman: University of Oklahoma Press, 1995), 120–21.

27. Ruth M. Underhill, *Papago Woman* (New York: Holt, Rinehart and Winston, 1979), 92.
28. Perdue, *Cherokee Women*, 29.
29. Cora Du Bois and Dorothy Demetracopoulou, "Wintu Myths," *University of California Publications in American Archaeology and Ethnology* 28 (1931): 362.

8: THE PRINCIPLES OF NATIVE AMERICAN COUNSELING

1. The only indigenous American counseling method that is widely recognized is *Ho'oponopono*, the traditional Hawaiian spiritual counseling and family mediation process, in which prayer and forgiveness are key features. Most works on Hawaiian spirituality mention it. See Victoria E. Shook, *Ho'oponopono: Contemporary Uses of a Hawaiian Problem-Solving Process* (Honolulu: University of Hawaii Press, 1985).
2. David E. Jones, *Sanapia: Comanche Medicine Woman* (Prospect Heights, Ill.: Waveland Press, 1972), 74.
3. Jack Frederick Kilpatrick and Anna Gritts Kilpatrick, *Walk in Your Soul: Love Incantations of the Oklahoma Cherokees* (Dallas: Southern Methodist University Press, 1965), 9.
4. Thomas E. Mails, *Fools Crow: Wisdom and Power* (Tulsa, Okla.: Council Oak Books, 1991), 155.
5. For a superb textbook that explores the integration of indigenous and conventional mental health services, see *A Gathering of Wisdoms—Tribal Mental Health: A Cultural Perspective* (LaConner, Wash.: Swinomish Tribal Community, 1991). Eduardo and Bonnie Duran also offer an excellent example of multicultural approaches to psychotherapy in their book *Native American Postcolonial Psychology* (Albany: State University of New York Press, 1995).
6. Brian Campbell Broom, "Medicine and Story: A Novel Clinical Panorama Arising from a Unitary Mind/Body Approach to Physical Illness," *Advances in Mind-Body Medicine* 16, no. 3 (summer 2000): 161–62.
7. Steve Wall and Harvey Arden, *Wisdom Keepers: Meetings with Native American Spiritual Elders* (Hillsboro, Oreg.: Beyond Words Publishing, 1990), 106.
8. Viktor E. Frankl, *Man's Search for Meaning* (New York: Simon & Schuster, 1984), 98.
9. The relationship between patients' expectations and their health creates a serious ethical dilemma for Western physicians, who generally believe that honest disclosure is in the best interests of the patients. The quality of Western medical practice would benefit if more medical schools offered training in how to induce the placebo effect with good words and kind behavior and recommended that physicians use these tools whenever possible. Great healers can phrase a poor prognosis in a positive and hopeful way, without dodging the truth. See Joseph A. Carrese, M.D., Ph.D., and Lorna A. Rhodes, Ph.D., "Western Bioethics on the Navajo Reservation: Benefit or Harm?" *Journal of the American Medical Association* 274, no. 10 (1995): 826–29.
10. Robert A. Hahn, Ph.D., M.P.H., "Nocebos Contribute to Host of Ills," *Journal of the American Medical Association* 275, no. 5 (1996): 345–47.
11. Ibid., 345.
12. N. S. Yagwer, "Emotions as a Cause of Rapid and Sudden Death," *Archives of Neurology and Psychiatry* 36 (1936): 875.
13. Sorcerers want followers for an additional, malevolent, reason: they use them as a psychic shield, protection from negative forces meant for the sorcerer. "When bad medicine men have a curse returned [to them], their followers will have bad luck" (Russell Willier [Cree], quoted in David Young with Grant Ingram and Lise Swartz, *Cry of the Eagle* [Toronto: University of Toronto Press, 1989], 49).
14. I am certainly not assuming that in the modern world, it is easy or always possible to find work that is in perfect accord with one's spiritual gifts and ideals. I do believe, however, that spiritual people should be willing to sacrifice money and personal comfort for the sake of integrity. We need to find the kind of work and lifestyle that causes the least possible harm to ourselves, to others, and to the environment.
15. Sandra Ingerman, *Soul Retrieval* (San Francisco: HarperSanFrancisco, 1991).
16. Jay Miller, *Shamanic Odyssey: The Lushootseed Salish Journey to the Land of the Dead* (Menlo Park, Calif.: Ballena Press, 1988). According to Miller, the Lushootseed believe that a person has three

related faculties: mind, guardian spirits or powers, and soul, a concept intimately connected with life force and breath. For an overview of Native American beliefs about the soul, see Åke Hultkrantz, *Soul and Native Americans* (Woodstock, Conn.: Spring Publications, 1997). Jill Leslie McKeever Furst discusses pre-Columbian beliefs about the soul among the Aztecs, as well as numerous parallels to Native North American philosophy, in her brilliant book *The Natural History of the Soul in Ancient Mexico* (New Haven, Conn.: Yale University Press, 1995).

17. The full name of this condition is chronic fatigue and immune dysfunction syndrome (CFIDS). CFIDS is a serious, debilitating condition that causes recurrent pain, fatigue, depression, cognitive impairment, digestive problems, and weakened immunity. Like cancer, it does not have one simple cause. CFIDS is linked to viral infection (commonly in the herpes group, such as Epstein-Barr), exposure to high levels of chemical toxins (such as pesticides, antibiotics, heavy metals), and genetic predisposition—it often runs in families. Although CFIDS may go into short- or long-term remission, there is no known cure.

18. The goal of Taoism is to learn about the Tao, the Way of Nature, and ultimately, to become one with it. Interestingly, I have heard Cherokee elders speak about the importance of learning "the Way." "He understands the Way," War Eagle (Cherokee) said to me, when complimenting a medicine man.

19. Meyer Levin, *Classic Hassidic Tales* (New York: Penguin Books, 1975), 45–57. First published as *The Golden Mountain*, 1932.

20. Walter B. Cannon, " 'Voodoo' Death," *Psychosomatic Medicine* 19, no. 3 (1957): 182–90. Also see a further elaboration of Cannon's ideas in "Hex Death: Voodoo Magic or Persuasion?" by Clifton K. Meador, M.D., of Vanderbilt University School of Medicine, *Southern Medical Journal* 85, no. 3 (1992): 244–47. Meador cites examples of how the persuasive power of the words and actions can cause death. He concludes, "The phenomena of hexing and persuasion are worthy of further careful and unbiased scientific observations."

21. Richard A. Kirkpatrick, M.D., "Witchcraft and Lupus Erythematosus," *Journal of the American Medical Association* 245, no. 19 (1981): 1937.

22. Larry Dossey, M.D., *Be Careful What You Pray For . . . You Just Might Get It* (New York: HarperCollins, 1997).

23. "Man Acquitted in Death of Bearwalker," *News from Indian Country* 11, no. 12 (late June 1997).

24. Annemarie Shimony, "Eastern Woodlands: Iroquois of Six Nations," in *Witchcraft and Sorcery of the American Native Peoples*, ed. Deward E. Walker Jr. (Moscow: University of Idaho Press, 1989), 152.

25. Because hair and nails may be vulnerable to wandering malevolent spirits, followers of Native Spirituality burn or dispose of them very carefully rather than tossing them outside or anywhere that they might be seen or easily taken.

26. Shimony, "Eastern Woodlands," 146.

27. Quoted by Abraham Conklin, Ponca spiritual leader, in "All Roads Are Good," *Native Peoples* (fall 1994): 42.

28. The Four Noble Truths are:
    1. Suffering and imperfection are realities of life.
    2. Suffering is caused by self-centered desire.
    3. Suffering can be made to cease.
    4. The way to end suffering is by following the Noble Eightfold Path, which means applying the principles of moderation, mindfulness, and integrity to every aspect of one's life, particularly to understanding, thought, speech, action, livelihood, effort, mindfulness, and concentration.

29. I make no claim to be practicing the Lushootseed "Spirit Canoe Healing Ceremony," though the ceremony I received in personal vision may bear some resemblance to it.

30. Marc Simmons, *Witchcraft in the Southwest: Spanish and Indian Supernaturalism on the Rio Grande* (Lincoln: University of Nebraska Press, 1974), 141.

31. "The Ancient Wisdom in Shamanic Cultures," an interview with Michael Harner by Gary Doore, *American Theosophist* (November 1985): 330.

9: CULTIVATING THE GOOD MIND:
A COUNSELOR'S GARDENING TOOLS

1. *Developing Healthy Communities: Fundamental Strategies for Health Promotion* (Lethbridge, Alberta, Canada: Four Worlds Development Press, 1985), 5.

2. Four Worlds Development Project, *The Sacred Tree* (Lethbridge, Alberta, Canada: Four Worlds Development Press, 1984), 51.

3. Swinomish Tribal Mental Health Project, *A Gathering of Wisdoms—Tribal Mental Health: A Cultural Perspective* (LaConner, Wash.: Swinomish Tribal Community, 1991), 80.

4. Ann Fienup-Riordan, *Boundaries and Passages: Rule and Ritual in Yup'ik Eskimo Oral Tradition* (Norman: University of Oklahoma Press, 1994), 209.

5. Adolf Hungry Wolf, *A Good Medicine Collection: Life in Harmony with Nature* (Summertown, Tenn.: Book Publishing Co., 1990), no page numbers.

6. Evan T. Pritchard, *No Word for Time: The Way of the Algonquin People* (Tulsa, Okla.: Council Oak Books, 1997), 69.

7. There are, of course, exceptions to this convention, including black Southern Baptists and individual Christians, who may have a more exuberant style of praying.

8. Pat Moffitt Cook, *Shaman, Jhankri and Néle: Music Healers of Indigenous Cultures* (Roslyn, N.Y.: Ellipsis Arts, 1997), 32.

9. Maureen Trudelle Schwarz, *Navajo Lifeways: Contemporary Issues, Ancient Knowledge* (Norman: University of Oklahoma Press, 2001), 142. Chinese Buddhists similarly identify tears and laughter as signs of empathy. The Chinese Buddhist Goddess of Compassion is called Guan Shi Yin, literally, "She Who Hears the World's Cries and Laughter."

10. Jim Northrup, *The Rez Road Follies* (Minneapolis: University of Minnesota Press, 1997). The first two jokes quoted are from page 12, the last from page 2.

11. Steven M. Sultanoff, Ph.D., "Survival of the Witty-est: Creating Resilience through Humor," *Therapeutic Humor* 11, no. 5 (1997): 1–2. The journal is published by the American Association for Therapeutic Humor, 222 S. Meramec, Suite 303, St. Louis, MO 63105.

12. Jim Mitchell, Ph.D., "Taking It to the Limit: The Role of Humor in Surviving Extreme Situations," *Humor & Health Journal* 5, no. 6 (1996): 5. The journal is published by the Humor & Health Institute, P.O. Box 16814, Jackson, MS 39236-6814.

13. Ibid., 8.

14. Joseph R. Dunn, Ph.D., "The HA, HA, HA Prescription: An Interview with Clifford Kuhn, M.D.," *Humor & Health Journal* 6, no. 5 (1997): 69–78.

15. Barton Wright, *Clowns of the Hopi: Tradition Keepers and Delight Makers* (Flagstaff, Ariz.: Northland Publishing, 1994), 2.

16. Patty Wooten, R.N., *Compassionate Laughter: Jest for Your Health* (Salt Lake City: Commune-a-Key Publishing, 1996), 7–9.

17. Cited in Allen Klein's *The Healing Power of Humor: Techniques for Getting through Loss, Setbacks, Upsets, Disappointments, Difficulties, Trials, Tribulations, and All That Not-So-Funny Stuff* (Los Angeles: Tarcher, 1989), 19.

18. "PNI Research Summary" (based on the research of Dr. Lee S. Berk of Loma Linda University's School of Medicine and Public Health), *Humor & Health Journal* 5, no. 5 (1996): 6.

19. Rod A. Martin, Ph.D., and James P. Dobbin, M.A., "Sense of Humor, Hassles, and Immunoglobulin A: Evidence for a Stress-Moderating Effect of Humor," *International Journal of Psychiatry in Medicine* 18, no. 2 (1988): 93–105; and Kathleen M. Dillon, Ph.D., Brian Minchoff, and Katherine H. Baker, Ph.D., "Positive Emotional States and Enhancement of the Immune System," *International Journal of Psychiatry in Medicine* 15, no. 1 (1985–1986): 13–18.

20. Lee S. Berk, Dr.PH., M.P.H., "The Laughter-Immune Connection: New Discoveries," *Humor & Health Journal* 5, no. 5 (1996): 1–5.

21. Lee S. Berk, D.H.Sc., M.P.H., et al., "Neuroendocrine and Stress Hormone Changes During Mirthful Laughter," *American Journal of Medical Sciences* 298, no. 6 (1989): 390–96.

22. Ibid.

23. In Mexico, *curanderas* and *curanderos* use ordinary chicken eggs as diagnostic tools. The healer waves an egg through a patient's aura. The egg is broken open, and the healer looks at the yolk for

any symbols of witchcraft. The egg may also be used to draw out and cleanse the patient of destructive forces.

24. William Wildschut, *Crow Indian Medicine Bundles*, 2d ed. (1927; reprint, New York: Museum of the American Indian Heye Foundation, 1975), 106.

25. Donald Sandner, M.D., *Navaho Symbols of Healing: A Jungian Exploration of Ritual, Image, and Medicine* (Rochester, Vt.: Healing Arts Press, 1991), 33.

26. Frances Densmore, *Teton Sioux Music and Culture,* Bureau of American Ethnology, bulletin 61 (Washington, D.C.: Smithsonian Institution, 1918), 249.

27. Anthony F. C. Wallace, *The Death and Rebirth of the Seneca* (New York: Random House, 1972), 59.

28. See Barbara Tedlock's "Zuni and Quiché Dream Sharing and Interpreting" in the work she edited, *Dreaming: Anthropological and Psychological Interpretations* (Santa Fe, N.M.: School of American Research Press, 1992), 105–31. Creative people in all cultures recognize that dream experiences are not bound by time or the linear sequence of events. Mozart would sometimes dream-hear an entire symphony at once yet remember it in all of its linear, waking-consciousness detail. Precognitive dreams may not involve projecting the mind into the future but, rather, accessing a realm in which all events are present simultaneously.

29. Wallace, *Death and Rebirth of the Seneca*, 71.

30. "The symbols act as transformers, their function being to convert libido from a 'lower' into a 'higher' form" (*Symbols of Transformation*, Bollingen Series 20, vol. 5 [New York: Pantheon Books, 1956], 232).

31. Jeanne Achterberg, "Imagery—Health Care, Mind-Body Plasticity, and Overcoming the Constraints of Individual Differences in Imagery Ability" (San Francisco: Saybrook Institute Residential Conference class notes, June 24–27, 1998), 9.

32. L. B. Boyer et al., "Comparisons of the Shamans and Pseudoshamans of the Apaches of the Mescalero Indian Reservation: A Rorschach Study," *Journal of Projective Techniques* 28 (1964): 179. The results of this study are especially impressive considering that Boyer's writings demean Apache culture and have a tone of white intellectual and moral superiority. He characterized Apache people as "dependent" and "irresponsible." In "Folk Psychiatry of the Apaches," published in Ari Kiev's *Magic, Faith, and Healing: Studies in Primitive Psychiatry Today* (New York: Macmillan, 1964), Boyer says that the roles of medicine person and sorcerer are displaced representations of the omnipotence and omniscience of good and bad parents.

33. Richard Noll, "Mental Imagery Cultivation as a Cultural Phenomenon: The Role of Visions in Shamanism," *Current Anthropology* 26 (1985): 443–52.

34. Ian Wickramaskera, "Secrets Kept from the Mind but Not the Body or Behavior: The Unsolved Problems of Identifying and Treating Somatization and Psychophysiological Disease," *Advances in Mind-Body Medicine* 14, no. 2 (1998): 81–98. Here, I am comparing moderately high hypnotizability to moderately low hypnotizability. Other factors being equal, the highs tend to be healthier and to have greater facility at self-regulation. Extreme highs and extreme lows, however, are both at greater risk for disease or for transforming psychological stress into disease symptoms—the former because they are too suggestible, the latter because they are likely to deny their emotions. Extremes of credulity and skepticism are maladaptive and limit the ability to cope with stress.

10: MASSAGE AND ENERGY THERAPIES

1. Mariana Caplan, *Untouched: The Need for Genuine Affection in an Impersonal World* (Prescott, Ariz.: Hohm Press, 1998), xxiii.

2. Robert H. Lowie, *The Crow Indians* (New York: Rinehart, 1935), 62–63.

3. Ake Hultkrantz, *Shamanic Healing and Ritual Drama* (New York: Crossroad, 1992), 91.

4. George Horse Capture, ed., *The Seven Visions of Bull Lodge* (Ann Arbor, Mich.: Bear Claw Press, 1980), 86–88.

5. Virgil J. Vogel, *American Indian Medicine* (Norman: University of Oklahoma Press, 1982), 187.

6. James Mooney, *Myths of the Cherokee and Sacred Formulas of the Cherokees* (1888; reprint, Nashville, Tenn.: Charles and Randy Elder—Booksellers, 1982), 346.

7. Ibid., 365. Cherokee healers also treat jaundice by pouring a tea blended of wild cherry bark and other herbs on the heated stones of the Sweat Lodge. Wild cherry bark is a common ingredient in Cherokee blood tonics. This herb should only be taken in recommended doses and under the supervision of an experienced herbalist. Wild cherry bark contains small amounts of hydrocyanic acid, a cyanidelike poison.

8. Trudy Griffin-Pierce, *Earth Is My Mother, Sky Is My Father: Space, Time and Astronomy in Navajo Sandpainting* (Albuquerque: University of New Mexico Press, 1992), 43. This book is a beautiful and sensitive introduction to the Diné worldview.

9. See Dr. Burr's *The Fields of Life: Our Links with the Universe* (New York: Ballantine Books, 1972).

10. Healers represented various modalities, including therapeutic touch, European "bioenergy" healing, qigong, and Native American medicine. I was able to produce unusual data while practicing either of the latter two methods. In one experiment involving Native American healing, I imagined fanning a patient, whom I had not met and who was in another room in the building, with a swan's wing. She had no way of knowing what I was thinking. Yet during a recorded interview that took place immediately after the session, she told one of the researchers that she had felt "white feathers" all over her body. I didn't know about this correspondence until a year later, when I read the written report. In several sessions, there was a measurable correlation between my feeling of healing energy coming from a certain direction and electrical spikes recorded on the copper panel in that direction.

One of the outstanding scientists to analyze the Menninger data was William A. Tiller, Ph.D, professor emeritus and former chair of the Department of Materials Science and Engineering at Stanford University. See his *Science and Human Transformation: Subtle Energies, Intentionality and Consciousness* (Walnut Creek, Calif.: Pavior Publishing, 1997). For peer-reviewed journal articles, see Elmer E. Green, Ph.D., et al., "Anomalous Electrostatic Phenomena in Exceptional Subjects," *Subtle Energies* 2, no. 3 (1991): 69–94, and "Gender Differences in a Magnetic Field," *Subtle Energies* 3, no. 2 (1992): 65–103. Also see William Tiller, Ph.D., et al., "Toward Explaining Anomalously Large Body Voltage Surges on Exceptional Subjects," *Journal of Scientific Exploration* 9, no. 3 (1995): 331–50.

11. Experiments conducted at Chinese medical schools, universities, and both military and public hospitals show that qigong healers can emit natural energy (*qi*) from their hands to influence biological processes. For example, they can:

- Shrink malignant brain tumors in mice. (Tonjian Zhao with Caixi Li and Qianhong Xu, "Investigation of Effects of External Energy Waiqi (Emitted Qi) on Gliomas of Mice," *Proceedings of the Third National Academic Conference on Qigong Science* [Guangzhou, China, 1990], 87.)
- Increase survival time among mice infected with leukemia. (Lidong Zhou et al., "Mechanisms of the Anti-tumor Effect of Qigong Waiqi [Emitted Qi]," *Proceedings of the Third National Academic Conference on Qigong Science*, 88.)
- Normalize blood sugar levels in diabetic rats. (Lida Feng, Juqiing Qian, and Liaomin Peng, "An Observation of the Effects of Emitted Qi on Diabetes Mellitus," *Proceedings of the Third World Conference for Academic Exchange of Medical Qigong* [Beijing, 1996], 104.)
- Prevent a dish of cultured rat neurons (not illiterate rat neurons!) from being damaged by normally destructive biochemicals (hydroxyl free radicals). (Yipeng Tang et al., "Protective Effect of Emitted Qi on the Primary Culture of Neurocytes in Vitro against Free Radical Damage," *Proceedings of the Second World Conference for Academic Exchange of Medical Qigong* [Beijing, 1993], 100.)

12. Thomas Buckley, "Doing Your Thinking," in *I Become Part of It: Sacred Dimensions of Native American Life*, ed. D. M. Dooling and Paul Jordan-Smith (San Francisco: HarperSanFrancisco, 1989), 37.

13. Basil Johnston, *Ojibway Heritage* (New York: Columbia University Press, 1976), 15.

14. Bear Heart with Molly Larkin, *The Wind Is My Mother: The Life and Teachings of a Native American Shaman* (New York: Clarkson Potter, 1996), 96.

15. Editors of Time-Life Books, *Keepers of the Totem* (Alexandria, Va.: Time-Life, 1993), 105.

16. Edith Turner, *The Hands Feel It: Healing and Spirit Presence among a Northern Alaskan People*

(De Kalb: Northern Illinois University Press, 1996), 33. To speak of the alignment and positioning of the internal organs makes good scientific sense. We know that internal organs are held in place by fascia, connective tissue, and various factors—such as poor posture, shallow breathing, or emotional stress—can change the tension in fascial tissue, moving the organs. When the organs are out of place, they function less efficiently. In Rolfing, a Western method of deep tissue massage, fascia is pressed and stretched in order to realign bodily structures and return the organs to their natural positions. Osteopathic physicians also use massage techniques to affect organ position and health.

Turner's description of how organs "maintain" spirit is virtually identical to the beliefs of ancient Chinese Taoists. In Taoist philosophy, the organs are considered the dwelling place of the souls. (We each have yang and yin, masculine and feminine, souls.) When the organs are healthy, the souls abide. When the organs are unhealthy, the souls flee. To ensure health, therapies must address both the physical and spiritual aspects of disease. See my book *The Way of Qigong: The Art and Science of Chinese Energy Healing* (New York: Ballantine Books, 1999) and my audio course and study guide *Taoism: Essential Teachings of the Way and Its Power* (Boulder, Colo.: Sounds True, 1998) for further information about Taoist healing practices.

17. Mooney, *Myths of the Cherokee and Sacred Formulas of the Cherokees*, 351.
18. These techniques have extraordinary parallels in China. In 1980, a seventy-year-old Taoist abbot, Huang Gengshi, Ph.D., told me that to be an effective healer, one must prepare oneself with spiritual exercises. He told me that before attempting to transmit *qi*, "healing energy," through his hands, he warmed his hands over a ritual fire in which secret talismans had been burned. Taoists apply clockwise and counterclockwise circles identically to Native Americans. Clockwise circles "tonify," or add energy. Counterclockwise circles "sedate," or reduce excess energy. See my video course and study guide *Qi Healing: Energy Medicine Techniques to Heal Yourself and Others* (Boulder, Colo.: Sounds True, 2000).
19. Jay Miller, *Shamanic Odyssey* (Menlo Park, Calif.: Ballena Press, 1988), 45.
20. Richard Katz, *Boiling Energy: Community Healing among the Kalahari Kung* (Cambridge, Mass.: Harvard University Press, 1982), 110.
21. Robert H. Ruby and John A. Brown, *John Slocum and the Indian Shaker Church* (Norman: University of Oklahoma Press, 1996), 79.
22. I had a personal experience of Brad's shaking power at the 1997 Common Boundary conference on healing and spirituality in Washington, D.C. Brad Keeney and I had both been invited to present lectures. Although we had not been introduced, as soon as our eyes met, we recognized each other. We walked immediately toward each other and embraced with a simultaneous exclamation of "Brother!" My wife was standing nearby and was astonished to see me enthusiastically renew a friendship with a stranger! Brad and I had what the Chinese call *yuan fen*, "destined affinity."

The next day, while eating lunch in the conference hotel restaurant, we discovered remarkable similarities in our spiritual paths. I had trained in Zulu medicine for five years with a student of the Zulu holy man Vusamazulu Credo Mutwa ("Baba"), but unlike Brad, I had never met Baba myself. On the other hand, Brad was interested in the life and teachings of a departed Cree holy man, Grandfather Albert Lightning, and was learning about him from his son. I knew *Mosom*, Grandfather, personally and treasure the beautiful teachings he shared with me.

On the last day of the conference, Brad asked me if he could give me a "gift from the Kalahari." Although I didn't know what he had in mind, I accepted. Brad and I found a quiet corner of the hotel. He placed one of his hands on my upper back and the other opposite on my upper chest. He began to shake vigorously and apparently involuntarily throughout his entire body. His face, shoulders, torso, and feet were vibrating with some invisible power, like a wave that was continuously cresting in his body and crashing and rippling in his fingertips. I felt the trembling power pass through me. Brad whispered African prayers in my ear, which I knew were prayers of blessing and protection.

While receiving this beautiful "gift," I was transported to the Kalahari. I saw the tribal people with whom he had danced; I viewed their villages and landscape. I was in Africa as truly as if I had opened my eyes and found myself physically there.
23. Thomas Waterman, *The Shake Religion of Puget Sound: Smithsonian Annual Report for 1922* (Washington, D.C.: Smithsonian Institution, 1924), 505.

24. Ruby and Brown, *John Slocum and the Indian Shaker Church*, 81.
25. Claude E. Schaeffer, "Blackfoot Shaking Tent," Glenbow-Alberta Institute Occasional Papers (Calgary, Alberta: Glenbow-Alberta Institute, 1969), 6–7.
26. See Brenda Fowler's *Iceman: Uncovering the Life and Times of a Prehistoric Man Found in an Alpine Glacier* (New York: Random House, 2000) for a detailed and engrossing discussion of the Iceman discovery.
27. Josie Glausiusz, "The Ice Man Healeth," *Discover,* February 2000, 16.
28. Thomas E. Mails, *Secret Native American Pathways* (Tulsa, Okla.: Council Oak Books, 1988), 296.
29. Melvin R. Gilmore, *Uses of Plants by the Indians of the Missouri River Region* (1919; reprint, Lincoln: University of Nebraska Press, 1977), 93.
30. James Willard Schultz, *Recently Discovered Tales of Life among the Indians* (Missoula, Mont.: Mountain Press Publishing Co., 1988), 63.
31. Adolf Hungry Wolf, *Teachings of Nature: Good Medicine Book No. 14* (Invermere, British Columbia: Good Medicine Books, 1975), 16.
32. Herbert Benson, M.D., and David P. McCallie Jr., "Angina Pectoris and the Placebo Effect," *New England Journal of Medicine* 300, no. 25 (June 21, 1979), 1424–29.
33. Hilda Neihardt and Lori Utecht, eds., *Black Elk Lives: Conversations with the Black Elk Family* (Lincoln: University of Nebraska Press, 2000), 141.
34. F. G. Speck, *Midwinter Rites of the Cayuga Long House* (Philadelphia: University of Pennsylvania Press, 1949), 110.
35. Peter M. Knudtson, *The Wintun Indians of California and Their Neighbors* (Happy Camp, Calif.: Naturegraph Publishers, 1977), 63.
36. Ann Fienup-Riordan, *The Living Tradition of Yup'ik Masks: Agayuliyararput—Our Way of Making Prayer* (Seattle: University of Washington Press, 1996), 191.
37. Personal communication, Taoist abbot Huang Gengshi, 1977.
38. Mooney, *Myths of the Cherokee and Sacred Formulas of the Cherokees*, 358. Although Mooney was unable to identify this herb, which the medicine man described as "yellow rooted grass," recent Cherokee herbals identify it as either yellow dock (*Rumex crispus*, or *Dalonige unasdedla* in Cherokee), traditionally used as an astringent and a disinfectant for skin sores, or yellow root (Latin name, *Xanthorhiza simplicissima*, or *Dalanei* in Cherokee), a gargle for mouth ulcers and pyorrhea. In *The Green Pharmacy* (Emmaus, Pa.: Rodale Press, 1997), 438, botanist and former U.S. Department of Agriculture researcher James A. Duke, Ph.D., writes that yellow dock is a potent antibiotic and antibacterial.
39. Karl H. Schlesier, *The Wolves of Heaven* (Norman: University of Oklahoma Press, 1987), 15.
40. Bear Heart with Larkin, *The Wind Is My Mother*, 96.
41. David E. Jones, *Sanapia: Comanche Medicine Woman* (Prospect Heights, Ill.: Waveland Press, 1984), 50.
42. A. L. Kroeber, *Handbook of the Indians of California* (New York: Dover Publications, 1976), 424.
43. Chinese acupuncturists treat both back pain and hemorrhoids by pricking points on the lower back. Nigerian Igbo healers rub a turtle shell on the back to relieve back pain.
44. Exodus 28: 17–21 describes twelve stones, symbolizing the twelve tribes of Israel, in the breastplate of the high priest of the Jews. Several of them are crystalline quartzes, including agate, amethyst, onyx, and jasper. Jewish scholars believe that the twelve stones had mystical properties that inspired the priest to prophetic statements on the Day of Atonement (Yom Kippur). Popular early European books on the healing properties of stones include the sixth-century Latin work *De virtutibus lapidum* (On the powers of stones), by Damigeron, and Albertus Magnus's (d. 1279) *Book of Secrets*, published in the sixteenth century in England, where it remained an influential work throughout the Elizabethan period. See Michael R. Best and Frank H. Brightman, eds., *The Book of Secrets of Albertus Magnus: Of the Virtues of Herbs, Stones and Certain Beasts, Also a Book of the Marvels of the World* (London: Oxford University Press, 1973).
45. C. Norman Shealy, M.D., Ph.D., et al., "Non-pharmaceutical Treatment of Depression Using a Multimodal Approach," *Subtle Energies* 4, no. 2 (1993): 125–34. Also see Dr. Shealy's *Miracles Do Happen: A Physician's Experience with Alternative Medicine* (Rockport, Mass.: Element Books, 1995), 203–4.

46. The technique is called CES, cranial electrical stimulation, and it is often helpful for depression. It raises blood levels of beta-endorphins (associated with positive moods) and serotonin (often low in depression), which enhances feelings of security, self-worth, calm, and resilience.

47. Brain-wave synchronization using 10-hertz photostimulation.

48. My elders taught me to keep quartz in a pouch or, when placed on an altar, covered with a cloth. It is taken out of its covering only when the healer is in a calm and clear state of mind and when it is actually needed. Quartz should be used cautiously because it can amplify an angry mood as well as a positive prayer.

49. John G. Neihardt, *Black Elk Speaks: Being the Life Story of a Holy Man of the Oglala Sioux* (New York: Morrow, 1932), 204–5.

11: THE PALEOLITHIC POSTURE

1. Stanley Krippner and Jürgen Kremer published a critique of Dr. Goodman's work in the journal *ReVision* ("Trance Postures," *ReVision* 16, no. 4 [spring 1994]: 173–82). The authors contend that Goodman does not present sufficient evidence for the past or present existence of trance postures among indigenous cultures. Perhaps the approximately twenty-six postures that Goodman has identified in worldwide indigenous art represent not trance postures but animal imitation, preparations for tribal ceremonies, or just pragmatic and customary postures that are used for other activities such as prayer, drug ingestion, or conversation. The authors attempted to replicate Goodman's results on three occasions by directing students to hold trance postures and then scientifically analyzing their reported experiences with psychological scales and questionnaires. They did not find a consistent correlation between the reports of the test subjects and Goodman's descriptions of the expected effects of the postures.

Dr. Goodman has admirably defended her position in her unpublished paper "Some Critical Comments on 'Trance Postures' by Jürgen Kremer and Stanley Krippner." She notes that it may be impossible to conclusively answer questions about the past practice of trance postures because of the lack of written records. She does cite, however, several examples of continuing present practice among the Matsigenka Indians of east Peru, shamans of Uzbekistan, Australian aborigines, and African diviners. She also sees evidence of trance posture in Native American folk tales and art.

I believe that there is merit to both the critique and Goodman's response. According to Goodman's published works, trance postures shape human experience and may be as essential a feature of trance induction as drumming, dancing, or other ritual activities. She discusses the postures as features of healing, divination, and spiritual transformation. Although it is unlikely that the trance postures were ever practiced as a formalized or decontextualized exercise, as Goodman teaches them in workshops and classes, this does not lessen their value. Postures tap into common aspects of human physiology and consciousness, helping both Western and non-Western people to renew their experience of the Sacred. Kremer and Krippner are right that "Goodman may have unearthed a human potential not used previously in this particular way."

The answer to the question of "whether Goodman has rediscovered lost practices or developed a new ritual behavior" hinges on how we define *practices*. Trance postures are certainly part of ritual behaviors. In the 1920s, Knud Rasmussen (1879–1933) wrote in one of his classic descriptions of Greenland spiritual traditions, "There were also certain positions which the shaman had to adopt at particular moments. If the shaman was to journey through the air, the handle of the drum had to rest against his big toe at the moment he was to rush out of the house" ("An Angmagssalik Shaman's Magic Drum Seance, Edited from Notes Left by Knud Rasmussen," *Shaman's Drum* 49 [summer 1998]: 63–64). Among the Tsimshian, ritual postures were associated with four secret shamanic societies. Scholar John Cove gives a brief description of these postures, drawing on earlier manuscripts of William Beynon: "A person belonging to *mitla* [Dancers] would hold right hand over heart and left hand extended as far as elbow with forearm raised. A person belonging to the *xgedem* [Cannibals] would have right hand over heart and left hand fully extended. *Nuhlim:* a person belonging to this group [Dog Eaters] would extend both hands upraised" (John Cove, *Shattered Images: Dialogues and Meditations on Tsimshian Narratives*, Carleton University Library

Series 139 [Ottawa, Ontario: Carleton University Library, 1987], 255). Clearly, these postures are linked with trance experience. They were "practiced" but only in a specific cultural context.

Some of Goodman's postures are "snapshots" taken in the midst of action, such as a ritual dance or a hunter's supplication. Their representations in rock art are also stills of significant or repeated postural motifs. The fact that these postures may not have been deliberately or regularly practiced as unmoving poses does not lessen their importance within those ceremonies or to the experience of trance.

Does the altered state of consciousness cause one to hold the body in a certain fashion, or does the altered posture induce a change of consciousness? You can start from either end. When I studied the Feldenkrais technique of postural and neurological education, I was fascinated to discover that merely imitating the movements associated with prayer in various religions evokes changes in consciousness. Each type of movement—whether it be Buddhist bowing, Jewish chanting (while rocking the body), or Sufi twirling—awakens an expanded, reverent, and distinct state of mind.

The link between posture and consciousness was probably intuitively understood by most hunter-gatherers. When people stand perfectly still for long periods of time while observing nature and waiting for prey, their minds change. They become the forest, the wind, the animals they hunt. The ancient Chinese explored these principles in considerable detail and have always used static postures, sometimes individually held for an hour at a time, to induce changes in consciousness. According to Chinse Taoism, expertise in healing, martial arts, and meditation requires physical and mental stability.

The most important and inspiring defense Goodman makes of her work is a transpersonal one. Goodman wonders about the validity of test results in a classroom or laboratory versus results achieved when postures are practiced with the *purpose* of contacting a spiritual or an alternate reality. Goodman clearly accepts the validity of an alternate reality:

> In our seventeen years of work with ritual-posture complex, we experienced over and over again that when we first tried a new posture, the "other side" enthusiastically awarded us the richest of details. . . . [W]e do not approach the spirits in the manner of a SWAT team—or a psychological test team, which is pretty much the same thing—but rather invite them respectfully to work with us.
>
> Felicitas D. Goodman, "Some Critical Comments on *Trance Postures* by Jürgen Kremer and Stanley Krippner," an unpublished paper sent to me by Dr. Goodman, 1994, 23.

2. Charles V. W. Brooks, *Sensory Awareness: The Rediscovery of Experiencing* (New York: Viking, 1974), 229–30.

3. Karl W. Luckert, *The Navajo Hunter Tradition* (Tucson: University of Arizona Press, 1975), 63.

4. Ibid.

5. For an excellent discussion of this and other bodily positions in Algonquin rock art, see Joan M. Vastokas and Romas K. Vastokas, *Sacred Art of the Algonkians: A Study of the Peterborough Petroglyphs* (Peterborough, Ontario: Mansard Press, 1973).

6. Peter Nabokov, *Indian Running: Native American History and Tradition* (Santa Fe, N.M.: Ancient City Press, 1981), 144–45.

7. H. Henrietta Stockel, *Women of the Apache Nation: Voices of Truth* (Reno: University of Nevada Press, 1991), 41.

8. Maureen Trudelle Schwarz, *Molded in the Image of Changing Woman: Navajo Views on the Human Body and Personhood* (Tucson: University of Arizona Press, 1997), 10.

9. Alex Stacoff with Jürg Steger, Edgar Stüssi, and Christoph Reinschmidt, "Lateral Stability in Sideward Cutting Movements," *Medicine and Science in Sports and Exercise* 28, no. 3 (1996): 350–58.

    Steven E. Robbins and Gerard J. Gouw, "Athletic Footwear: Unsafe Due to Perceptual Illusions," *Medicine and Science in Sports and Exercise* 23, no. 2 (1991): 217–24, and "Athletic Footwear and Chronic Overloading," *Sports Medicine* 9, no. 2 (1990): 76–85.

    Udaya Bhaskara Rao and Benjamin Joseph, "The Influence of Footwear on the Prevalence of Flat Foot," *Journal of Bone and Joint Surgery* 74B, no. 4 (1992): 525–27.

    Steven E. Robbins and Adel M. Hanna, "Running-Related Injury Prevention through Barefoot Adaptations," *Medicine and Science in Sports and Exercise* 19, no. 2 (1987): 148–56.

Steele F. Stewart, "Footgear—Its History, Uses and Abuses," *Clinical Orthopaedics and Related Research* 88 (1972): 119–30.

Samuel B. Shulman, "Survey in China and India of Feet That Have Never Worn Shoes," *Journal of the National Association of Chiropodists* 49 (1949): 26–30.

Also see www.barefooters.org.

10. Robbins and Gouw, "Athletic Footwear," cited in www.unshod.org.

11. Ibid.

12. For a succinct description of warrior power and spiritual practices among the Yurok, see Thomas Buckley, "Yurok Doctors and the Concept of 'Shamanism,' " in *California Indian Shamanism*, ed. Lowell John Bean (Menlo Park, Calif.: Ballena Press, 1992), 117–55. "Certain men acquired guardian spirits that imbued them with extra-ordinary bravery and fighting skills through vision questing in power-places" (p. 128).

12: UNFOLDING THE MYSTERY: SWEAT LODGE AND SACRED PIPE

1. Frank Waters, *Masked Gods: Navajo and Pueblo Ceremonialism* (New York: Ballantine Books, 1950), 324.

2. Sandra Ingerman, *Medicine for the Earth: How to Transform Personal and Environmental Toxins* (New York: Three Rivers Press, 2000), 265.

3. The details and spiritual/ethical implications of this ritual are detailed in Ingerman's inspiring book. I personally witnessed a cup of water mixed with ammonium hydroxide, a common pollutant, change from a deadly pH level of 12 to a nonfatal level of 9 after a one-hour ceremony. A non-prayed-for control, kept isolated in another room under identical conditions of temperature and light, remained unchanged. Chemists claim that such a transformation is impossible, yet it happens, and Ingerman has repeated the experiment, with similarly impressive results, many times. Interestingly, the transformation only occurs when a group of people perform the ritual. A single person is ineffective. We need one another to transform the world and to survive. What a wonderful teaching!

4. Malidoma Patrice Somé, *Ritual: Power, Healing and Community* (Portland, Oreg.: Swan Raven & Company, 1993), 90.

5. Joseph Campbell, *Myths to Live By* (New York: Viking, 1972), 98.

6. Perhaps the story of Abraham and Isaac illustrates that God's command was not meant to be followed but, rather, to remind people of the dangers of blind faith. The great author and humanitarian Elie Wiesel writes in *Messengers of God: Biblical Portraits and Legends* (New York: Simon & Schuster, 1976), "All things considered, Abraham was perhaps wrong in obeying, or even in making believe that he was obeying." Abraham was participating in an injustice by "including Isaac in an equation he could not comprehend, by playing with Isaac's suffering . . ." (p. 94). Wiesel also discusses another dimension of the story: Isaac, *Yitzhak* in Hebrew, means "he who will laugh." Isaac survives a horrific trauma; he probably spent the rest of his life haunted by images of his holocaust, yet he laughs. The lesson? "[T]hat it is possible to suffer and despair an entire lifetime and still not give up the art of laughter. . . . [H]e [Isaac] remained capable of laughter. And in spite of everything, he did laugh" (p. 97).

7. Arval Looking Horse, "The Sacred Pipe in Modern Life," in *Sioux Indian Religion: Tradition and Innovation*, ed. Raymond J. DeMallie and Douglas R. Parks (Norman: University of Oklahoma Press, 1987), 69.

8. Robert S. McPherson, "Of Metaphors and Learning: Navajo Teachings for Today's Youth," *American Indian Quarterly* 22, no. 4 (fall 1998): 461.

9. James Mooney has the clearest description of the river purification ceremony. ("The Cherokee River Cult," *Journal of American Folk-Lore* 13 [1900]: 1–10.) The river is addressed as "Long Man," *Yunwi Gunahita*, a giant whose head is in the mountains and whose feet extend to the lowlands or valleys.

At regular intervals, usually at each recurring new moon, it is customary among the more religiously disposed of the old conservatives, for the whole family to go down together at daybreak, and fasting, to the river and stand with bare feet just touching the water, while the priest, or, if properly instructed, the father of the household, stands behind them and recites a prayer for each in turn, after which they plunge in and bathe their whole bodies in the river.

Alternately, river water can be dipped in the hands and sprinkled on the body. Mooney states that going to water was part of every important tribal function. It was (and still is) used to confer blessings, health, and longevity and during "conjuring" rituals, such as invocations recited near a river, to combat sorcery and neutralize the power of nightmares.

Going to water was practiced all year long. If the river were frozen, a hole would be broken in the ice. I have a Cherokee friend who plunged every day of his youth. As a result, today, at age fifty, he is healthy and strong and has an extraordinary tolerance to cold. I have walked with him in zero-degree (Fahrenheit) temperatures, I shivering in my down parka and he comfortably sweating in his T-shirt!

10. The *mikvah*, the ritual purification bath of the Jews, is also referred to as a womb for spiritual rebirth. It is taken before important ceremonies and as a monthly purification after menstruation. Rabbi Aryeh Kaplan writes, "In many ways, the mikvah represents the womb. When a person immerses, it is as if he has momentarily returned to the womb. Then, when he emerges, it is as if he were reborn. He is then like a completely new person" (*Made in Heaven: A Jewish Wedding Guide* [Brooklyn, N.Y.: Moznaim Publishing Corp., 1983], 77).

11. Harold Littlebird, *On Mountain's Breath* (Santa Fe, N.M.: Tooth of Time Books, 1982), 11. Littlebird has produced exceptional audiotapes of his poetry and songs, including: *The Road Back In: Song and Poetry of Remembrance* (Peralta, N.M.: Littlebird Studios, 1987) and *A Circle Begins: Poetry and Song by Harold Littlebird* (Peralta, N.M.: Littlebird Studios, 1985). They may be ordered from Harold Littlebird, 6 Buskirk Lane, Peralta, NM 87042.

12. Information on the Maricopa from Time-Life Books, *The Way of the Warrior* (Alexandria, Va.: Time-Life Books, 1993), 104–7.

13. Jay Miller, ed., *Mourning Dove: A Salishan Autobiography* (Lincoln: University of Nebraska Press, 1990), 36.

14. One does not, however, generally enter the *Temazcal* during menstruation. See the essay "Temazcal," by Dr. Horacio Rojas Alba, of the Instituto Mexicano de Medicinas Tradicionales, published on the Web in *Tlahui-Medic* 2, no. 2 (1996), www.tlahui.com/medic/medic2/index.html, a Web site about traditional and alternative medicines in Mexico.

15. A good example is the Huaqing Hot Springs near Xi'an, in central China. It was built into a resort during the Western Zhou dynasty (1027–771 B.C.), was a favorite spa during the Tang dynasty (A.D. 618–907), and is still enjoyed today.

16. See Joseph Bruchac's excellent book *The Native American Sweat Lodge: History and Legends* (Freedom, Calif.: Crossing Press, 1993).

17. See Carmen Blacker, *The Catalpa Bow: A Study of Shamanistic Practices in Japan* (London: George Allen & Unwin, 1975), 317–18.

18. Robert L. Hall, *An Archaeology of the Soul: North American Indian Belief and Ritual* (Urbana: University of Illinois Press, 1997), 125–26.

19. Jeanne Achterberg, *Imagery in Healing: Shamanism and Modern Medicine* (Boston: Shambhala Publications, 1985), 34. Also see Leon Chaitow, N.D., D.O., *Antibiotic Crisis: Antibiotic Alternatives* (London: HarperCollins, 1998), 170–74.

20. Dr. Chaitow discusses the benefits as well as some of the dangers of heat therapy in his book (*Antibiotic Crisis*, 173). As a medical treatment, it should be supervised by a physician. I am personally heat-sensitive and easily develop heat exhaustion if I am under a hot summer sun for more than a half hour. Yet, strangely, I do not experience this problem in the Sweat Lodge.

21. Ralph W. Moss, Ph.D., *Cancer Therapy: The Independent Consumer's Guide to Non-Toxic Treatment and Prevention* (Brooklyn, N.Y.: Equinox Press, 1992), 377.

22. Philip L. Hooper, M.D., "Hot-Tub Therapy for Type 2 Diabetes Mellitus," letter to the editor, *New England Journal of Medicine* 341, no. 12 (1999): 924–25.

23. Some Lakota believe that the Itazipco—literally, "No Bows" (often called by their French name, "Sans Arcs")—were given the Pipe because they were so destitute that they didn't even have bows and arrows: the Great Spirit pitied them and gave them the Sacred Pipe for spiritual sustenance. I

heard a different explanation from a very wise, non-Lakota elder and pipe carrier: the No Bows were thus called because, *by choice*, they hunted with primitive weapons such as the spear and at-latl. Because they valued simplicity and were against technology—perhaps their medicine people foresaw its future misuse—they were the proper caretakers for the Pipe.

24. Joseph Epes Brown, ed., *The Sacred Pipe: Black Elk's Account of the Seven Rites of the Oglala Sioux* (Norman: University of Oklahoma Press, 1953), 5–6. The quote in the next sentence is from page 7.

25. Some Europeans call the pipe a calumet, from the medieval French *chalamel* or *chalumeau*, mean-ing "reed." The Lakota term for a sacred pipe, *Canunpa*, is becoming increasingly common in English.

26. Peter J. Powell, *Sweet Medicine: The Continuing Role of the Sacred Arrows, the Sun Dance, and the Sacred Buffalo Hat in Northern Cheyenne History*, vol. 1 (Norman: University of Oklahoma Press, 1969), 120.

27. Keewaydinoquay, "*Mukwah Miskomin or Kinnickinnick*, 'Gift of the Bear,' " unpublished manu-script, 1977, 16, kindly sent to me by Grandmother "Kee."

28. William M. Thackeray, *Sketches and Travels in London* (1856).

13: TOBACCO: WICKED WEED OR GIFT OF THE GODS?

1. Belief in the Little People is widespread in Native North America. The Blackfoot of Montana say that the spirit of tobacco *is* a Little Person. Men and their wives plant the tobacco seeds together. At the end of the planting season, the man places a stick in the center of their plot on which he ties a pair of tiny moccasins and a pouch of tobacco seeds, gifts for the Little People.

2. Francis Robicsek, *The Smoking Gods: Tobacco in Maya Art, History, and Religion* (Norman: University of Oklahoma Press, 1978), 31.

3. An exceptional organization that educates people about the culture, history, and dangers of to-bacco is the Traditional Native American Tobacco Seed Bank and Education Program (TNAT). TNAT also provides Native Americans with native tobacco leaves and seeds at no cost, as long as they agree to use the tobacco respectfully and in a traditional manner. TNAT, University of New Mexico, 1717 Lomas Blvd. NE, Albuquerque, NM 87131.

4. Julian Lang, "The Divine Origin of Tobacco," *Winds of Change* 12, no. 3 (summer 1997): 57. Reprinted from *News from Native California* 9, no. 3 (spring 1996).

5. For example, a medicine person trained in conjuring may turn a person from evil to good, influ-ence court decisions, or make a hunter more successful.

6. Donald M. Bahr et al., eds., *Piman Shamanism and Staying Sickness* (Tucson: University of Arizona Press, 1974), 198.

7. Vladimir N. Basilov, "Chosen by the Spirits," in *Shamanic Worlds: Rituals and Lore of Siberia and Central Asia*, ed. Marjorie Mandelstam Balzer (Armonk, N.Y.: M. E. Sharpe, 1997), 11.

8. Sarangerel, *Chosen by the Spirits: Following Your Shamanic Calling* (Rochester, Vt.: Destiny Books, 2001), 170.

9. R. Gordon Wasson, *Soma: Divine Mushroom of Immortality* (New York: Harcourt, Brace & World, 1968), 333. Perhaps the most striking example of a parallel medicinal application of tobacco is found in the medicine of India, *Ayurveda*. Tobacco was carried to India by Portuguese sailors, pre-sumably without instructions for its use. Tobacco was quickly accepted by Indian folk medicine. The smoke was blown in the ear for earaches, over swollen joints to reduce pain, and on the gums for toothache—exactly as tobacco had been used by Native Americans. A tobacco poultice was used to treat insect bites, swellings, and skin diseases. Again, this is astonishingly similar to to-bacco's use by Native Americans. See Robert E. Svoboda, *Ayurveda: Life, Health and Longevity* (New York: Penguin, 1992), 216.

10. Some African tribes use tobacco in a fashion similar to Native Americans. The Igbo of Nigeria pray to their *agbara*, "protecting spirits," to empower *utaba* (*Nicotiana tabacum*) before they apply the leaves to dental cavities.

11. Jean Nicot, *Dictionnaire Franco-Latin* (Paris: 1573), 478.

12. Svoboda, *Ayurveda*, 216.

13. As an isolated chemical, the nicotine in tobacco is extremely dangerous. If the nicotine in one small cigar were extracted and injected into an adult's body, it would kill him. Two drops (60–120 milligrams) placed on the skin is equally deadly.

14. Robert Freedman, M.D., et al., "Schizophrenia and Nicotinic Receptors," *Harvard Review of Psychiatry* 2, no. 4 (1994): 189.

15. James H. Austin, M.D., *Zen and the Brain: Toward an Understanding of Meditation and Consciousness* (Cambridge, Mass.: MIT Press, 1998), 169.

16. The connection between tobacco and hallucinogens is recognized by the Indians of Central America and the Amazon. Mexican Tarahumara Indians consider tobacco the most important shamanic aid next to peyote and more powerful than datura. Amazonian tribal healers commonly add tobacco to brews containing the powerful hallucinogenic vine *ayahuasca* and believe that although ayahuasca aids shamanic vision, tobacco is the true source of their power. See Jonathan Ott, *Pharmacotheon: Entheogenic Drugs, Their Plant Sources and History* (Kennewick, Wash.: Natural Products Co., 1996), 373–74.

17. John B. Little, M.D., et al., "Distribution of Polonium in Pulmonary Tissues of Cigarette Smokers," *New England Journal of Medicine* 273 (December 16, 1965): 1350, and John B. Little and Edward P. Radford Jr., "Polonium 210 in Bronchial Epithelium of Cigarette Smokers," *Science* 155 (February 3, 1967): 606.

18. Marie Brady, R.T., "Radiologic Technologist Examines Radioactivity from Cigarette Smoke," an interview with Gustave F. Kilthau, M.R.T., *Nurse Week/Health Week*, June 1, 1996, p. 2.

19. Tobaccos grown in less contaminated environments and without high-phosphate fertilizers have a much lower polonium concentration. Tobaccos grown in India, for example, have less than 20 percent the polonium of American tobaccos. This may help explain why some tobaccos cause less cancer.

20. John B. Little, Ann R. Kennedy, and Robert B. McGandy, "Lung Cancer Induced in Hamsters by Low Doses of Alpha Radiation from Polonium-210," *Science* 188 (May 16, 1975): 737–38. Also see the same authors' "Effect of Dose Distribution on the Induction of Experimental Lung Cancer by Alpha Radiation," *Health Physics* 35 (November 1978): 595–606.

21. See the works cited in notes 17 and 20. Additional evidence can be found in:
    - Edward P. Radford Jr. and Vilma R. Hunt, "Polonium-210: A Volatile Radioelement in Cigarettes," *Science* 143 (January 17, 1964): 247–49.
    - Edward P. Radford Jr. and Vilma R. Hunt, "Cigarettes and Polonium-210," *Science* 144 (April 24, 1964): 366–67.
    - Edward P. Radford Jr., Vilma R. Hunt, and John B. Little, "Carcinogenicity of Tobacco-Smoke Constituents," *Science* 165 (July 18, 1969): 312.
    - Edward A. Martell, "Tobacco Radioactivity and Cancer in Smokers," *American Scientist* 63 (July–August 1975): 404–12.
    - Edward P. Radford and Edward A. Martell, "Polonium-210: Lead-210 Ratios as an Index of Residence Times of Insoluble Particles from Cigarette Smoke in Bronchial Epithelium," in *Inhaled Particles*, vol. 4, ed. W. H. Walton (Oxford, U.K.: Pergamon Press, 1977), 567–81.
    - Michael Castleman, "Are Cigarettes Radioactive?" *Medical Self-Care* 10 (fall 1980): 20–23.

14: PLANT PEOPLE: THE HEALING POWER OF HERBS

1. See the classic and enjoyable works of Peter Tompkins and Christopher Bird, *The Secret Life of Plants* (New York: HarperCollins, 1989), and *Secrets of the Soil: New Solutions for Restoring Our Planet* (Anchorage, Alaska: Earthpulse Press, 1998).

2. Ralph S. Solecki, "Shanidar IV: A Neanderthal Flower Burial in Northern Iraq," *Science* 190 (1975): 880–81.

3. The Sumerians lived in Mesopotamia, on the delta flats of the Tigris and Euphrates Rivers, generally considered the birthplace of Western civilization. Interestingly, more than 95 percent of their writings deal with economic matters—receipts, bills of sale, partnership agreements, wills, and

wages. The West's economic obsession goes back that far! See Samuel Noah Kramer's *Sumerian Mythology: A Study of Spiritual and Literary Achievement in the Third Millennium* B.C., rev. ed. (Philadelphia: University of Pennsylvania Press, 1998).

4. Natural antibiotics are far more common than most people suspect. The journal *Economic Botany* reported that when 2,222 plants were tested, some antimicrobial properties were found in 1,362 of them. (L. G. Nickell, "Antimicrobial Activity of Vascular Plants," *Economic Botany* 13 [1959]: 281–318.)

5. Henry S. Burrage, ed., *Early English and French Voyages* (New York: Charles Scribner's Sons, 1906), 75.

6. Logan Clendening, *Source Book of Medical History* (New York: Paul B. Hoeber, Inc., 1942), 464. Although the Native Americans did not know about vitamin C, they followed a diet that prevented its depletion. Natural Indian remedies for scurvy were common and were frequently adopted by non-Indians. During the California gold rush of 1849, prospectors drank Indian spruce tea to prevent scurvy.

7. In the 1840s, John Hoxsey, a horse breeder in southern Illinois, saw one of his prize stallions cure its tumorous growth by deliberately eating certain plants in the pasture. He combined those herbs with others to create three medications, one taken internally that contained burdock, red clover, licorice, and other herbs that have a long history of usage among Native Americans, and two others applied externally, like a topical ointment, to burn off skin tumors. One of the external formulas includes bloodroot, used topically for dermatological conditions and skin cancer by the Cherokee, Haudenosaunee, and many other tribes. In *When Healing Becomes a Crime: The Amazing Story of the Hoxsey Cancer Clinics and the Return of Alternative Therapies* (Rochester, Vt.: Healing Arts Press, 2000), author and filmmaker Kenny Ausubel writes, "Because 1840 Illinois was also Indian country at the western frontier of the nation, John Hoxsey most likely had contact with Native American healers who used herbs extensively and maintained wide-ranging continental trade routes that brought remote plants into general circulation" (p. 193). It is thus reasonable to assume that Hoxsey learned about some of the herbs in his formulas from Native healers. Hoxsey successfully treated other horses with cancer and became known for his gift of healing. He passed the formula on to his descendants. His grandson, veterinarian John C. Hoxsey, used the formula to treat animal and, sometimes, human tumors.

John's son, Harry Hoxsey (1901–1974), continued the family tradition with work on human cancer patients. He opened several cancer clinics, and at the peak of his popularity in the 1950s, the self-educated healer directed seventeen clinics throughout the United States. Hoxsey's unorthodox methods put him in conflict with the American Medical Association and the Food and Drug Administration. In spite of frequent successes, including the long-term survival of many "terminal" patients, the courts ruled that the only legal ways to treat cancer were surgery, radiation, and chemotherapy. In 1960, all Hoxsey clinics were shut down. One Hoxsey clinic, called "The Bio-Medical Clinic," still functions today in Tijuana, Mexico. (In the United States, the first major review of Hoxsey patient records did not occur until 1999, and a comprehensive study of the Hoxsey method has yet to be conducted!)

Essiac tea was named and popularized by a Canadian nurse, Rene M. Caisse (1888–1978). *Essiac* is *Caisse* spelled backward. In 1922, while working as a surgical nurse at Sisters of Providence Hospital in Haileybury, Ontario, Caisse met an eighty-year-old female patient who had a scar on her breast, the only visible sign of a breast cancer she had thirty years earlier. The woman told Nurse Caisse that she had rejected her doctor's recommendation for a mastectomy and instead consulted an Anishinabe medicine man who prescribed an herbal "holy drink" twice a day. Her cancer had gradually diminished in size and disappeared. The medicine man gave the woman the formula, and she gave it to Caisse.

In the mid-1930s, Caisse left her nursing job to open a cancer clinic in Bracebridge, Ontario, north of Toronto, where she treated patients with the drink, now renamed Essiac tea. She also began commuting regularly to Chicago, where she treated cancer patients at the Tumor Clinic of Northwestern University Medical School. In 1939, when the Canadian Royal Cancer Commission investigated Essiac, there were so many patient witnesses that a massive hotel ballroom had to be used as a waiting room. Today, patients continue to report incredible results, including cures from advanced cancers of the bladder, breast, and prostate. In his *Herbs against Cancer: History and*

Controversy (Brooklyn, N.Y.: Equinox Press, 1998), Ralph W. Moss, Ph.D., cites an unpublished Israeli study of 162 cancer patients treated with Essiac. Fifty percent of the patients experienced relief from the side effects of chemotherapy; tumors regressed in 20 percent; and 2.5 percent were completely cured on Essiac alone.

Essiac tea contains traditional Native American herbs that, individually, demonstrate verifiable effects against cancer, including burdock and sheep sorrel. It has avoided legal censure because, unlike the Hoxsey formula, Essiac is very gentle, has low toxicity, and is generally considered safe to take without supervision. Today, it is available at most health food stores in North America, marketed as a gentle "body purifier" that helps the body heal itself. As with the Hoxsey formula, it has not been adequately evaluated in the clinic or laboratory.

I believe that science will never fully verify the efficacy of the Hoxsey formula, Essiac, or other herbal cures taken in whole or in part from Native peoples. The herbs were originally gathered and used with prayer. From the Native viewpoint, when a traditional herbal formula is published and popularized, its power is diluted. The healing power of herbs is also adversely affected when they are objects of negative thinking produced by economic and power struggles between healers and medical or governmental institutions.

For insight into the Hoxsey and Essiac formulas and controversies surrounding them, see the two excellent books cited earlier: Ralph W. Moss's *Herbs against Cancer* and Kenny Ausubel's *When Healing Becomes a Crime*.

8. Virgil J. Vogel, *American Indian Medicine* (Norman: University of Oklahoma Press, 1970), 267.

9. Jews were notable exceptions. Their religion requires bathing regularly and washing the hands before eating.

10. Alev Lytle Croutier, *Taking the Waters: Spirit, Art, Sensuality* (New York: Abbeville Press, 1992), 96.

11. Ivan Illich, *Medical Nemesis: The Expropriation of Health* (New York: Random House, 1976), 156–57.

12. "For more than a century, analysis of disease trends has shown that the environment is the primary determinant of the state of general health of any population" (Illich, *Medical Nemesis*, 17). There is no need to repeat here the evidence Illich presents from works in medical anthropology and epidemiology. In *Betrayal of Trust: The Collapse of Global Public Health*, Pulitzer Prize–winning journalist Laurie Garrett writes that in the United Kingdom, infectious diseases declined by 87 percent between 1838 and 1949, before antibiotics were introduced. "The same can be said for the United States," she writes, "where less than 4 percent of the total improvement in life expectancy since the 1700s can be credited to twentieth century advances in medical care" (p. 18).

13. One of the best-known laws prohibiting Native American religions was the "Rules for Indian Courts," issued August 27, 1892, by the U.S. commissioner of Indian affairs, Thomas J. Morgan. Included in this ruling is article 4(a):

> Dances, etc.—Any Indian who shall engage in the sun dance, scalp dance, or war dance, or any other similar feast, so called, shall be deemed guilty of an offense, and upon conviction thereof shall be punished for the first offense by the withholding of his rations for not exceeding ten days or by imprisonment for not exceeding ten days. . . .

The sentences became more severe with repeated offenses. Article 4(c) condemns *all* Native spiritual practices:

> Practices of medicine men.—Any Indian who shall engage in the practices of so-called medicine men, or who shall resort to any artifice or device to keep the Indians of the reservation from adopting and following civilized habits and pursuits, or shall adopt any means to prevent the attendance of children at school, or shall use any arts of a conjurer to prevent Indians from abandoning their barbarous rites and customs, shall be deemed guilty of an offense. . . .

Conviction of a first offense required ten to thirty days' imprisonment.

The federal government demonstrated mild tolerance of Native spirituality in 1934, when another commissioner of Indian affairs, John Collier, issued a policy statement, "Indian Religious Freedom and Indian Culture" (Bureau of Indian Affairs circular 2970), that advised no interference with "Indian religious life or ceremonial expression." The federal government made no guarantee of Native Americans' First Amendment rights, the freedom of worship pledged by the U.S.

Constitution, until the "American Indian Religious Freedom Act," passed by joint resolution of Congress in 1978. Yet even today, Native people are often denied access to their sacramental herbs (such as peyote) and to their sacred sites, which they are unable to protect from tourism, mining, or other forms of development.

In Canada, the "Potlatch laws," passed in 1884–1885, prohibited the "wasteful" and "degrading" custom of Potlatches, ceremonial gift giving, as well as the Winter Spirit Dances and other Native spiritual performances or activities. Offenders received two months in prison, and the goods seized, including many beautiful works of art, ended up in Canadian and United States museums. The Potlatch laws were not repealed until 1951.

14. See Maureen K. Lux, *Medicine That Walks: Disease, Medicine, and Canadian Plains Native People, 1880–1940* (Toronto, Ontario: University of Toronto Press, 2001). Lux, a postdoctoral fellow at the Hannah Institute for the History of Medicine, shows, convincingly, that the epidemics would not have been as devastating to Native populations if not accompanied by the deadly Euro-American assault on Native culture.

15. David Wallace Adams, *Education for Extinction: American Indians and the Boarding School Experience, 1875–1928* (Lawrence: University Press of Kansas, 1995), 133.

16. Amadeo M. Rea, *Folk Mammalogy of the Northern Pimans* (Tucson: University of Arizona Press, 1998), 31.

17. James W. Herrick, *Iroquois Medical Botany* (Syracuse, N.Y.: Syracuse University Press, 1995), 69.

18. Jennie Goodrich, Claudia Lawson, and Vana Parrish Lawson, *Kashaya Pomo Plants* (Berkeley, Calif.: Heyday Books, 1980), 20.

19. Mohegan author Gladys Tantaquidgeon divides Leni-Lenape herbal medicines into two categories: simple and compound. Simple remedies contain 1 to 3 herbs. Compound remedies contain 7 to 20 plant parts. The Leni-Lenape healer Wi-tapa-nóxwe, "Walks with Daylight," sometimes used as many as 14 plants. (Gladys Tantaquidgeon, *Folk Medicine of the Delaware and Related Algonkian Indians* [Harrisburg: Pennsylvania Historical and Museum Commission, 1972], 29.) Although most formulas use few plants, Alex Johnston mentions a notable exception: a Cree formula used to attract a member of the opposite sex that contains 120 to 130 plant species. (Alex Johnston, *Plants and the Blackfoot* [Lethbridge, Alberta: Lethbridge Historical Society, 1987], 13.)

20. Myers was of Scotch-Irish ancestry, but Native by training and through marriage. See the inspiring chapter on Myers's life by James Green, "Kwi-tsi-tsa-las: Portrait of an Herbalist," in *American Herbalism: Essays on Herbs and Herbalism by Members of the American Herbalist Guild,* ed. Michael Tierra, O.M.D. (Freedom, Calif.: Crossing Press, 1992), 69–84.

21. Paul B. Hamel and Mary U. Chiltoskey, *Cherokee Plants and Their Uses—A 400 Year History* (Sylva, N.C.: Herald Publishing Co., 1975), 5.

22. Johnston, *Plants and the Blackfoot,* 13.

23. James Mooney, *Myths of the Cherokee* (1888; reprint, Nashville, Tenn.: Charles and Randy Elder—Booksellers, 1982), 252.

24. Frances Densmore, *Uses of Plants by the Chippewa Indians: Forty-fourth Annual Report of the Bureau of American Ethnology to the Secretary of the Smithsonian Institution, 1926–1927* (Washington, D.C.: United States Government Printing Office, 1928), 323. An abridged version of the report may be found in *How Indians Use Wild Plants for Food, Medicine and Crafts* (New York: Dover, 1974).

25. This story was also published in a moving book. Tehanetorens, *Legends of the Iroquois* (Summertown, Tenn.: Book Publishing Co., 1998).

26. Keewaydinoquay, "*Mukwah Miskomin or Kinnickinnick,* 'Gift of the Bear,' " unpublished manuscript, 1977, kindly sent to me by Grandmother "Kee."

27. Tis Mal Crow, *Native Plants, Native Healing: Traditional Muskogee Way* (Summertown, Tenn.: Native Voices, 2001), 39–51.

28. James A. Duke, Ph.D., *The Green Pharmacy* (Emmaus, Pa.: Rodale Press, 1997), 449.

29. Andrew Weil, M.D., *Health and Healing* (Boston: Houghton Mifflin, 1983), 100.

30. For an interesting discussion of the colors and properties of Cherokee plants, see noted herbalist David Winston's "Nvwote: Cherokee Medicine and Ethnobotany," in *American Herbalism: Essays on Herbs and Herbalism by Members of the American Herbalist Guild,* ed. Michael Tierra, O.M.D. (Freedom, Calif.: Crossing Press, 1992), 89.

31. Spirits drunk without spirit lead to frenzied possession rather than spiritual communion. A Tsistsistas friend tells me that he used to visit bars and, while completely sober, observe the drunks to learn about spirit possession.

32. "World's Plants in Danger," *Earth Island Journal: International Environmental News* (summer 1998): 16.

33. Alan Ereira, *The Elder Brothers* (New York: Knopf, 1992), 224.

APPENDIX B: MEETINGS WITH REMARKABLE ELDERS

1. Andrew Dreadfulwater, "We'll Have Hats with Feathers in Them . . . But We Won't Be No Indians," *Interculture* (Montreal: Centre Interculturel Monchanin) 17, no. 4, issue 85 (October–December 1984): 23.

2. Seneca Indian Historical Society/Wolf Clan Teaching Lodge, P.O. Box 2313, Orange Park, FL 32067-2313.

3. The change in War Eagle's level of fluency is a mystery. It may be an example of what psychologists call "state-dependent memory," a hidden or repressed memory that returns only when certain conditions are present. As a child, War Eagle was probably fluent in Cherokee; the vision may have helped him to access and open a forgotten chamber in his mind.

4. War Eagle never stated that he wrote this poem, and I have been unable to verify its origin. His wife believes it was written by War Eagle but cannot be absolutely certain.

5. During the years that Ingwe lived in California, I had not yet been initiated into Yoruba and KyKongo traditions—blessings I later received thanks to two dear African sisters: Daphne and Kay Lynne.

6. After power-feeding the *libretta,* I visited and studied with Nonoy three or four weeks each year for the next three years.

7. Among the southeastern tribes, including the Cherokee, about 80 percent of the people identify themselves as Christian. Some practice both the traditional religion and Christianity, but many feel that the two are mutually exclusive and adhere to one or the other.

8. On March 4, 1999, Lahe'ena'ea Gay, thirty-nine years old, was tragically kidnapped and murdered by leftist rebels in Arauca State, Colombia, about two hundred miles from Bogotá. Also murdered were her two colleagues, Ingrid Washinawatok (Menominee Nation, Wisconsin), forty-one, and Terence Freitas, twenty-four. The three had spent a week with Colombia's U'wa tribe, helping them to organize schools and to preserve their traditional culture. I, along with so many others, mourn the loss of these courageous champions of indigenous rights.

9. Queen Emma was born Emma Rooke (1838–1885), granddaughter of an English mariner on her father's side and descended from a brother of King Kamehameha I on her mother's. In 1856, she married Kamehameha IV (Alexander Liholiho) and became known as Queen Emma.

10. The most common type of Igbo healer is called the *dibia*, the "diviner," who, as a priest of Agwu, the God of Communication and Divination, interprets hidden meanings of events and things in the present, past, or future. The *dibia* may also work as an herbalist or a bone-setter.

— NATIVE AMERICAN RESOURCES —

SELECT BIBLIOGRAPHY

The category "Native American" includes only books about the Native peoples of North America, including Greenland. You can find Central and South American Indian and Native Hawaiian works in "Global Healing Traditions."

GENERAL NATIVE AMERICAN CULTURE AND VALUES

Awiakta, Marilou. *Selu: Seeking the Corn-Mother's Wisdom.* Golden, Colo.: Fulcrum Publishing, 1993.

Beck, Peggy V., and Anna L. Walters. *The Sacred: Ways of Knowledge, Sources of Life.* Tsaile (Navajo Nation), Ariz.: Navajo Community College Press, 1977.

Brown, Dee. *Bury My Heart at Wounded Knee.* New York: Holt, Rinehart and Winston, 1970.

Buhner, Stephen Harrod. *One Spirit, Many Peoples: A Manifesto for Earth Spirituality.* Niwot, Colo.: Roberts Rinehart Publishers, 1997.

Cajete, Gregory, Ph.D. *Look to the Mountain: An Ecology of Indigenous Education.* Durango, Colo.: Kivakí Press, 1994.

Campbell, Joseph. *The Way of the Seeded Earth, Part 2: Mythologies of the Primitive Planters: The Northern Americas.* Vol. 2 of *Historical Atlas of World Mythology.* New York: Harper & Row, 1989.

Cooper, Thomas W. *A Time before Deception: Truth in Communication, Culture, and Ethics.* Santa Fe, N.M.: Clear Light Publishers, 1998.

Cox, Beverly, and Martin Jacobs. *Spirit of the Harvest: North American Indian Cooking.* New York: Stewart, Tabori & Chang, 1991.

Deloria, Vine, Jr. *For This Land: Writings on Religion in America.* New York: Routledge, 1999.

———. *God Is Red: A Native View of Religion.* Golden, Colo.: Fulcrum Publishing, 1994.

Deloria, Vine, Jr. and Daniel R. Wildcat. *Power and Place: Indian Education in America.* Golden, Colo.: Fulcrum Resources, 2001.

Dickason, Olive Patricia. *Canada's First Nations: A History of Founding Peoples from Earliest Times.* Norman: University of Oklahoma Press, 1992.

Dooling, D. M., and Paul Jordan-Smith, eds. *I Become Part of It: Sacred Dimensions of Native American Life.* San Francisco: HarperSanFrancisco, 1989.

Dunsmore, Roger. *Earth's Mind.* Albuquerque: University of New Mexico Press, 1997.

Eaton, Evelyn. *Snowy Earth Comes Gliding.* Independence, Calif.: Draco Foundation, 1974.

Griffin-Pierce, Trudy. *Native Americans: Enduring Cultures and Traditions.* New York: Friedman/Fairfax Publishers, 1996.

Hall, Robert L. *An Archaeology of the Soul: North American Indian Belief and Ritual.* Urbana: University of Illinois Press, 1997.

Harrod, Howard L. *The Animals Came Dancing: Native American Sacred Ecology and Animal Kinship.* Tucson: University of Arizona Press, 2000.

Harvey, Karen D., and Lisa D. Harjo. *Indian Country: A History of Native People in America.* Golden, Colo.: Fulcrum Publishing, 1994.

Hill, Tom, and Richard W. Hill Sr., eds. *Creation's Journey: Native American Identity and Belief.* Washington, D.C.: Smithsonian Institution Press, 1994.

Hoxie, Frederick E.; Peter C. Mancall; and James H. Merrell, eds. *American Nations: Encounters in Indian Country, 1850 to the Present.* New York: Routledge, 2001.

Irwin, Lee, ed. *Native American Spirituality: A Critical Reader.* Lincoln: University of Nebraska Press, 2000.

Josephy, Alvin M., Jr. *500 Nations: An Illustrated History of North American Indians.* New York: Knopf, 1994.

Lane, Phil, project coordinator. *The Sacred Tree.* Lethbridge, Alberta: Four Worlds Development Press, 1984.

Laubin, Gladys, and Reginald Laubin. *Indian Dances of North America: Their Importance to Indian Life.* Norman: University of Oklahoma Press, 1977.

Littlebird, Larry. *Hunting Sacred: Everything Listens.* Santa Fe, N.M.: Western Edge Press, 2001.

McMillan, Alan D. *Native Peoples and Cultures of Canada.* Vancouver, B.C.: Douglas & McIntyre, 1995.

Moquin, Wayne, and Charles Van Doren, eds. *Great Documents in American Indian History.* New York: Da Capo Press, 1995.

Morey, Sylvester M., and Olivia L. Gilliam, eds. *Respect for Life: The Traditional Upbringing of American Indian Children.* Garden City, N.Y.: Waldorf Press, n.d. (approx. 1974).

Niezen, Ronald. *Spirit Wars: Native North American Religions in the Age of Nation Building.* Berkeley: University of California Press, 2000.

Pringle, Heather. *In Search of Ancient North America: An Archaeological Journey to Forgotten Cultures.* New York: Wiley, 1996.

Ross, Rupert. *Dancing with a Ghost: Exploring Indian Reality.* Toronto, Ontario: Reed Books Canada, 1992.

———. *Returning to the Teachings: Exploring Aboriginal Justice.* Toronto, Ontario: Penguin Books, 1996.

Sullivan, Lawrence E., ed. *Native Religions and Cultures of North America: Anthropology of the Sacred.* New York: Continuum Publishing, 2000.

Taiaiake, Alfred. *Peace, Power, Righteousness: An Indigenous Manifesto.* Don Mills, Ontario: Oxford University Press, 1999.

Thomas, David Hurst, et al. *The Native Americans: An Illustrated History.* Atlanta: Turner Publishing, 1993.

Weatherford, Jack. *Indian Givers: How Indians of the Americas Transformed the World.* New York: Ballantine Books, 1988.

———. *Native Roots: How the Indians Enriched America.* New York: Ballantine Books, 1991.

Weaver, Jace, ed. *Native American Religious Identity: Unforgotten Gods.* Maryknoll, N.Y.: Orbis Books, 1998.

Wells, Ronald Austin. *The Honor of Giving: Philanthrophy in Native America.* Indianapolis: Indiana University Center on Philanthropy, 1998.

Winch, Terence, ed. *All Roads Are Good: Native Voices on Life and Culture.* Washington, D.C.: Smithsonian Institution Press, 1994.

REGIONAL NATIVE AMERICAN CULTURE

Basso, Keith H. *Wisdom Sits in Places: Landscape and Language among the Western Apache.* Albuquerque: University of New Mexico Press, 1996.

Bean, Lowell John. *Mukat's People: The Cahuilla Indians of Southern California.* Berkeley: University of California Press, 1972.

Benton-Banai, Edward. *The Mishomis Book: The Voice of the Ojibway.* Hayward, Wis.: Indian Country Communications, 1988.

Bierwert, Crisca. *Brushed by Cedar, Living by the River: Coast Salish Figures of Power.* Tucson: University of Arizona Press, 1999.

Brightman, Robert. *Grateful Prey: Rock Cree Human-Animal Relationships.* Berkeley: University of California Press, 1993.

Debo, Angie. *And Still the Waters Run: The Betrayal of the Five Civilized Tribes.* Norman: University of Oklahoma Press, 1940. Reissue ed., Princeton, N.J.: Princeton University Press, 1972.

Densmore, Frances. *Teton Sioux Music and Culture.* Washington, D.C.: Bureau of American Ethnology, Smithsonian Institution, 1918. Reprint, Lincoln: University of Nebraska Press, 1992.

Diamond, Beverley; M. Sam Cronk; and Franziska von Rosen. *Visions of Sound: Musical Instruments of First Nations Communities in Northeastern America.* Chicago: University of Chicago Press, 1994.

Dusenberry, Verne. *The Montana Cree: A Study in Religious Persistence.* Norman: University of Oklahoma Press, 1962.

Ewers, John C. *The Blackfeet: Raiders on the Northwestern Plains.* Norman: University of Oklahoma Press, 1958.

Fienup-Riordan, Ann. *Boundaries and Passages: Rule and Ritual in Yup'ik Eskimo Oral Tradition.* Norman: University of Oklahoma Press, 1994.

Fletcher, Alice C., and Francis La Flesche. *The Omaha Tribe.* 2 vols. Washington, D.C.: Bureau of American Ethnology, 1911. Reprint, Lincoln: University of Nebraska Press, 1992.

Frey, Rodney. *The World of the Crow Indians: As Driftwood Lodges.* Norman: University of Oklahoma Press, 1987.

———, ed. *Stories That Make the World: Oral Literature of the Indian Peoples of the Inland Northwest.* Norman: University of Oklahoma Press, 1995.

Griffin-Pierce, Trudy. *Earth Is My Mother, Sky Is My Father: Space, Time, and Astronomy in Navajo Sandpainting.* Albuquerque: University of New Mexico Press, 1992.

Grinnell, George Bird. *The Cheyenne Indians: Their History and Ways of Life.* 2 vols. Lincoln: University of Nebraska Press, 1972.

Howard, James H. *The Ponca Tribe.* Lincoln: University of Nebraska Press, 1995.

Hudson, Charles. *The Southeastern Indians.* Knoxville: University of Tennessee Press, 1976.

Jennings, Francis. *The Invasion of America: Indians, Colonialism, and the Cant of Conquest.* New York: Norton, 1975.

Johnston, Basil. *The Manitous: The Spiritual World of the Ojibway.* New York: HarperCollins, 1995.

Knudtson, Peter M. *The Wintun Indians of California and Their Neighbors.* Happy Camp, Calif.: Naturegraph Publishers, 1977.

Kroeber, A. L. *The Arapaho.* New York: Bulletin of the American Museum of Natural History, 1902, 1904, and 1907. Reprint, Lincoln: University of Nebraska Press, 1983.

———. *Handbook of the Indians of California.* Bulletin 78 of the Bureau of American Ethnology. Washington, D.C.: U.S. Government Printing Office, 1925. Reprint, New York: Dover, 1976.

Lowie, Robert H. *The Crow Indians.* New York: Reinhart, 1935. Reprint, Lincoln: University of Nebraska Press, 1983.

Mandelbaum, David G. *The Plains Cree: An Ethnographic, Historical, and Comparative Study.* New York: American Museum of Natural History, 1940. Reprint, Regina, Saskatchewan: Canadian Plains Research Center, 1979.

Marriott. *The Ten Grandmothers: Epic of the Kiowas.* Norman: University of Oklahoma Press, 1945.

McNeley, James Kale. *Holy Wind in Navajo Philosophy.* Tucson: University of Arizona Press, 1981.

Medicine Crow, Joseph. *From the Heart of the Crow Country: The Crow Indians' Own Stories.* New York: Crown, 1992.

Miller, Jay. *Lushootseed Culture and the Shamanic Odyssey: An Anchored Radiance*. Lincoln: University of Nebraska Press, 1999.

———. *Tsimshian Culture: A Light through the Ages*. Lincoln: University of Nebraska Press, 1997.

Neel, David. *The Great Canoes: Reviving a Northwest Coast Tradition*. Seattle: University of Washington Press, 1995.

Nelson, Richard K. *Make Prayers to the Raven: A Koyukon View of the Northern Forest*. Chicago: University of Chicago Press, 1983.

Ortiz, Alfonso. *The Tewa World: Space, Time, Being and Becoming in a Pueblo Society*. Chicago: University of Chicago Press, 1969.

Perdue, Theda. *Nations Remembered: An Oral History of the Cherokees, Chickasaws, Choctaws, Creeks, and Seminoles in Oklahoma, 1865–1907*. Norman: University of Oklahoma Press, 1993.

Powell, Peter J. *Sweet Medicine: The Continuing Role of the Sacred Arrows, the Sun Dance, and the Sacred Buffalo Hat in Northern Cheyenne History*. 2 vols. Norman: University of Oklahoma Press, 1969.

Pritchard, Evan T. *No Word for Time: The Way of the Algonquin People*. Tulsa, Okla.: Council Oak Books, 1997.

Rasmussen, Knud. *Across Arctic America: Narrative of the Fifth Thule Expedition*. New York: G. P. Putnam's Sons, 1927. Reprint, Fairbanks: University of Alaska Press, 1999.

Rawls, James J. *Indians of California: The Changing Image*. Norman: University of Oklahoma Press, 1984.

Rea, Amadeo M. *Folk Mammalogy of the Northern Pimans*. Tucson: University of Arizona Press, 1998.

Reichard, Gladys A. *Navaho Religion: A Study of Symbolism*. New York: Bollingen Foundation, 1950.

Ruby, Robert H., and John A. Brown. *Dreamer Prophets of the Columbia Plateau: Smohala and Skolaskin*. Norman: University of Oklahoma Press, 1989.

———. *Indians of the Pacific Northwest*. Norman: University of Oklahoma Press, 1981.

Sando, Joe S. *Pueblo Nations: Eight Centuries of Pueblo Indian History*. Santa Fe, N.M.: Clear Light Publishers, 1992.

Schlesier, Karl H. *The Wolves of Heaven: Cheyenne Shamanism, Ceremonies, and Prehistoric Origins*. Norman: University of Oklahoma Press, 1987.

Schwarz, Maureen Trudelle. *Molded in the Image of Changing Woman: Navajo Views on the Human Body and Personhood*. Tucson: University of Arizona Press, 1997.

———. *Navajo Lifeways: Contemporary Issues, Ancient Knowledge*. Norman: University of Oklahoma Press, 2001.

Smyth, Willie, and Esmé Ryan, eds. *Spirit of the First People: Native American Music Traditions of Washington State*. Seattle: University of Washington Press, 1999.

Tehanetorens. *Legends of the Iroquois*. Summertown, Tenn.: Book Publishing Co., 1998.

Thomas, Chief Jacob, with Terry Boyle. *Teachings from the Longhouse*. Toronto, Ontario: Stoddart Publishing, 1994.

Tooker, Elisabeth. *An Ethnography of the Huron Indians, 1615–1649*. Syracuse, N.Y.: Syracuse University Press, 1991.

Trenholm, Virginia Cole. *The Arapahoes, Our People*. Norman: University of Oklahoma Press, 1970.

Trenholm, Virginia Cole, and Maurine Carley. *The Shoshonis: Sentinels of the Rockies*. Norman: University of Oklahoma Press, 1964.

Trigger, Bruce G. *The Children of Aataentsic: A History of the Huron People to 1660*. Montreal, Québec: McGill-Queen's University Press, 1976.

Tukummiq and Tom Lowenstein. *The Things That Were Said of Them: Shaman Stories and Oral Histories of the Tikigaq People*. Berkeley: University of California Press, 1992.

Underhill, Ruth Murray. *Singing for Power: The Song Magic of the Papago Indians of Southern Arizona*. Berkeley: University of California Press, 1938.

Wallace, Anthony F. C. *The Death and Rebirth of the Seneca*. New York: Vintage Books, 1969.

Wallace, Paul A. W. *The White Roots of Peace*. Philadelphia: University of Pennsylvania Press, 1946.

Waters, Frank. *Book of the Hopi*. New York: Penguin Books, 1963.

———. *Masked Gods: Navaho and Pueblo Ceremonialism*. New York: Ballantine Books, 1950.

Wilson, Chesley Goseyun; Ruth Longcor Harnisch Wilson; and Bryan Burton. *When the Earth Was Like New: Western Apache Songs and Stories*. Danbury, Conn.: World Music Press, 1994.

Wilson, Edmund. *Apologies to the Iroquois*. Syracuse, N.Y.: Syracuse University Press, 1959.

FACTS OF LIFE: CHALLENGES AND DEMOGRAPHICS

Adams, David Wallace. *Education for Extinction: American Indians and the Boarding School Experience, 1875–1928*. Lawrence: University Press of Kansas, 1995.

Deloria, Vine, Jr. *Behind the Trail of Broken Treaties: An Indian Declaration of Independence*. Austin: University of Texas Press, 1974.

———. *Custer Died for Your Sins: An Indian Manifesto*. Norman: University of Oklahoma Press, 1969.

———, ed. *American Indian Policy in the Twentieth Century*. Norman: University of Oklahoma Press, 1985.

Grinde, Donald A., and Bruce E. Johansen. *Ecocide of Native America: Environmental Destruction of Indian Lands and Peoples*. Santa Fe, N.M.: Clear Light Publishers, 1995.

Matthiessen, Peter. *Indian Country*. New York: Viking Press, 1979.

———. *In the Spirit of Crazy Horse*. New York: Viking Press, 1980.

Pevar, Stephen L. *The Rights of Indians and Tribes: The Basic ACLU Guide to Indian and Tribal Rights*. Carbondale: Southern Illinois University Press, 1992.

Russell, George. *Native American FAQs Handbook*. Phoenix: Russell Publications, 2000.

Steiner, Stan. *The Vanishing White Man*. Norman: University of Oklahoma Press, 1976.

Thornton, Russell. *American Indian Holocaust and Survival: A Population History since 1492*. Norman: University of Oklahoma Press, 1987.

White, Richard. *The Roots of Dependency: Subsistence, Environment, and Social Change among the Choctaws, Pawnees, and Navajos*. Lincoln: University of Nebraska Press, 1983.

NATIVE AMERICAN HEALING AND INDIGENOUS SCIENCE

Bahr, Donald M., et al. *Piman Shamanism and Staying Sickness*. Tucson: University of Arizona Press, 1974.

Bean, Lowell John. *California Indian Shamanism*. Menlo Park, Calif.: Ballena Press, 1992.

Bopp, Michael, Ph.D. *Developing Healthy Communities: Fundamental Strategies for Health Promotion*. Lethbridge, Alberta: Four Worlds Development Project, 1985.

Bruchac, Joseph. *The Native American Sweat Lodge: History and Legends*. Freedom, Calif.: Crossing Press, 1993.

Cajete, Gregory. *Native Science: Natural Laws of Interdependence*. Santa Fe, N.M.: Clear Light Publications, 2000.

———, ed. *A People's Ecology: Explorations in Sustainable Living—Health, Environment, Agriculture, Native Traditions*. Santa Fe, N.M.: Clear Light Publications, 1999.

Duran, Eduardo, and Bonnie Duran. *Native American Postcolonial Psychology*. Albany: State University of New York Press, 1995.

Eaton, Evelyn. *I Send a Voice*. Wheaton, Ill.: Theosophical Publishing House, 1978.

Erdoes, Richard. *Crying for a Dream: The World through Native American Eyes*. Santa Fe, N.M.: Bear & Company, 1990.

Howard, James H., with Willie Lena. *Oklahoma Seminoles: Medicines, Magic, and Religion*. Norman: University of Oklahoma Press, 1984.

Johnston, Basil. *Ojibway Ceremonies*. Lincoln: University of Nebraska Press, 1982.

———. *Ojibway Heritage*. New York: Columbia University Press, 1976.

Kavasch, E. Barrie, and Karen Baar. *American Indian Healing Arts: Herbs, Rituals, and Remedies for Every Season of Life*. New York: Bantam Books, 1999.

Kilpatrick, Jack Frederick, and Anna Gritts Kilpatrick. *Run toward the Nightland: Magic of the Oklahoma Cherokees*. Dallas: Southern Methodist University Press, 1967.

Lake, Medicine Grizzlybear. *Native Healer: Initiation into an Ancient Art*. Wheaton, Ill.: Quest Books, 1991.

Lewis, Thomas H. *The Medicine Men: Oglala Sioux Ceremony and Healing*. Lincoln: University of Nebraska Press, 1990.

Looks for Buffalo Hand, Floyd. *Learning Journey on the Red Road*. Toronto, Ontario: Learning Journey Communications, 1998.

Lyon, William S. *Encyclopedia of Native American Healing*. New York: Norton, 1996.

Mehl-Madrona, Lewis. *Coyote Medicine*. New York: Scribner, 1997.

Miller, Jay. *Shamanic Odyssey: The Lushootseed Salish Journey to the Land of the Dead*. Menlo Park, Calif.: Ballena Press, 1988.

Mooney, James. *Sacred Formulas of the Cherokees*. Washington, D.C.: Bureau of American Ethnology, 7th Annual Report, 1885–1886, 1891.

Nabokov, Peter. *Indian Running: Native American History and Tradition*. Santa Fe, N.M.: Ancient City Press, 1981.

Paper, Jordan. *Offering Smoke: The Sacred Pipe and Native American Religion*. Moscow: University of Idaho Press, 1988.

Peat, F. David. *Lighting the Seventh Fire: The Spiritual Ways, Healing, and Science of the Native American*. New York: Birch Lane Press, 1994.

Ruby, Robert H., and John A. Brown. *John Slocum and the Indian Shaker Church*. Norman: University of Oklahoma Press, 1996.

Sandner, Donald, M.D. *Navaho Symbols of Healing: A Jungian Exploration of Ritual, Image, and Medicine*. Rochester, Vt.: Healing Arts Press, 1991.

Smith, Huston, and Reuben Snake, eds. *One Nation under God: The Triumph of the Native American Church*. Santa Fe, N.M.: Clear Light Publishers, 1996.

Stewart, Omer C. *Peyote Religion: A History*. Norman: University of Oklahoma Press, 1987.

Swinomish Tribal Mental Health Project. *A Gathering of Wisdoms—Tribal Mental Health: A Cultural Perspective*. LaConner, Wash.: Swinomish Tribal Community, 1991.

Turner, Edith. *The Hands Feel It: Healing and Spirit Presence among a Northern Alaskan People*. DeKalb: Northern Illinois University Press, 1996.

Vogel, Virgil J. *American Indian Medicine*. Norman: University of Oklahoma Press, 1970. Reprint, Norman: University of Oklahoma Press, 1990.

Waldram, James B. *The Way of the Pipe: Aboriginal Spirituality and Symbolic Healing in Canadian Prisons*. Peterborough, Ontario: Broadview Press, 1997.

Dreams, Visions, and Rock Art

Because dreams and visions are often sources of healing power and healing guidance, the books in this section may be considered a subcategory of "Native American Healing." I also include books about Native American rock art, the record of the visions, symbols, history, and culture of the ancient people of Turtle Island.

Applegate, Richard B. *Atishwin: The Dream Helper in South-Central California*. Socorro, N.M.: Ballena Press, 1978.

Barasch, Marc Ian. *Healing Dreams: Exploring the Dreams That Can Transform Your Life*. New York: Penguin Putnam, 2000.

Conway, Thor. *Painted Dreams: Native American Rock Art*. Minocqua, Wis.: North Word Press, 1993.

Gackenbach, Jayne, and Stephen LaBerge, eds. *Conscious Mind, Sleeping Brain: Perspectives on Lucid Dreaming*. New York: Plenum Press, 1988.

Irwin, Lee. *The Dream Seekers: Native American Visionary Traditions of the Great Plains*. Norman: University of Oklahoma Press, 1994.

Kelen, Leslie, and David Sucec. Photographs by Craig Law et al. *Sacred Images: A Vision of Native American Rock Art*. Layton, Utah: Gibbs Smith, 1996.

Krippner, Stanley, Ph.D., ed. *Dreamtime and Dreamwork: Decoding the Language of the Night*. Los Angeles: Tarcher, 1990.

LaBerge, Stephen, Ph.D. *Lucid Dreaming*. New York: Ballantine Books, 1985.

Tedlock, Barbara, ed. *Dreaming: Anthropological and Psychological Interpretations*. Santa Fe, N.M.: School of American Research Press, 1992.

Turpin, Solveig A., ed. *Shamanism and Rock Art in North America*. San Antonio, Tex.: Rock Art Foundation, 1994.

Ullman, Montague, M.D., and Stanley Krippner, Ph.D., with Alan Vaughan. *Dream Telepathy: Experiments in Nocturnal ESP*. Baltimore: Penguin Books, 1973.

Van de Castle, Robert L., Ph.D. *Our Dreaming Mind*. New York: Ballantine Books, 1995.

Vastokas, Joan M., and Romas K. Vastokas. *Sacred Art of the Algonkians: A Study of the Peterborough Petroglyphs*. Peterborough, Ontario: Mansard Press, 1973.

Whitley, David S. *The Art of the Shaman: Rock Art of California*. Salt Lake City: University of Utah Press, 2000.

WOMEN'S MEDICINE

Albers, Patricia, and Beatrice Medicine, eds. *The Hidden Half: Studies of Plains Indian Women*. Lanham, Md.: University Press of America, 1983.

Buckley, Thomas, and Alma Gottlieb, eds. *Blood Magic: The Anthropology of Menstruation*. Berkeley: University of California Press, 1988.

Jacasum, John Paul, ed. *Omushkegowuk Women's Traditional Practices Project: Restoring the Balance.* Timmins, Ontario: Ojibway and Cree Cultural Centre, 2000.

Klein, Laura F., and Lillian A. Ackerman, eds. *Women and Power in Native North America.* Norman: University of Oklahoma Press, 1995.

Lake, Tela Star Hawk. *Hawk Woman Dancing with the Moon.* New York: M. Evans and Company, 1996.

Paper, Jordan. *Through the Earth Darkly: Female Spirituality in Comparative Perspective.* New York: Continuum Publishing, 1997.

Perdue, Theda. *Cherokee Women: Gender and Culture Change, 1700–1835.* Lincoln: University of Nebraska Press, 1998.

Peters, Virginia Bergman. *Women of the Earth Lodges: Tribal Life on the Plains.* Norman: University of Oklahoma Press, 1995.

Powers, Marla N. *Oglala Women: Myth, Ritual, and Reality.* Chicago: University of Chicago Press, 1986.

Spittal, Wm. Guy, ed. *Iroquois Women: An Anthology.* Ohsweken, Ontario: Iroqrafts, 1990.

Stockel, H. Henrietta. *Women of the Apache Nation: Voices of Truth.* Reno: University of Nevada Press, 1991.

St. Pierre, Mark, and Tilda Long Soldier. *Walking in the Sacred Manner: Healers, Dreamers, and Pipe Carriers—Medicine Women of the Plains Indians.* New York: Touchstone, 1995.

THE SORCERER'S APPRENTICE

Kluckhohn, Clyde. *Navaho Witchcraft.* Boston: Beacon Press, 1944.

Simmons, Marc. *Witchcraft in the Southwest: Spanish and Indian Supernaturalism on the Rio Grande.* Lincoln: University of Nebraska Press, 1974.

Walker, Deward E., Jr., ed. *Witchcraft and Sorcery of the American Native Peoples.* Moscow: University of Idaho Press, 1989.

Watson, Lyall. *Dark Nature: A Natural History of Evil.* New York: HarperCollins, 1995.

BIOGRAPHIES AND AUTOBIOGRAPHIES

Bear Heart with Molly Larkin. *The Wind Is My Mother: The Life and Teachings of a Native American Shaman.* New York: Clarkson Potter, 1996.

Black Elk, Wallace H., and William S. Lyon. *Black Elk: The Sacred Ways of a Lakota.* San Francisco: Harper & Row, 1990.

Boyd, Doug. *Mad Bear: Spirit, Healing, and the Sacred in the Life of a Native American Medicine Man.* New York: Simon & Schuster, 1994.

———. *Rolling Thunder.* New York: Dell Publishing, 1974.

Catches, Pete S., Sr. *Sacred Fireplace* (Oceti Wakan): *Life and Teachings of a Lakota Medicine Man.* Santa Fe, N.M.: Clear Light Publishers, 1999.

Coel, Margaret. *Chief Left Hand: Southern Arapaho*. Norman: University of Oklahoma Press, 1981.

Fawcett, Melissa Jayne. *Medicine Trail: The Life and Lessons of Gladys Tantaquidgeon*. Tucson: University of Arizona Press, 2000.

Fikes, Jay C., ed. *Reuben Snake: Your Humble Serpent: Indian Visionary and Activist*. Santa Fe, N.M.: Clear Light Publishers, 1996.

Harney, Corbin. *The Way It Is: One Water . . . One Air . . . One Mother Earth*. Nevada City, Calif.: Blue Dolphin Publishing, 1995.

Horse Capture, George, ed. *The Seven Visions of Bull Lodge*. Ann Arbor, Mich.: Bear Claw Press, 1980.

Johansen, Bruce E., and Donald A. Grinde Jr. *The Encyclopedia of Native American Biography: Six Hundred Life Stories of Important People, from Powhatan to Wilma Mankiller*. New York: Da Capo Press, 1997.

Jones, David E. *Sanapia: Comanche Medicine Woman*. Prospect Heights, Ill.: Waveland Press, 1972.

Keeney, Bradford, Ph.D., ed. *Lakota Yuwipi Man: Gary Holy Bull*. Philadelphia: Ringing Rocks Press, 1999.

Lame Deer, John (Fire), and Richard Erdoes. *Lame Deer, Seeker of Visions*. New York: Washington Square Press, 1972.

Linderman, Frank B. *Plenty-Coups: Chief of the Crows*. Lincoln: University of Nebraska Press, 1930.

Mails, Thomas E. *Fools Crow*. Garden City, N.Y.: Doubleday, 1979.

Mankiller, Wilma, and Michael Wallis. *Mankiller: A Chief and Her People*. New York: St. Martin's Press, 1993.

Miller, Jay, ed. *Mourning Dove: A Salishan Autobiography*. Lincoln: University of Nebraska Press, 1990.

Mohatt, Gerald, and Joseph Eagle Elk. *The Price of a Gift: A Lakota Healer's Story*. Lincoln: University of Nebraska Press, 2000.

Neeley, Bill. *The Last Comanche Chief: The Life and Times of Quanah Parker*. New York: Wiley, 1995.

Neihardt, John G. *Black Elk Speaks: Being the Life Story of a Holy Man of the Oglala Sioux*. Lincoln: University of Nebraska Press, 1932.

Newcomb, Franc Johnson. *Hosteen Klah: Navaho Medicine Man and Sand Painter*. Norman: University of Oklahoma Press, 1964.

Stands in Timber, John, and Margot Liberty. *Cheyenne Memories*. Lincoln: University of Nebraska Press, 1967.

Utley, Robert M. *The Lance and the Shield: The Life and Times of Sitting Bull*. New York: Ballantine Books, 1993.

Yellowtail, Thomas. *Yellowtail: Crow Medicine Man and Sun Dance Chief—An Autobiography as Told to Michael Oren Fitzgerald*. Norman: University of Oklahoma Press, 1991.

VOICES OF THE ELDERS

Cardinal, Harold, and Walter Hildebrandt. *Treaty Elders of Saskatchewan: Our Dream Is That Our Peoples Will One Day Be Clearly Recognized as Nations*. Calgary, Alberta: University of Calgary Press, 2000.

Johnson, Sandy, and Dan Budnik. *The Book of Elders: The Life Stories and Wisdom of Great American Indians*. New York: HarperCollins, 1994.

Margolin, Malcolm, ed. *The Way We Lived: California Indian Stories, Songs and Reminiscences*. Berkeley, Calif.: Heyday Books, 1993.

Meili, Dianne. *Those Who Know: Profiles of Alberta's Native Elders*. Edmonton, Alberta: NeWest Press, 1991.

Neel, David. *Our Chiefs and Elders*. Vancouver: University of British Columbia Press, 1992.

Thorpe, Dagmar. *People of the Seventh Fire: Returning Lifeways of Native America*. Ithaca, N.Y.: Akwe:kon Press, 1996.

Wall, Steve, and Harvey Arden. *Travels in Stone Canoe: The Return to the Wisdomkeepers*. New York: Simon & Schuster, 1998.

———. *Wisdomkeepers: Meetings with Native American Spiritual Elders*. Hillsboro, Oreg.: Beyond Words Publishing, 1990.

NATIVE HERBAL MEDICINE

Cochran, Wendell. *Cherokee Medicinal Herbs*. Park Hill, Okla.: Cross Cultural Education Center, 1984.

Cowan, Eliot. *Plant Spirit Medicine*. Newberg, Oreg.: Blue Water Publishing, 1995.

Crow, Tis Mal. *Native Plants, Native Healing: Traditional Muskogee Way*. Summertown, Tenn.: Book Publishing Co, 2001.

Curtin, L.S.M. *By the Prophet of the Earth: Ethnobotany of the Pima*. Tucson: University of Arizona Press, 1949.

Densmore, Frances. *How Indians Use Wild Plants for Food, Medicine and Crafts*. New York: Dover, 1974.

Dumire, William W., and Gail D. Tierney. *Wild Plants of the Pueblo Province: Exploring Ancient and Enduring Uses*. Santa Fe: Museum of New Mexico Press, 1995.

Erichsen-Brown, Charlotte. *Medicinal and Other Uses of North American Plants: A Historical Survey with Special Reference to the Eastern Indian Tribes*. New York: Dover, 1989.

Gilmore, Melvin R. *Uses of Plants by the Indians of the Missouri River Region*. Lincoln: University of Nebraska Press, 1977.

Goodrich, Jennie; Claudia Lawson; and Vana Parrish Lawson. *Kashya Pomo Plants.* Berkeley, Calif.: Heyday Books, 1980.

Gunther, Erna. *Ethnobotany of Western Washington: The Knowledge and Use of Indigenous Plants by Native Americans.* Seattle: University of Washington Press, 1945.

Hamel, Paul B., and Mary U. Chiltoskey. *Cherokee Plants and Their Uses—A 400 Year History.* Sylva, N.C.: Herald Publishing Co., 1975.

Herrick, James W. *Iroquois Medical Botany.* Syracuse, N.Y.: Syracuse University Press, 1995.

Howarth, David, and Kahlee Keane. *Native Medicines.* Alvena, Saskatchewan: Root Woman & Dave, 1995.

Hungry Wolf, Adolf. *Teachings of Nature.* Skookumchuck, B.C.: Good Medicine Books, 1989.

Johnston, Alex. *Plants and the Blackfoot.* Lethbridge, Alberta: Lethbridge Historical Society, 1987.

Kavasch, E. Barrie. *American Indian Earth Sense: Herbaria of Ethnobotany and Ethnomycology.* Washington, Conn.: Birdstone Publishers, 1996.

Kay, Margarita Artschwager. *Healing with Plants in the American and Mexican West.* Tucson: University of Arizona Press, 1996.

Keewaydinoquay. *Puhpohwee for the People: A Narrative Account of Some Uses of Fungi among the Ahnishinaabeg.* DeKalb: Northern Illinois University, 1998.

Kindscher, Kelly. *Medicinal Wild Plants of the Prairie: An Ethnobotanical Guide.* Lawrence: University Press of Kansas, 1992.

Marles, Robin J., et al. *Aboriginal Plant Use in Canada's Northwest Boreal Forest.* Vancouver: University of British Columbia Press, 2000.

Mayes, Vernon O., and Barbara Bayless Lacy. *Nanise': A Navajo Herbal—One Hundred Plants from the Navajo Reservation.* Tsaile, Ariz.: Navajo Community College Press, 1989.

Moerman, Daniel E. *Native American Ethnobotany.* Portland, Oreg.: Timber Press, 1998.

Rea, Amadeo M. *At the Desert's Green Edge: An Ethnobotany of the Gila River Pima.* Tucson: University of Arizona Press, 1997.

Tantaquidgeon, Gladys. *Folk Medicine of the Delaware and Related Algonkian Indians.* Harrisburg: Pennsylvania Historical and Museum Commission, 1977.

Turner, Nancy J. *Plant Technology of First Peoples in British Columbia.* Vancouver: University of British Columbia Press, 1998.

Winter, Joseph C., ed. *Tobacco Use by Native North Americans: Sacred Smoke and Silent Killer.* Norman: University of Oklahoma Press, 2000.

WESTERN HERBAL MEDICINE

Blumenthal, Mark, ed. *Herbal Medicine: Expanded Commission E Monographs.* Austin, Tex.: American Botanical Council, 2000.

Castleman, Michael. *The Healing Herbs: The Ultimate Guide to the Curative Powers of Nature's Medicines*. New York: Bantam Books, 1991.

Duke, James A., Ph.D. *The Green Pharmacy: New Discoveries in Herbal Remedies for Common Diseases and Conditions from the World's Foremost Authority on Healing Herbs*. Emmaus, Pa.: Rodale Press, 1997.

Foster, Steven. *Forest Pharmacy: Medicinal Plants in American Forests*. Durham, N.C.: Forest History Society, 1995.

Foster, Steven, and Varro E. Tyler, Ph.D. *Tyler's Honest Herbal*. Binghamton, N.Y.: Haworth Press, 1999.

Gladstar, Rosemary. *Rosemary Gladstar's Family Herbal: A Guide to Living Life with Energy, Health, and Vitality*. North Adams, Mass.: Storey Books, 2001.

Hoffmann, David. *The Herbal Handbook: A User's Guide to Medical Herbalism*. Rochester, Vt.: Healing Arts Press, 1987.

———. *The New Holistic Herbal*. 3d ed. Rockport, Mass.: Element Press, 1990.

Miller, Lucinda G., Pharm.D., and Wallace J. Murray, Ph.D. *Herbal Medicinals: A Clinician's Guide*. Binghamton, N.Y.: Haworth Press, 1998.

Moore, Michael. *Medicinal Plants of the Mountain West*. Santa Fe: Museum of New Mexico Press, 1979.

Moss, Ralph W., Ph.D. *Herbs against Cancer: History and Controversy*. Brooklyn, N.Y.: Equinox Press, 1998.

Mowrey, Daniel B., Ph.D. *Guaranteed Potency Herbs: Next Generation Herbal Medicine*. New Canaan, Conn.: Keats Publishing, 1990.

———. *The Scientific Validation of Herbal Medicine*. N.P.: Cormorant Books, 1986.

St. Claire, Debra. *The Herbal Medicine Cabinet: Preparing Natural Remedies at Home*. Berkeley, Calif.: Celestial Arts, 1997.

Sumner, Judith. *The Natural History of Medicinal Plants*. Portland, Oreg.: Timber Press, 2000.

Tierra, Michael, C.A., N.D. *Planetary Herbology*. Santa Fe, N.M.: Lotus Press, 1988.

———. *The Way of Herbs*. New York: Pocket Books, 1983.

Willard, Terry, Ph.D. *Edible and Medicinal Plants of the Rocky Mountains and Neighboring Territories*. Calgary, Alberta: Wild Rose College of Natural Healing, 1992.

Wood, Matthew. *The Book of Herbal Wisdom*. Berkeley, Calif.: North Atlantic Books, 1997.

———. *Seven Herbs: Plants as Teachers*. Berkeley, Calif.: North Atlantic Books, 1986.

THE POWER, BEAUTY, AND PLIGHT OF NATURE

Abram, David. *The Spell of the Sensuous*. New York: Vintage Books, 1996.

Ausubel, Kenny. *Restoring the Earth: Visionary Solutions from the Bioneers*. Tiburon, Calif.: H. J. Kramer, 1997.

Bekoff, Marc. *Strolling with Our Kin: Speaking for and Respecting Voiceless Animals*. New York: Lantern Books, 2000.

Bekoff, Marc, ed. *The Smile of a Dolphin: Remarkable Accounts of Animal Emotions*. New York: Discovery Books, 2000.

Berry, Thomas. *The Dream of the Earth*. San Francisco: Sierra Club Books, 1988.

Berry, Wendell. *Another Turn of the Crank: Essays by Wendell Berry*. Washington, D.C.: Counterpoint, 1995.

————. *The Unsettling of America: Culture and Agriculture*. San Francisco: Sierra Club Books, 1977.

Brown, Lester, R.; Michael Renner; Christopher Flavin; and the Worldwatch Institute. *Vital Signs: The Environmental Trends That Are Shaping Our Future*. New York: Norton, published yearly.

Brown, Tom, Jr., with William Jon Watkins. *The Tracker: The True Story of Tom Brown, Jr., as Told to Jon Watkins*. New York: Berkley Books, 1978.

Brown, Tom, Jr., with William Owen. *The Search: The Continuing Story of the Tracker Tom Brown, Jr., with William Owen*. New York: Berkley Books, 1980.

Cohen, Michael J. *As If Nature Mattered: A Naturalist Guided Tour through Hidden Valleys of Your Mind*. Sharon, Conn.: National Audubon Society Expedition Institute, 1986.

————. *How Nature Works: Regenerating Kinship with Planet Earth*. Walpole, N.H.: Stillpoint Publishing, 1988.

Colborn, Theo; Dianne Dumanoski; and John Peterson Myers. *Our Stolen Future: Are We Threatening Our Fertility, Intelligence, and Survival?—A Scientific Detective Story*. New York: Penguin Books, 1996.

Cousineau, Phil. *The Art of the Pilgrimage: The Seeker's Guide to Making Travel Sacred*. Berkeley, Calif.: Conari Press, 1998.

Ereira, Alan. *The Elder Brothers*. New York: Knopf, 1992.

Ewen, Alexander, ed. *Voice of Indigenous Peoples: Native People Address the United Nations*. Santa Fe, N.M.: Clear Light Publishers, 1994.

French, Hilary. *Vanishing Borders: Protecting the Planet in the Age of Globalization*. New York: Norton, 2000.

Gallagher, Carole. *American Ground Zero: The Secret Nuclear War*. Cambridge, Mass.: MIT Press, 1993.

Gallagher, Winifred. *The Power of Place: How Our Surroundings Shape Our Thoughts, Emotions, and Actions*. New York: HarperCollins, 1993.

Goodall, Jane. *Reason for Hope: A Spiritual Journey*. New York: Warner Books, 1999.

Gore, Al. *Earth in the Balance: Ecology and the Human Spirit*. New York: Houghton Mifflin, 1992.

Gulliford, Andrew. *Sacred Objects and Sacred Places: Preserving Tribal Traditions*. Boulder: University Press of Colorado, 2000.

Hallendy, Norman. *Inuksuit: Silent Messengers of the Arctic*. Toronto, Ontario: Douglas & McIntyre, 2000.

Hartmann, Thom. *The Last Hours of Ancient Sunlight: Waking Up to Personal and Global Transformation*. New York: Three Rivers Press, 1998.

Hawken, Paul. *The Ecology of Commerce: A Declaration of Sustainability*. New York: HarperCollins, 1993.

Heidlebaugh, Tom, with the Tribal Communities of the Pacific Northwest. *One with the Watershed: A Salmon Homecoming Story-Based Curriculum for Primary Environmental Education*. Olympia, Wash.: Northwest Indian Fisheries Commission, n.d.

Henley, Thom. *Rediscovery: Ancient Pathways, New Directions; Outdoor Activities Based on Native Traditions*. Vancouver, B.C.: Lone Pine Publishing, 1996.

High Country News. *Western Water Made Simple*. Washington, D.C.: Island Press, 1987.

Ingerman, Sandra. *Medicine for the Earth: How to Transform Personal and Environmental Toxins*. New York: Three Rivers Press, 2000.

LaChapelle, Dolores. *Sacred Land, Sacred Sex—Rapture of the Deep: Concerning Deep Ecology and Celebrating Life*. Silverton, Colo.: Finn Hill Arts, 1988.

LaDuke, Winona. *All Our Relations: Native Struggles for Land and Life*. Cambridge, Mass.: South End Press, 1999.

Lopez, Barry Holstun. *Of Wolves and Men*. New York: Scribner, 1978.

Lovelock, James. *The Ages of Gaia: A Biography of Our Living Earth*. New York: Bantam Books, 1988.

Mander, Jerry. *In the Absence of the Sacred: The Failure of Technology and the Survival of the Indian Nations*. San Francisco: Sierra Club Books, 1991.

Mander, Jerry, and Edward Goldsmith, eds. *The Case against the Global Economy and for a Turn toward the Local*. San Francisco: Sierra Club Books, 1996.

Meeker, Joseph W. *The Comedy of Survival: In Search of an Environmental Ethic*. Los Angeles: Guild of Tutors Press, 1972.

———. *Minding the Earth: Thinly Disguised Essays on Human Ecology*. Alameda, Calif.: Latham Foundation, 1988.

Payne, Roger. *Among Whales*. New York: Dell, 1995.

Raffensperger, Carolyn, and Joel Tickner, eds. *Protecting Public Health and the Environment: Implementing the Precautionary Principle*. Washington, D.C.: Island Press, 1999.

Rezendes, Paul. *The Wild Within: Adventures in Nature and Animal Teachings*. New York: Penguin Putnam, 1998.

Ryley, Nancy. *The Forsaken Garden: Four Conversations on the Deep Meaning of Environmental Illness*. Wheaton, Ill.: Quest Books, 1998.

Schumacher, E. F. *Small Is Beautiful: Economics as If People Mattered*. New York: Harper & Row, 1973.

Shepard, Paul. *Coming Home to the Pleistocene*. Washington, D.C.: Island Press, 1998.

———. *The Tender Carnivore and the Sacred Game*. Athens: University of Georgia Press, 1973.

Shepard, Paul, and Barry Sanders. *The Sacred Paw: The Bear in Nature, Myth, and Literature*. New York: Viking Penguin, 1985.

Shiva, Vandana. *Monocultures of the Mind: Perspectives on Biodiversity and Biotechnology*. New York: Zed Books, 1993.

Snyder, Gary. *The Practice of the Wild*. San Francisco: North Point Press, 1990.

Swan, James A. *Sacred Places: How the Living Earth Seeks Our Friendship*. Santa Fe, N.M.: Bear & Company, 1990.

Tompkins, Peter, and Christopher Bird. *The Secret Life of Plants*. New York: HarperCollins, 1989.

———. *Secrets of the Soil: New Solutions for Restoring Our Planet*. Anchorage, Alaska: Earthpulse Press, 1998.

GLOBAL HEALING TRADITIONS: SPIRITUAL, INDIGENOUS, AND SHAMANIC

Avila, Elena, R.N., M.S.N., with Joy Parker. *Woman Who Glows in the Dark: A Curandera Reveals Traditional Aztec Secrets of Physical and Spiritual Health*. New York: Penguin Putnam, 1999.

Balzer, Marjorie Mandelstam, ed. *Shamanic Worlds: Rituals and Lore of Siberia and Central Asia*. Armonk, N.Y.: M. E. Sharpe, 1997.

Blacker, Carmen. *The Catalpa Bow: A Study of Shamanistic Practices in Japan*. London: George Allen & Unwin, 1975.

Bray, David Kaonohiokala, and Douglas Low. *The Kahuna Religion of Hawaii*. Garberville, Calif.: Borderland Sciences, 1960.

Calderón, Eduardo, et al. *Eduardo el Curandero: The Words of a Peruvian Healer*. Richmond, Calif.: North Atlantic Books, 1982.

Campbell, Joseph. *The Way of the Animal Powers. Vol. 1 of Historical Atlas of World Mythology*. San Francisco: Harper & Row, 1983.

———. *The Way of the Seeded Earth, Part 1: The Sacrifice. Vol. 2 of Historical Atlas of World Mythology*. New York: Harper & Row, 1988.

Cohen, Kenneth S. *The Way of Qigong: The Art and Science of Chinese Energy Healing*. New York: Ballantine Books, 1999.

Cook, Pat Moffitt. *Shaman, Jhankri and Néle: Music Healers of Indigenous Cultures*. Book and compact disc. Roslyn, N.Y.: Ellipsis Arts, 1997.

Davies, Stevan L. *Jesus the Healer: Possession, Trance, and the Origins of Christianity*. New York: Continuum Publishing, 1995.

Doore, Gary, ed. *Shaman's Path: Healing, Personal Growth, and Empowerment*. Boston: Shambhala Publications, 1988.

Eliade, Mircea. *Shamanism: Archaic Techniques of Ecstasy*. Princeton, N.J.: Princeton University Press, 1964.

Furst, Peter T. *Hallucinogens and Culture*. San Francisco: Chandler & Sharp, 1976.

Furst, Peter T., ed. *Flesh of the Gods: The Ritual Use of Hallucinogens*. New York: Praeger Publishers, 1972.

Goodman, Felicitas D. *Where Spirits Ride the Wind: Trance Journeys and Other Ecstatic Experiences*. Bloomington: Indiana University Press, 1990.

Gore, Belinda. *Ecstatic Body Postures*. Santa Fe, N.M.: Bear & Company, 1995.

Green, Edward C. *Indigenous Theories of Contagious Disease*. Walnut Creek, Calif.: Sage Publications, 1999.

Gutmanis, June. *Kahuna La'au Lapa'au: The Practice of Hawaiian Herbal Medicine*. Honolulu: Island Heritage, 1976.

Halifax, Joan. *Shamanic Voices: A Survey of Visionary Narratives*. New York: Dutton, 1979.

Harden, M. J. *Voices of Wisdom: Hawaiian Elders Speak*. Kula, Hawaii: Aka Press, 1999.

Harner, Michael. *The Way of the Shaman*. 3d ed. San Francisco: Harper & Row, 1990.

Harner, Michael, ed. *Hallucinogens and Shamanism*. New York: Oxford University Press, 1973.

Heinze, Ruth-Inge. *Shamans of the 20th Century*. New York: Irvington Publishers, 1991.

Ingerman, Sandra. *Soul Retrieval: Mending the Fragmented Self*. San Francisco: Harper & Row, 1991.

Kakar, Sudhir. *Shamans, Mystics and Doctors: A Psychological Inquiry into India and Its Healing Traditions*. New York: Knopf, 1982.

Katz, Richard. *Boiling Energy: Community Healing among the Kalahari Kung*. Cambridge, Mass.: Harvard University Press, 1982.

————. *The Straight Path: A Story of Healing and Transformation in Fiji*. Reading, Mass.: Addison-Wesley, 1993.

Katz, Richard; Megan Biesele, and Verna St. Denis. *Healing Makes Our Hearts Happy: Spirituality and Cultural Transformation among the Kalahari Ju/'hoansi*. Rochester, Vt.: Inner Traditions, 1997.

Keeney, Bradford. *Shaking Out the Spirits: A Psychotherapist's Entry into the Healing Mysteries of Global Shamanism*. Barrytown, N.Y.: Station Hill Press, 1994.

Keeney, Bradford, Ph.D., ed. *Kalahari Bushmen Healers*. Philadelphia: Ringing Rocks Press, 1999.

Kharitidi, Olga, M.D. *Entering the Circle: The Secrets of Ancient Siberian Wisdom Discovered by a Russian Psychiatrist*. New York: HarperCollins, 1996.

Krippner, Stanley, and Alberto Villodo. *The Realms of Healing*. Millbrae, Calif.: Celestial Arts, 1976.

Lamb, F. Bruce. *The Story of Manuel Córdova-Rios: Wizard of the Upper Amazon*. 3d ed. Berkeley, Calif.: North Atlantic Books, 1971.

Larsen, Stephen. *The Shaman's Doorway: Opening Imagination to Power and Myth*. Barrytown, N.Y.: Station Hill Press, 1988.

Lawlor, Robert. *Voices of the First Day: Awakening in the Aboriginal Dreamtime*. Rochester, Vt.: Inner Traditions, 1991.

Leonard, Linda Schierse. *Creation's Heartbeat: Following the Reindeer Spirit*. New York: Bantam Books, 1995.

Markides, Kyriacos C. *The Magus of Strovolos: The Extraordinary World of a Spiritual Healer*. New York: Penguin Books, 1985.

Matthews, Caitlín, and John Matthews. *The Encyclopaedia of Celtic Wisdom*. Boston: Element Books, 1994.

Matthews, John. *The Celtic Shaman: A Handbook*. Boston: Element Books, 1992.

Mutwa, Credo Vusamazulu. *Song of the Stars: The Lore of a Zulu Shaman*. Barrytown, N.Y.: Station Hill Openings, 1996.

Myerhoff, Barbara G. *Peyote Hunt: The Sacred Journey of the Huichol Indians*. Ithaca, N.Y.: Cornell University Press, 1974.

Nunn, John F. *Ancient Egyptian Medicine*. Norman: University of Oklahoma Press, 1996.

Ortiz de Montellano, Bernard R. *Aztec Medicine, Health, and Nutrition*. Rutgers, N.J.: Rutgers University Press, 1990.

Pennick, Nigel. *Celtic Sacred Landscapes*. London: Thames & Hudson, 1996.

Perera, Victor, and Robert D. Bruce. *The Last Lords of Palenque: The Lacondon Mayas of the Mexican Rain Forest*. Boston: Little, Brown, 1982.

Prechtel, Martín. *Secrets of the Talking Jaguar: A Mayan Shaman's Journey to the Heart of the Indigenous Soul*. New York: Penguin Putnam, 1998.

Pukui, Mary Kawena; E. W. Haertig, M.D.; and Catherine A. Lee. *Nana I Ke Kumu (Look to the Source)*. Vols. 1 and 2. Honolulu: Queen Lili'uokalani Children's Center, 1972, 1979.

Robicsek, Francis. *The Smoking Gods: Tobacco in Maya Art, History, and Religion*. Norman: University of Oklahoma Press, 1978.

Somé, Malidoma Patrice. *Of Water and the Spirit: Ritual, Magic, and Initiation in the Life of an African Shaman*. New York: Penguin, 1994.

———. *Ritual: Power, Healing and Community*. Portland, Oreg.: Swan Raven & Co., 1993.

Stoller, Paul, and Cheryl Olkes. *In Sorcery's Shadow*. Chicago: University of Chicago Press, 1987.

Trotter, Robert T., II, and Juan Antonio Chavira. *Curanderismo: Mexican American Folk Healing*. Athens: University of Georgia Press, 1981.

Turnbull, Colin M. *The Forest People*. New York: Simon & Schuster, 1961.

Van Der Post, Laurens. *A Mantis Carol*. Washington, D.C.: Island Press, 1975.

Ventocilla, Jorge; Heraclio Herrera; and Valerio Núñez. *Plants and Animals in the Life of the Kuna*. Austin: University of Texas Press, 1995.

Voigt, Anna, and Nevill Drury. *Wisdom from the Earth: The Living Legacy of the Aboriginal Dreamtime*. Boston: Shambhala, 1998.

Walsh, Roger N., M.D., Ph.D. *The Spirit of Shamanism*. Los Angeles: Tarcher, 1990.

Watson, Lyall. *Lightning Bird: The True Story of One Man's Journey into Africa's Past*. New York: Simon & Schuster, 1982.

Wilbert, Johannes. *Tobacco and Shamanism in South America*. New Haven, Conn.: Yale University Press, 1987.

Worrall, Ambrose A., and Olga N. Worrall. *The Gift of Healing: A Personal Story of Spiritual Therapy*. Columbus, Ohio: Ariel Press, 1985.

HEALING HUMOR

Adams, Patch, M.D., with Maureen Mylander. *Gesundheit! Bringing Good Health to You, the Medical System, and Society through Physician Service, Complementary Therapies, Humor, and Joy*. Rochester, Vt.: Healing Arts Press, 1993.

Barry, Dave. *Dave Barry Turns 40*. New York: Ballantine Books, 1990.

———. *Stay Fit and Healthy until You're Dead*. Emmaus, Pa.: Rodale Press, 1985.

Klein, Allen. *The Healing Power of Humor*. Los Angeles: Tarcher, 1989.

Northrup, Jim. *The Rez Road Follies*. Minneapolis: University of Minnesota Press, 1997.

Sinclair, Peter. *The Universe Is Made of Stories . . . and Other Stories: Tales from Alex's Restaurant*. High Point, N.C.: Plan Nine Publishing, 2001.

Wooten, Patty, R.N. *Compassionate Laughter: Jest for Your Health*. Salt Lake City: Commune-a-Key Publishing, 1996.

Humor Journals

Humor & Health Journal
P.O. Box 16814
Jackson, MI 39236

Therapeutic Humor
222 S. Meramec, Suite 303
St. Louis, MO 63105

HEALING AND CONSCIOUSNESS: COMPLEMENTARY AND ALTERNATIVE MEDICINE, SPIRITUAL HEALING, AND PARAPSYCHOLOGY

Achterberg, Jeanne. *Imagery in Healing: Shamanism and Modern Medicine.* Boston: Shambhala Publications, 1985.

Achterberg, Jeanne, Ph.D.; Barbara Dossey, R.N., M.S., F.A.A.N.; and Leslie Kolkmeier, R.N., M.Ed. *Rituals of Healing: Using Imagery for Health and Wellness.* New York: Bantam Books, 1994.

Alternative Medicine: Expanding Medical Horizons. NIH Publication 94–066. Washington, D.C.: National Institutes of Health, 1992.

Austin, James H., M.D. *Zen and the Brain: Toward an Understanding of Meditation and Consciousness.* Cambridge, Mass.: MIT Press, 1998.

Ausubel, Kenny. *When Healing Becomes a Crime: The Amazing Story of the Hoxsey Cancer Clinics and the Return of Alternative Therapies.* Rochester, Vt.: Healing Arts Press, 2000.

Barasch, Marc Ian. *The Healing Path: A Soul Approach to Illness.* New York: Penguin Books, 1993.

Benor, Daniel J., M.D. *Healing Research.* Vol. 1, *Spiritual Healing: Scientific Validation of a Healing Revolution.* Southfield, Mich.: Vision Publications, 2001.

Borysenko, Joan, Ph.D. *Minding the Body, Mending the Mind.* New York: Bantam, 1988.

————. *A Woman's Book of Life: The Biology, Psychology, and Spirituality of the Feminine Life Cycle.* New York: Riverhead Books, 1996.

Brooks, Charles V. W. *Sensory Awareness: The Rediscovery of Experiencing.* New York: Viking Press, 1974.

Broughton, Richard S., Ph.D. *Parapsychology: The Controversial Science.* New York: Ballantine Books, 1991.

Campbell, Don. *The Mozart Effect: Tapping the Power of Music to Heal the Body, Strengthen the Mind, and Unlock the Creative Spirit.* New York: Avon Books, 1997.

Caplan, Mariana, M.A. *Untouched: The Need for Genuine Affection in an Impersonal World.* Prescott, Ariz.: Hohm Press, 1998.

Cardeña, Etzel; Steven Jay Lynn; and Stanley Krippner, eds. *Varieties of Anomalous Experience.* Washington, D.C.: American Psychological Association, 2000.

Carper, Jean. *Food—Your Miracle Medicine: How Food Can Prevent and Cure Over 100 Symptoms and Problems.* New York: HarperCollins, 1993.

Chopra, Deepak, M.D. *Ageless Body, Timeless Mind: The Quantum Alternative to Growing Old.* New York: Crown, 1993.

————. *Quantum Healing*. New York: Bantam Books, 1989.

Classen, Constance; David Howes; and Anthony Synnott. *Aroma: The Cultural History of Smell*. New York: Routledge, 1994.

Colbin, Annemarie. *Food and Healing*. New York: Ballantine Books, 1986.

Cousins, Norman. *Anatomy of an Illness as Perceived by the Patient: Reflections on Healing and Regeneration*. New York: Norton, 1979.

————. *Head First: The Biology of Hope and the Healing Power of the Human Spirit*. New York: Penguin Books, 1989.

————. *The Healing Heart*. New York: Avon Books, 1983.

Dossey, Barbara Montgomery, et al. *Holistic Nursing: A Handbook for Practice*. Gaithersburg, Md.: Aspen Publishers, 1995.

Dossey, Larry, M.D. *Be Careful What You Pray For . . . You Just Might Get It*. San Francisco: HarperSanFrancisco, 1997.

————. *Healing beyond the Body: Medicine and the Infinite Reach of the Mind*. Boston: Shambhala Publications, 2001.

————. *Healing Words: The Power of Prayer and the Practice of Medicine*. San Francisco: HarperSanFrancisco, 1993.

————. *Meaning and Medicine: Lessons from a Doctor's Tales of Breakthrough and Healing*. New York: Bantam Books, 1991.

Eaton, S. Boyd, M.D.; Marjorie Shostak; and Melvin Konner, M.D., Ph.D. *The Paleolithic Prescription: A Program of Diet and Exercise and a Design for Living*. New York: Harper & Row, 1988.

Frank, Jerome D., Ph.D., M.D., and Julia B. Frank, M.D. *Persuasion and Healing: A Comparative Study of Psychotherapy*. 3d ed. Baltimore: Johns Hopkins University Press, 1991.

Frankl, Viktor E. *Man's Search for Meaning*. New York: Simon & Schuster, 1984.

Fried, Robert, Ph.D. *The Breath Connection: How to Reduce Psychosomatic and Stress-Related Disorders with Easy-to-Do Breathing Exercises*. New York: Plenum Press, 1990.

Fuhrman, Joel, M.D. *Fasting and Eating for Health: A Medical Doctor's Program for Conquering Disease*. New York: St. Martin's Press, 1995.

Goleman, Daniel. *Emotional Intelligence*. New York: Bantam, 1995.

Goleman, Daniel, Ph.D., and Joel Gurin, eds. *Mind-Body Medicine*. Yonkers, N.Y.: Consumer Reports Books, 1993.

Green, Elmer, and Alyce Green. *Beyond Biofeedback*. New York: Dell, 1978.

Hover-Kramer, Dorothea. *Healing Touch: A Resource for Health Care Professionals*. Albany, N.Y.: Delmar Publishers, 1996.

Howes, David. *The Varieties of Sensory Experience: A Sourcebook in the Anthropology of the Senses*. Toronto, Ontario: University of Toronto Press, 1991.

Jahn, Robert G., and Brenda J. Dunne. *Margins of Reality: The Role of Consciousness in the Physical World*. New York: Harcourt Brace & Co., 1987.

Jonas, Wayne M.D., and Jeffrey Levin, Ph.D., eds. *Essentials of Complementary and Alternative Medicine*. Baltimore: Lippincott, Williams & Wilkins, 1999.

Krieger, Dolores, Ph.D., R.N. *Accepting Your Power to Heal: The Personal Practice of Therapeutic Touch*. Santa Fe, N.M.: Bear & Company, 1993.

———. *The Therapeutic Touch: How to Use Your Hands to Help or Heal*. Englewood Cliffs, N.J.: Prentice-Hall, 1979.

Krippner, Stanley, and Patrick Welch. *Spiritual Dimensions of Healing: From Native Shamanism to Contemporary Health Care*. New York: Irvington Publishers, 1992.

Larson, David B., M.D., M.S.P.H., and Susan S. Larson, M.A.T. *The Forgotten Factor in Physical and Mental Health: What Does the Research Show? An Independent Study Seminar*. Arlington, Va.: National Institute for Healthcare Research, 1992.

Laskow, Leonard, M.D. *Healing with Love: A Physician's Breakthrough Mind/Body Medical Program for Healing Yourself and Others*. New York: HarperCollins, 1992.

Leshan, Lawrence, Ph.D. *Beyond Technique: Psychotherapy for the 21st Century*. Northvale, N.J.: Jason Aronson, 1996.

———. *The Medium, the Mystic, and the Physicist: Toward a General Theory of the Paranormal*. New York: Viking, 1974.

Levin, Jeff, Ph.D. *God, Faith, and Health: Exploring the Spirituality-Healing Connection*. New York: Wiley, 2001.

Levin, Jeffrey S., ed. *Religion in Aging and Health: Theoretical Foundations and Methodological Frontiers*. Thousand Oaks, Calif.: Sage Publications, 1994.

Lown, Bernard, M.D. *The Lost Art of Healing*. New York: Houghton Mifflin, 1996.

Macrae, Janet. *Therapeutic Touch: A Practical Guide*. New York: Knopf, 1995.

McGarey, Gladys, M.D., with Jess Stearn. *The Physician Within You: Medicine for the Millennium*. Deerfield Beach, Fla.: Health Communications, 1997.

Motz, Julie. *Hands of Life: Use Your Body's Own Energy Medicine for Healing, Recovery, and Transformation*. New York: Bantam Books, 1998.

Murphy, Michael. *The Future of the Body: Explorations into the Further Evolution of Human Nature*. New York: Putnam, 1992.

Murphy, Michael, and Steven Donovan. *The Physical and Psychological Effects of Meditation: A Review of Contemporary Research with a Comprehensive Bibliography, 1931–1996*. 2d ed. Sausalito, Calif.: Institute of Noetic Sciences, 1997.

Naparstek, Belleruth. *Staying Well with Guided Imagery*. New York: Warner Books, 1994.

———. *Your Sixth Sense: Awakening Your Psychic Potential*. New York: HarperCollins, 1997.

Northrup, Christiane, M.D. *Women's Bodies, Women's Wisdom: Creating Physical and Emotional Health and Healing*. New York: Bantam, 1994.

Ornish, Dean, M.D. *Dr. Dean Ornish's Program for Reversing Heart Disease: The Only System Scientifically Proven to Reverse Heart Disease without Drugs or Surgery*. New York: Ballantine Books, 1990.

———. *Love and Survival: The Scientific Basis for the Healing Power of Intimacy*. New York: HarperCollins, 1998.

Ornstein, Robert, Ph.D., and David Sobel, M.D. *The Healing Brain: Breakthrough Discoveries about How the Brain Keeps Us Healthy*. New York: Simon & Schuster, 1987.

Oschman, James L. *Energy Medicine: The Scientific Basis*. London: Harcourt Publishers, 2000.

Pauling, Linus. *How to Live Longer and Feel Better*. New York: Freeman, 1986.

Pelletier, Kenneth R. *Mind as Healer, Mind as Slayer*. New York: Dell, 1977.

———. *Sound Mind, Sound Body: A New Model for Lifelong Health*. New York: Simon & Schuster, 1994.

Pert, Candace B., Ph.D. *Molecules of Emotions: Why You Feel the Way You Feel*. New York: Scribner, 1997.

Pfeiffer, Carl C., Ph.D., M.D. *Mental and Elemental Nutrients: A Physician's Guide to Nutrition and Health Care*. New Canaan, Conn.: Keats Publishing, 1975.

———. *Nutrition and Mental Illness: An Orthomolecular Approach to Balancing Body Chemistry*. Rochester, Vt.: Healing Arts Press, 1987.

Radin, Dean, Ph.D. *The Conscious Universe: The Scientific Truth of Psychic Phenomena*. New York: HarperCollins, 1997.

Remen, Rachel Naomi, M.D. *Kitchen Table Wisdom: Stories That Heal*. New York: Riverhead Books, 1996.

Rubik, Beverly. *Life at the Edge of Science*. Philadelphia: Institute for Frontier Science, 1996.

Sapolsky, Robert M. *Why Zebras Don't Get Ulcers: A Guide to Stress, Stress-Related Diseases, and Coping*. New York: Freeman, 1994.

Schmid, Ronald F., N.D. *Native Nutrition: Eating According to Ancestral Wisdom*. Rochester, Vt.: Healing Arts Press, 1987.

Sears, Barry, Ph.D. *The Zone: A Dietary Road Map*. New York: HarperCollins, 1995.

Shealy, C. Norman, M.D., Ph.D. *Miracles Do Happen: A Physician's Experience with Alternative Medicine*. Rockport, Mass.: Element Books, 1995.

———. *Third Party Rape: The Conspiracy to Rob You of Health Care*. St. Paul: Galde Press, 1993.

Singh, Ranji N., Ph.D. *Self-Healing: Powerful Techniques*. London, Ontario: Health Psychology Associates, 1998.

Spiegel, David, M.D. *Living Beyond Limits*. New York: Ballantine Books, 1993.

Targ, Russell, and Jane Katra, Ph.D. *Miracles of Mind: Exploring Nonlocal Consciousness and Spiritual Healing*. Novato, Calif.: New World Library, 1998.

Tart, Charles T., ed. *Altered States of Consciousness.* 3d ed. New York: HarperCollins, 1990.

Temoshok, Lydia, Ph.D., and Henry Dreher. *The Type C Connection: The Mind-Body Link to Cancer and Your Health*. New York: Penguin, 1992.

Thondup, Tulku. *The Healing Power of Mind: Simple Meditation Exercises for Health, Well-Being, and Enlightenment*. Boston: Shambhala Publications, 1998.

Tiller, William A., Ph.D. *Science and Human Transformation: Subtle Energies, Intentionality and Consciousness*. Walnut Creek, Calif.: Pavior Publishing, 1997.

Walford, Roy L., M.D. *The 120-Year Diet: How to Double Your Vital Years*. New York: Simon & Schuster, 1986.

Weil, Andrew, M.D. *Health and Healing: Understanding Conventional and Alternative Medicine*. Boston: Houghton Mifflin, 1983.

———. *Spontaneous Healing: How to Discover and Enhance Your Body's Natural Ability to Maintain and Heal Itself.* New York: Knopf, 1995.

Williams, Dr. Roger J. *Nutrition against Disease*. New York: Bantam Books, 1981.

Complementary and Alternative Medicine Journals

Advances in Mind-Body Medicine
InnoVision Communications
169 Saxony Road, Suite 104
Encinitas, CA 92024
(866) 828-2962 or (760) 633-3910

Alternative Therapies in Health and Medicine
P.O. Box 627
Holmes, PA 19043
(800) 345-8112 or (610) 532-4700

Herbalgram: The Journal of the American Botanical Council and the Herb Research Foundation
American Botanical Council
P.O. Box 201660
Austin, TX 78720-1660
(800) 373-7105 or (512) 331-8868

Journal of Alternative and Complementary Medicine: Research on Paradigm, Practice, and Policy
Mary Ann Liebert, Inc.
2 Madison Ave.
Larchmont, NY 10538-1962
(800) M-LIEBERT or (914) 834-3100

Journal of the American Society for Psychical Research
American Society for Psychical Research
5 W. 73d St.
New York, NY 10023

Journal of Scientific Exploration
Society of Scientific Exploration
P.O. Box 5848
Stanford, CA 94309-5848

Noetic Sciences Review
Institute of Noetic Sciences
P.O. Box 909
Sausalito, CA 94966-0909
(800) 383-1394 or (415) 331-5650

Subtle Energies
International Society for the Study of Subtle Energy and Energy Medicine
11005 Ralston Road, Suite 100D
Arvada, CO 80004
(303) 425-4625

Townsend Letter for Doctors & Patients
Townsend Letter Group
911 Tyler St.
Port Townsend, WA 98368
(360) 385-6021

STAYING INFORMED:
NATIVE AMERICAN NEWSPAPER

News from Indian Country
Indian Country Communications
8558N Country Road K
Hayward, WI 54843

JOURNALS: NATIVE AMERICAN AND
INDIGENOUS CULTURE

American Indian Quarterly
University of Nebraska Press
P.O. Box 880484
Lincoln, NE 68588-0484

Bulletin of Primitive Technology
Society of Primitive Technology
P.O. Box 905
Rexburg, ID 83440

Cultural Survival Quarterly
96 Mount Auburn St.
Cambridge, MA 02138

Indigenous Woman
Indigenous Women's Network
P.O. Box 2967
Rapid City, SD 57709-2967

Native Americas
Akwe:kon Press
300 Caldwell Hall
Ithaca, NY 14853

Native Peoples Magazine
P.O. Box 18449
Anaheim, CA 92817-9913

News from Native California
P.O. Box 9145
Berkeley, CA 94709

Shaman's Drum: A Journal of Experiential Shamanism
P.O. Box 97
Ashland, OR 97520

Tribal College Journal of American Indian Higher Education
P.O. Box 720
Mancos, CO 81328

Winds of Change
AISES
5661 Airport Road
Boulder, CO 80301-2339

INDIAN COUNTRY TRAVEL GUIDES

Cantor, George. *North American Indian Landmarks: A Traveler's Guide*. Detroit: Visible Ink Press, 1993.

Eagle/Walking Turtle. *Indian America: A Traveler's Companion*. 4th ed. Santa Fe, N.M.: John Muir Publications, 1995.

Folsom, Franklin, and Mary Elting Folsom. *America's Ancient Treasures: A Guide to Archeological Sites and Museums in the United States and Canada*. 4th ed. Albuquerque: University of New Mexico Press, 1993.

Gattuso, John, ed. *Insight Guides: Native America*. Singapore: Höfer Press, 1992.

Halliday, Jan. *Native Peoples of Alaska: A Traveler's Guide to Land, Art, and Culture*. Seattle: Sasquatch Books, 1998.

Halliday, Jan, and Gail Chehak, in cooperation with the Affiliated Tribes of Northwest Indians. *Native Peoples of the Northwest*. Seattle: Sasquatch Books, 1996.

Maine Indian Basketmakers Alliance. *A Wabanaki Guide to Maine*. Old Town, Maine: Maine Indian Basketmakers Alliance, 2001.

McLaren, Deborah. *Rethinking Tourism and Ecotravel: The Paving of Paradise and What You Can Do to Stop It*. Hartford, Conn.: Kumarian Press, 1998.

Rozema, Vicki. *Footsteps of the Cherokees: A Guide to the Eastern Homelands of the Cherokee Nation*. Winston-Salem, N.C.: John F. Blair, Publisher, 1995.

Native American Tourism Services

In addition to the following organizations, you may call tribal agencies directly to ask if they have tourism services. Many tribes welcome the opportunity to educate and entertain guests while generating revenue for the tribe. Remember, however, that when you visit tribal land, you are in a foreign country, and the people who live there determine where and when you may visit. Some tribal ceremonies and sacred sites may be closed to tourists.

Affiliated Tribes of Northwest Indians
4211 200th St. SW, Suite 107
Linwood, WA 98036
(425) 774-5419

Alaska Heritage Tours
2525 C St., #405
Anchorage, AK 99503
(877) 258-6877 or (907) 265-4500

Alliance of Tribal Tourism Advocates
P.O. Box 234
Lower Brule, SD 57690
(605) 473-5301

Arizona American Indian Tourism Association
P.O. Box 22218
Flagstaff, AZ 86002
(520) 523-7320

Avant Garde Travel
P.O. Box 123
Dove Creek, CO 81324
(831) 648-3539 or (970) 677-3600

California Native American Cultural Tourism Association
2220 N. Catalina St.
Los Angeles, CA 90027
(213) 666-2428

Crow Canyon Archaeological Center
23390 Road K
Cortez, CO 81321
(800) 422-8975

Indian Country Tourism
P.O. Box 788
Louisville, CO 80027
(303) 661-9819

Journeys into American Indian Territories
P.O. Box 929
Westhampton Beach, NY 11978
(800) 458-2632 or (631) 878-8655

New Mexico Indian Tourism Association
2401 12th St. NW, Suite 212N
Albuquerque, NM 87104
(505) 246-1668

Nunavut Tourism
P.O. Box 1450
Iqaluit, Nunavut
Canada X0A 0H0
(800) 491-7910 or (867) 979-6551

Native American Music

Drumbeat Indian Arts, Inc.
4143 N. 16th St., Suite 6
Phoenix, AZ 85016
(602) 266-4823

Indian House
P.O. Box 472-A
Taos, NM 87571
(800) 748-0522 or (505) 776-2953

Silver Wave Records
P.O. Box 7943
Boulder, CO 80306
(303) 443-5617

Smithsonian Folkways Records
Center for Folklife Programs & Cultural Studies
955 L'Enfant Plaza 2600
Smithsonian Institution
Washington, DC 20560
(202) 287-3262

Traditional Healing, Science, and Culture: Educational Resources

The following organizations support Native American or indigenous education and culture. Contact them to offer support and to find out about outreach programs that may be open to the general public.

American Indian College Fund
8333 Greenwood Blvd.
Denver, CO 80221
(800) 776-3863 or (303) 426-8900

American Indian Science & Engineering Society (AISES)
5661 Airport Blvd.
Boulder, CO 80301-2339
(303) 939-0023

The Buffalo Trust
826 Camino de Monterey, Suite 86
Santa Fe, NM 87505
(505) 982-1215

Cultural Survival
96 Mount Auburn St.
Cambridge, MA 02138
(617) 441-5400

Diné College, Office of Continuing Education
P.O. Box 731
Tuba City, AZ 86045
(520) 283-6321

The Foundation for Shamanic Studies

P.O. Box 1939

Mill Valley, CA 94942

(This organization conducts research, offers training, publishes a members-only magazine, and helps to preserve shamanic traditions around the world.)

Four Worlds International Institute for Human and Community Development

347 Fairmont Blvd. S.

Lethbridge, Alberta T1K 7J8

Canada

(403) 320-7144

(This organization offers superb books, videos, and curriculum materials on community building and Native American culture.)

Be a Warrior for Peace

If you have benefited from the teachings in this book, then consider a concrete expression of your gratitude. Give something back to the Indian people. Be a warrior for peace by contributing to the Native American battle for justice and preservation of culture.

Please consider a regular financial donation to the following noble organizations.

THE NATIVE AMERICAN RIGHTS FUND

The Indian warriors of today carry briefcases and laptops, and their most common battlefield is the courtroom. The Native American Rights Fund (NARF) is a renowned leader in the ongoing fight to preserve Native American rights. NARF provides legal advice, representation, and research facilities to Indian tribes, organizations, and individuals. According to NARF publications, the five priorities of NARF are "(1) the preservation of tribal existence; (2) the protection of tribal natural resources; (3) the promotion of human rights; (4) the accountability of governments to Native Americans; and (5) the development of Indian law." NARF continues the important and *expensive* work of protecting tribal sovereignty, lands, water, and hunting and fishing rights and supporting education and religious freedom. Even the smallest donations are appreciated. Individuals who donate at least $500 annually may be invited to join the Peta Uha Council, a council of honored "fire keepers" who keep the light of justice burning.

The Native American Rights Fund

1506 Broadway

Boulder, CO 80302-6296

THE BUFFALO TRUST

According to an old Kiowa man, "The buffalo is more than an animal. It is the sun's shadow. Our lives are bound to it. If it lives, we live. If it dies, we die. It is our life and our living shield." The Buffalo Trust, founded by Pulitzer Prize–winning author N. Scott Momaday, is a nonprofit educational corporation designed to preserve and perpetuate Native

American living culture and cultural inheritance of the sacred. Momaday writes in the Buffalo Trust's Vision Statement:

> The Buffalo Trust will be a place, on sacred ground, where Indian people can come immediately into the presence of sacred matter—objects, stories, music, dances, feasts, ceremonies of all kinds. I envision the Buffalo Trust as a physical, geographic place, and eventually places, study centers; but the Buffalo Trust will also carry the experience of the sacred to Indian people wherever they are located, in outreach activities directed both to Indian audiences and broader audiences. The Buffalo Trust will afford opportunities for elders and medicine people to share their wisdom with others, for scholars to exchange ideas in an atmosphere of learning and participation, for Indian and non-Indian people to congregate freely in a spirit of celebration, goodwill, community, and reverence for the sacred and human being. Above all, the Buffalo Trust will provide experiences of sacred space where American Indian young people can and will regain that sense of the sacred that distinguishes them as the inheritors of a rich and venerable culture, that will throughout their lives enable them to know who they are in the spirit of their unique inheritance.

The Buffalo Trust
826 Camino de Monterey, Suite 86
Santa Fe, NM 87505

THE CRAZY HORSE MEMORIAL

In the sacred Black Hills, Lakota Nation (South Dakota), stands a visible testament to the power of shared visions. In 1943, the sculptor Korczak Ziolkowski received a letter from the Lakota chief Henry Standing Bear, which said, "My fellow Chiefs and I would like the White Man to know the Red Man had great heroes, too." Five years later, Korczak began the greatest sculptural undertaking the world has ever known, a 563-foot-high mountain carved into the image of the Lakota leader Crazy Horse. Crazy Horse points over his horse's mane, symbolically saying, "My lands are where my dead lie buried." When the project is completed, the outstretched arm will be almost as long as a football field. Mt. Rushmore's four presidents will be smaller than Crazy Horse's head, and the horse's head will be as tall as a twenty-two-story building. The project, still in progress, includes a permanent Native American museum, an Indian scholarship fund, and plans for a university and medical center. The Crazy Horse Memorial is entirely supported by grassroots organizations and donations. Korczak twice refused $10 million in government funding. This is a project by and for the People.

When Korczak died in October of 1982, the executive committee of the Oglala Sioux issued a resolution mourning his death and expressing their "great admiration and respect." The Six Nations Indian Museum (Onchiota, New York) stated in a similar resolution:

> WHEREAS, his passing is indeed an inestimable loss to all of us as a race, and we realize thereby that another of our GREAT who has many, many times brought honour to his Indian People, and of whom we are all proud, has taken the Sunset Trail. His passing is a loss to America and especially to Indian Peoples.

As a carver, a sculptor and a champion of Indian Peoples of America, the Great Spirit has dedicated none his equal. . . .

Korczak's family and numerous volunteers have continued his great work. To support the Crazy Horse Memorial or for more information, write:

Crazy Horse Grass Roots Club
Avenue of Chiefs
Crazy Horse, SD 57730-9506

~ OTHER WORKS BY ~ KENNETH COHEN

BOOK

The Way of Qigong: The Art and Science of Chinese Energy Healing (Ballantine Books)

AUDIO AND VIDEO COURSES

Published by Sounds True, (800) 333-9185 or (303) 665-3151

AUDIO

The Beginner's Guide to Feng Shui
Chi Kung Meditations
Healthy Breathing
The Power of Qi
The Practice of Qigong Healing and Meditation
Taoism: Essential Teachings of the Way and Its Power
Taoist Healing Imagery

VIDEO

Qigong: Traditional Chinese Exercises for Healing the Body, Mind, and Spirit
Qi Healing: Energy Medicine Techniques to Heal Yourself and Others

For Native American educational materials and a schedule of Ken Cohen's workshops and lectures, write to:

Sacred Earth Circle
P.O. Box 1727
Nederland, CO 80466
U.S.A.

— ABOUT THE AUTHOR —

Kenneth "Bear Hawk" Cohen, M.A., M.S.Th., is a health educator, traditional healer, and scholar of indigenous medicine. Although not ethnically Native American, he teaches with the blessings and support of traditional elders of many nations. Ken has been dedicated to indigenous ways for more than thirty years. He maintains close ties with his adoptive Cree family from Sturgeon Lake First Nation in Canada.

Kenneth Cohen is a leader in the dialogue between ancient wisdom and modern science. He was one of nine "exceptional healers" studied by the Menninger Institute and has lectured at medical schools, scientific conferences, and numerous universities. His sponsors have included the American Cancer Society, the Canadian Ministry of Health, the National Institute for the Clinical Application of Behavioral Medicine, and the International Society for the Study of Subtle Energy and Energy Medicine. Ken represented both Chinese and Native American medicine as a keynote speaker at the 1994 World Congress on Energy Medicine in Switzerland.

Kenneth was an apprentice to Cherokee spiritual teachers during the 1970s, and continued training with elders and healers throughout the 1980s. He is an initiate of the Red Cedar Circle (Si.Si.Wiss Medicine) and other medicine societies. In his quest for the common root of healing, Ken studied African medicine for five years with the Zulu healer Ingwe, in the lineage of the Holy Man, Vusamazulu Credo Mutwa, and was one of four North American students of a master diviner (*dibia*) of the Igbo Tribe, Nigeria. Ken was also initiated into healing traditions from the Philippines and Hawai'i.

To deepen his understanding of the world's spiritual traditions, Ken studied comparative religion at the New Seminary (New York City), where he was ordained as an Interfaith Minister and was the first graduate ever awarded both the ministry degree and advanced degree in spiritual therapy simultaneously. He is a member of the Association of Interfaith Ministers and is in demand as a lecturer for churches, seminaries, and theology conferences.

Kenneth is the author of the bestselling classic of Chinese medicine *The Way of Qigong: The Art and Science of Chinese Energy Healing*, as well as the popular Sounds True audio and video courses, and more than 200 journal articles on spirituality and health. He wrote the "Native American Medicine" chapter in *Essentials of Complementary and Alternative Medicine*, the first U.S. medical textbook to include Native American healing.

Ken lives with his family at 9,000 ft. elevation in the Rocky Mountains of Colorado.

~ INDEX ~